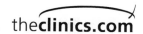

CHILD AND ADOLESCENT PSYCHIATRIC CLINICS OF NORTH AMERICA

Ethics

GUEST EDITOR
Mary Lynn Dell, MD, MTS, ThM

CONSULTING EDITOR
Harsh K. Trivedi, MD

January 2008 • Volume 17 • Number 1

SAUNDERS

An Imprint of Elsevier, Inc.
PHILADELPHIA   LONDON   TORONTO   MONTREAL   SYDNEY   TOKYO

W.B. SAUNDERS COMPANY
A Division of Elsevier Inc.

Elsevier Inc. • 1600 John F. Kennedy Boulevard • Suite 1800 • Philadelphia, Pennsylvania 19103-2899

http://www.childpsych.theclinics.com

CHILD AND ADOLESCENT PSYCHIATRIC CLINICS	**Volume 17, Number 1**
OF NORTH AMERICA	**ISSN 1056-4993**
January 2008	**ISBN-13: 978-1-4160-5864-9**
Editor: Sarah E. Barth	**ISBN-10: 1-4160-5864-8**

The ideas and opinions expressed in *Child and Adolescent Psychiatric Clinics of North America* do not necessarily reflect those of the Publisher. The Publisher does not assume any responsibility for any injury and/or damage to persons or property arising out of or related to any use of the material contained in this periodical. The reader is advised to check the appropriate medical literature and the product information currently provided by the manufacturer of each drug to be administered to verify the dosage, the method and duration of administration, or contraindications. It is the responsibility of the treating physician or other health care professional, relying on independent experience and knowledge of the patient, to determine drug dosages and the best treatment for the patient. Mention of any product in this issue should not be construed as endorsement by the contributors, editors, or the Publisher of the product or manufacturers' claims.

Child and Adolescent Psychiatric Clinics of North America (ISSN 1056-4993) is published quarterly by Elsevier Inc., 360 Park Avenue South, New York, NY 10010-1710. Months of issue are January, April, July, and October. Business and Editorial Offices: 1600 John F. Kennedy Boulevard, Suite 1800, Philadelphia, PA 19103-2899. Customer Service Offices: 6277 Sea Harbor Drive, Orlando, FL 32887-4800. Periodicals postage paid at New York, NY and additional mailing offices. Subscription prices are $220.00 per year (US individuals), $344.00 per year (US institutions), $113.00 per year (US students), $250.00 per year (Canadian individuals), $406.00 per year (Canadian institutions), $136.00 per year (Canadian students), $279.00 per year (international individuals), $406.00 per year (international institutions), and $136.00 per year (international students). International air speed delivery is included in all *Clinics* subscription prices. All prices are subject to change without notice. **POSTMASTER:** Send address changes to *Child and Adolescent Psychiatric Clinics of North America*, Elsevier Periodicals Customer Service, 6277 Sea Harbor Drive, Orlando, FL 32887-4800. **Customer Service: 1-800-654-2452 (US). From outside of the US, call 1-407-345-4000.**

Child and Adolescent Psychiatric Clinics of North America is covered in *Index Medicus, ISI, SSCI, Research Alert, Social Search, Current Contents,* and *EMBASE/Excerpta Medica.*

Printed in the United States of America.

CONSULTING EDITOR

HARSH K. TRIVEDI, MD, Bradley Hospital, Brown Medical School, East Providence, Rhode Island

CONSULTING EDITOR EMERITUS

ANDRÉS MARTIN, MD, MPH, Associate Professor of Child Psychiatry and Psychiatry, Yale Child Study Center, Yale University School of Medicine, New Haven; and Medical Director, Children's Psychiatric Inpatient Service, Yale New Haven Children's Hospital, New Haven, Connecticut

FOUNDING CONSULTING EDITOR

MELVIN LEWIS, MBBS, FRCPsych, DCH

GUEST EDITOR

MARY LYNN DELL, MD, MTS, ThM, Associate Professor of Psychiatry and Behavioral Sciences, and Faculty Fellow in Clinical Ethics, Emory University School of Medicine, Atlanta, Georgia

CONTRIBUTORS

NORMAN E. ALESSI, MD, Professor Emeritus, University of Michigan School of Medicine, Department of Psychiatry, Michigan

VINCENT A. ALESSI, Oberlin College, Oberlin, Ohio

LEE I. ASCHERMAN, MD, Professor and Director of Psychiatry, Division of Child and Adolescent Psychiatry, The University of Alabama at Birmingham; Chief of Services, The Children's Hospital of Alabama, Birmingham, Alabama

SIDNEY BLOCH, MD, PhD, Professor of Psychiatry, Department of Psychiatry and Center for Health and Society, University of Melbourne, St. Vincent's Hospital, Fitzroy, Melbourne, Australia

MARC E. DALTON, MD, MPH, Director of Pediatric Consultation Liaison Service and Emergency Psychiatry, Department of Psychiatry and Behavioral Sciences, Children's National Medical Center; Assistant Professor of Psychiatry, Behavioral Sciences and Pediatrics, George Washington University School of Medicine, Washington DC

MARY LYNN DELL, MD, MTS, ThM, Associate Professor of Psychiatry and Behavioral Sciences, Emory University School of Medicine, Atlanta, Georgia; Faculty Fellow in Clinical Ethics, Emory University School of Medicine, Atlanta, Georgia

DAVID RAY DEMASO, MD, Professor of Psychiatry and Pediatrics, Department of Psychiatry, Children's Hospital Boston, Boston, Massachusetts

ARDEN D. DINGLE, MD, Associate Professor, Psychiatry and Behavioral Sciences; Training Director, Child and Adolescent Psychiatry, Emory University School of Medicine, Atlanta, Georgia

JINGER G. HOOP, MD, MFA, Assistant Professor, Department of Psychiatry and Behavioral Medicine, Medical College of Wisconsin, Milwaukee, Wisconsin

PARAMJIT T. JOSHI, MD, Endowed Professor and Chair, Department of Psychiatry and Behavioral Sciences, Children's National Medical Center; and Professor of Psychiatry, Behavioral Sciences and Pediatrics, George Washington University School of Medicine, Washington DC

KATHY KINLAW, MDiv, Acting Director, John and Susan Wieland Center for Ethics, Emory University, Atlanta, Georgia

WILLIAM M. KLYKYLO, MD, Professor of Psychiatry and Director, Division of Child and Adolescent Psychiatry, Wright State University Boonshoft School of Medicine, Dayton, Ohio

CHRISTOPHER J. KRATOCHVIL, MD, Associate Professor of Psychiatry and Pediatrics, University of Nebraska Medical Center, Omaha, Nebraska

DEBORAH A. O'DONNELL, PhD, Assistant Professor, Department of Psychology, St. Mary's College of Maryland, St. Mary's City, Maryland

PATRICIA R. RECUPERO, JD, MD, Clinical Professor of Psychiatry, The Warren Alpert Medical School of Brown University; President/CEO, Butler Hospital, Providence, Rhode Island

JOSEPH M. REY, MD, PhD, Honorary Professor, Discipline of Psychological Medicine, University of Sydney, Sydney, Australia

LAURA WEISS ROBERTS, MD, MA, Professor and Chairman, Department of Psychiatry and Behavioral Medicine, Medical College of Wisconsin; Professor of Bioethics, Health Policy Institute, Medical College of Wisconsin, Milwaukee, Wisconsin

EDIE ROSENBERG, MBA, Department of Psychiatry, Children's Hospital Boston, Boston, Massachusetts

SAMUEL RUBIN, MD, Assistant Professor of Psychiatry, Division of Child and Adolescent Psychiatry, The University of Alabama at Birmingham, Birmingham, Alabama

DIANE H. SCHETKY, MD, Clinical Professor of Psychiatry, University of Vermont College of Medicine at Maine Medical Center, Rockport, Maine

CONTRIBUTORS

SANDRA B. SEXSON, MD, Professor, Psychiatry and Pediatrics; Division Chief and Training Director, Division of Child, Adolescent and Family Psychiatry; and Department of Psychiatry and Health Behavior Medical College of Georgia, Augusta, Georgia

WILLIAM R. SEXSON, MD, Associate Professor, Pediatrics/Neonatology; Faculty Fellow, Emory Center for Ethics; and Associate Dean for Clinical Affairs, Emory University School of Medicine; Atlanta, Georgia

ANGELA C. SMYTH, MD, Clinical Associate, Department of Child and Adolescent Psychiatry, University of Chicago, Chicago, Illinois

NERISSA SOH, BMedSc, MNutrDiet, PhD, Research Assistant to the Chair of Child and Adolescent Psychiatry, Child and Adolescent Mental Health Services, Service, Northern Sydney Central Coast Health, North Ryde, Australia

ADRIAN N. SONDHEIMER, MD, Research Teaching Specialist and (formerly) Associate Professor of Psychiatry, Division of Child and Adolescent Psychiatry, UMDNJ-New Jersey Medical School, Newark, New Jersey

MARGARET L. STUBER, MD, Jane and Marc Nathanson Professor, Psychiatry and Biobehavioral Medicine, Semel Institute at UCLA, David Geffen School of Medicine at UCLA; UCLA Department of Psychiatry & Biobehavioral Sciences, UCLA Neuropsychiatric Hospital, Los Angeles, California

BRIGETTE S. VAUGHAN, APRN, Department of Psychiatry, University of Nebraska Medical Center, Omaha, Nebraska

GARRY WALTER, MD, PhD, Professor of Child and Adolescent Psychiatry, University of Sydney, Sydney, Australia; Area Clinical Director, Child and Adolescent Mental Health Services, Northern Sydney Central Coast Health, North Ryde, Australia

Cover artwork Courtesy of Socorro Rivera G., Mexico City, Mexico

CONTENTS

> Familiarity with medical ethical theory and the history of bioethics
> is helpful for the understanding of the current state of bioethics, as
> well as possible future developments that will affect physicians
> and patients alike. This article reviews major schools of thought in
> bioethics and their relevance to clinical work with children,
> adolescents, and families. Child and adolescent psychiatrists need
> to be familiar with major ethical issues in general medicine,
> psychiatry, and pediatrics, in addition to those controversies that
> are more specific to their subspecialty. Employing a systematic
> approach for the identification and analysis of ethical concerns,
> such as the Four Topics Model of Jonsen and colleagues, improves
> child and adolescent psychiatrists' confidence that they are aware
> of ethical quandaries in practice and are addressing these issues in
> a transparent, well-informed manner.

> Core ethical principles for the conduct of psychotherapy with
> children and adolescents transcend times, trends, and jurisdictions.
> Advances in technology, variations in state law, and the evolution
> of federal law should stimulate consideration of how these ethical

principles apply to new situations; however, the guiding compass remains the psychotherapist's obligation to create and protect the integrity of the psychotherapeutic space to provide the child or adolescent the freedom to identify, examine, explore, and hopefully resolve the issues that bring one to treatment. Boundaries, privacy, confidentiality, and the patient's autonomy are components of this space. Together, they reflect a basic respect for the patient central to professional conduct and essential to any effective treatment process.

Please approve the following synopsis as it will appear in the table of contents: In child and adolescent psychiatry, medical records and professional communications raise important ethical concerns for the treating or consulting clinician. Although a distinction may be drawn between internal records (eg, medical records and psychotherapy notes) and external communications (eg, consultation reports and correspondence with pediatricians), several ethical principles apply to both types of documentation; however, specific considerations may vary, depending upon the context in which the records or communications were produced. Special care is due with regard to thoroughness and honesty, collaboration and cooperation, autonomy and dignity of the patient, confidentiality of the patient and family members, maintaining objectivity and neutrality, electronic communications media, and professional activities (eg, political advocacy). This article reviews relevant ethical concerns for child and adolescent psychiatrists with respect to medical records and professional communications, drawing heavily from forensic and legal sources, and offers additional recommendations for further reading for clarification and direction on ethical dilemmas.

Please approve the following synopsis as it will appear in the table of contents: This article examines the ways in which mental health services have been affected by managed care and describes how to address some of the ethical conflicts that have always existed, but have been transformed immeasurably. It outlines the ethical dilemmas between the competing values of mental health providers and managed care, as well as the practical ethical considerations related to confidentiality, billing, and coding. It suggests that there can be no real improvement for mental health providers in the ethical minefield of managed care until they stop focusing on how distressed they are about it and start dealing with the larger, systemic issues in psychiatry and American health care. The article concludes by noting that the only way to effect meaningful change in the health care system is to combine knowledge with advocacy and to proactively define the standards needed to make the necessary choices.

New Media and an Ethics Analysis Model for Child and Adolescent Psychiatry

Norman E. Alessi and Vincent A. Alessi

We and our patients are immersed in a mediascape that is unparalleled in history. It is a force of monumental proportion that for many youth competes with and has replaced parental, social, and cultural influences on their development. The ethical questions regarding this dynamic are frequently answered by little else than the application of vague and dated moral dictums based on "old media." To engender a comprehensive understanding of how "new media" interacts with our patients, we suggest a new perspective on the differentiation of old media from new media. Then, using our conceptual model of new media, we break down the ethical questions into the several overlapping ethical areas, these being media, professional, and bioethical. To aid in the application of the system of thought we provide a structured system of ethical analysis. Through these, we hope that this issue can be looked at with increased clarity and guidance within a framework for future thought.

Ethics and the Prescription Pad

Mary Lynn Dell, Brigette S. Vaughan, and Christopher J. Kratochvil

This article reviews the considerations that inform ethical psychotropic medication prescription processes at the clinical level with child and adolescent patients and their families or guardians. Physician attributes, cultural and religious factors, and the psychodynamic aspects of psychopharmacology are reviewed, in addition to the applications of basic ethical principles and concepts to the act of dispensing psychotropic medications. Attention is given to the processes of informed consent, assent, and challenges encountered to ethical prescribing for special populations such as children in foster care and juvenile justice systems. Ramifications of black box warnings and off label prescribing are discussed. Finally, the authors offer practical tips to guide clinicians in ethical psychopharmacologic management of their child and adolescent patients.

Conflicts of Interest Between Physicians and the Pharmaceutical Industry and Special Interest Groups

Diane H. Schetky

Health care in the United States is a tangled web of competing interest groups beneath which ethical conflicts of interest flourish.

Physicians, professional organizations, and academic medical centers must continually evaluate their relationships with the pharmaceutical industry as they relate to personal, professional, and institutional ethical values. This article explores the relevant pressing ethical issues and proposals for changing course and managing these potentially troublesome relationships.

Please approve the following synopsis as it will appear in the table of contents: Psychiatric research on children and adolescents is ethically justified by the need to reduce the burden that mental illnesses place on young people, their families, and society. Such research must be conducted with careful attention to the ethical principles of beneficence, justice, and respect for persons. Child and adolescent psychiatrists who collaborate on research trials or advise patients and families about research participation should consider nine domains when evaluating the ethical acceptability of particular protocols. These domains include scientific merit and design; expertise, commitment, and integrity; risks and benefits; confidentiality; participant selection and recruitment; informed consent and decisional capacity; incentives; institution and peer/professional review; and data presentation. Special ethical issues in child and adolescent psychiatry research concern the use of randomized, controlled treatment trials; the informed consent process for research involving adolescents; the therapeutic misconception; and conflicts of interest in physician referrals.

Please approve the following synopsis as it will appear in the table of contents: The ethics of publishing has received negligible attention in the child and adolescent psychiatry literature. We examine a range of ethical problems, including conflict of interest, bias, publishing fraudulent or inhumane research, redundant publication, plagiarism, concerns about authorship, insensitive use of language, and special issues about publishing research involving minors. Strategies to improve ethical standards of publishing are proposed.

The world as we know it is plagued with conflict, yet little attention is paid to the inherent ethical issues and challenges related to trauma work. It is important to be aware of these issues because they are bound to raise questions about how medical practitioners confer neutrality in the face of political agendas and war on one hand and maintain a commitment to a person's well-being on the other. When engaged in local, national, or international trauma work, cultural, ethnic, and political literacy is crucial, and an acknowledgment of one's subjectivity is paramount. There are contradictory points of view about practicing value-free psychiatry. Psychosocial programs should examine the long-term political consequences of their work as well as the short- and long-term humanitarian impact.

respectively, general psychiatry and child and adolescent psychiatry in the United States. Professional organizations set guidelines and standards for the expected behaviors of their members. To those ends, ethics committees were established by both the APA and the AACAP. This article describes how each of these organizations, via their committees, produced codes of ethics, and continuously provide relevant educational materials and advocacy efforts. It also reviews the APA ethics committee's responsibility for the evaluation of ethical complaints lodged against members. In closing, the article examines ethical dilemmas lurking on the horizon, beginning to be faced by the specialties and thus likely to be addressed by the committees.

FORTHCOMING ISSUES

RECENT ISSUES

ELSEVIER
SAUNDERS

Child Adolesc Psychiatric Clin N Am
17 (2008) xv–xvi

CHILD AND
ADOLESCENT
PSYCHIATRIC CLINICS
OF NORTH AMERICA

Foreword

On new beginnings. . .

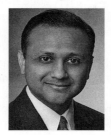

Harsh K. Trivedi, MD
Consulting Editor

You must be the change you want to see in the world.

—Mahatma Gandhi

As the incoming new Consulting Editor, I have spent much time thinking about this first foreword. My history with the *Clinics* actually predates the inception of the *Child and Adolescent Psychiatric Clinics of North America*. The *Clinics* and I first became acquainted when I was working as a weekend medical librarian at Lenox Hill Hospital on New York's Upper East Side during college. I remember being impressed by the aisles of neatly stacked color-coded, hardbound volumes that occupied nearly three aisles of book stacks; a collection with *Clinics* titles that covered more fields of medicine than I knew even existed at the time. I recall browsing the issues during breaks and lunch hours, remarking to myself about how great it was to have renowned authorities in the field guest edit and write topical review articles for application to clinical practice. Nearly two decades later, I now begin writing my first foreword as the Consulting Editor for one of those very *Clinics*.

I am fortunate that my start coincides with an issue dedicated to ethics. Much of my professional energies are devoted to my passion for mental health advocacy. Whether speaking to a mom about her child's care, to a teacher about a child's educational plan, to the mental health commissioner about children's access to appropriate levels of care, or to a United States Senator about mental health insurance coverage, I am acutely aware that there is a direct correlation between my ethical standing in society and the ability for others to accept and believe what I have to say. I thank Mary Lynn Dell for her thoughtful coverage of this topic. This is a crucial time in our field as many ethical issues have come to the forefront. It is my hope that this issue can serve as a primer to guide good clinical care and as the impetus for careful consideration of broader issues that impact our professionalism and our identity as a field.

Over the past year, much work has gone into ensuring a seamless transition in the editorship of the *Child and Adolescent Psychiatric Clinics of North America*. Careful attention was paid to ensuring that neither our contributors nor our readers were affected by this editorial change. I want to extend my sincere gratitude to Andrés Martin, who is leaving the *Clinics* to begin his editorship of the *Journal of the American Academy of Child and Adolescent Psychiatry*—the "Orange Journal." I thank Andrés for his guidance, support, and availability throughout this process and wish him success in his new role. I also thank Sarah Barth, our publisher at Elsevier, who is the true fabric of this publication and who has been the common thread between the two preceding Consulting Editors and myself.

On new beginnings, I am guided by a desire to create a *Clinics* that is indeed something that I would hope to receive in the mail: issues that are clinically relevant, timely in subject matter, and thoroughly useful. I extend a warm welcome to future guest editors and contributing authors with whom I will have the good fortune of working. As I look to continue building on the quality of these *Clinics*, I extend an open invitation to you to share your thoughts and to let me know how we can do better. Thank you and welcome.

Harsh K. Trivedi, MD
Bradley Hospital
Brown Medical School
1011 Veterans Memorial Parkway
East Providence, RI 02915, USA

E-mail address: harsh_trivedi@brown.edu

ELSEVIER
SAUNDERS

Child Adolesc Psychiatric Clin N Am
17 (2008) xvii–xix

CHILD AND
ADOLESCENT
PSYCHIATRIC CLINICS
OF NORTH AMERICA

Preface

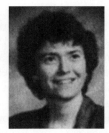

Mary Lynn Dell, MD, MTS, ThM
Guest Editor

Oh, my! how the world has changed!

—*Dr. Diane Schetky*

A little over a year ago, as I was contemplating topics and authors for this issue, I had a delightful and very productive brainstorming session over the telephone with Dr. Diane Schetky. When I mentioned that 12 years had passed since she had edited the only other issue of the *Child and Adolescent Psychiatric Clinics of North America* devoted to ethics, she exclaimed, "September of 1995?! Oh, my! How the world has changed!"

Indeed, the world in which our patients live and in which we practice medicine has changed radically over the last decade, and all indications point to future changes hurtling our way at a breakneck pace. The number of worlds in which we live and move and have our being also seems to be multiplying. In addition to local, state, national, and international political spheres, the arenas of technology, business, media and entertainment, ecology and the environment, and human genetics affect us daily. All of these worlds are relevant to pediatrics, emotions, behavior, educational institutions, recreation, and relationships, so all have meaning and importance to children, adolescents, families, and consequently, the field of child and adolescent psychiatry.

Keeping abreast of factual information has become increasingly daunting, demanding more of our professional and personal time, energy, and resources. Nevertheless, it is imperative that we set aside time to contemplate

doi:10.1016/j.chc.2007.08.004   *childpsych.theclinics.com*

some timeless and always-important questions. What are our responsibilities as clinicians working with individual children, families, and communities at this particular time and in our particular contexts? What do we as individuals, with our own personal backgrounds, education, training, experiences, and value systems, bring to our work? How do we incorporate new information and technology in the best interests of our patients? How do we strive to do the "right thing" for our patients in the midst of changing societal values, evolving health care systems, and turbulent economic and political climates?

These are a few of the questions that the authors of this issue attempt to address, wedding medical and psychiatric facts and the customs and traditions of our specialty with the wisdom that comes from actual clinical experience and practical problem solving. I believe that this collection can serve as a primer on ethics in child and adolescent psychiatry, an introduction and overview for trainees and younger clinicians, and a helpful refresher for more-seasoned practitioners who have come of age professionally since the discipline of bioethics has solidified as a necessary and helpful companion in our work.

In that spirit, this issue begins with an overview of the fields of general medical, pediatric, and psychiatric ethics, and commonly encountered schools of thought in bioethics. The piece also suggests the use of a helpful model, based on the work of ethicist Albert Jonsen, for use in systematic analysis and problem solving for clinical situations involving ethical quandaries.

The next five articles are grouped together based on their relevance to everyday clinical practice. Ascherman and Rubin review common ethical issues in child and adolescent psychotherapy. Recupero updates clinicians about ethical aspects of medical information and professional communications. Rosenberg and DeMaso spar with a "dubious guest" at our professional dinner table—managed care. The father and son duo of Alessi and Alessi proposes a framework for addressing very real ethical issues in the ever-multiplying virtual worlds of the new media. Dell, Vaughan, and Kratochvil consider the ever-expanding ethical aspects of psychotropic medication prescription for children and adolescents.

The remaining seven articles examine topics of broader and emerging interest to child and adolescent psychiatrists. Schetky reviews the influences of pharmaceutical companies and special interest groups on our profession. Hoop, Smyth, and Roberts translate the often-confusing principles of research ethics into practical language for clinicians working to understand new research reports and who care for children and families interested in participating in neuropsychiatric research and clinical trials. Walter, Rey, Soh, and Bloch discuss ethical aspects of scientific publication relevant to authors and readers alike. Joshi, Dalton, and McDonnell tackle the uncharted terrain of ethics in local, national, and international disaster psychiatry, including dilemmas of natural catastrophes and those due to human conflicts affecting children and families. Dingle and Stuber reflect on ethics education in child psychiatry across the continuum of medical student to practicing clinician and continuing medical education. Sexson and Sexson combine their experiences in pediatrics, psychiatry, and ethics in their article about child psychiatrists and health care institutional ethics committees. Finally, Sondheimer and Klykylo update us on the multi-faceted ethics activities of the American Psychiatric Association and the American Academy of Child and Adolescent Psychiatry.

As is the case for all edited volumes, space precludes including all topics that might be of interest and importance to the broad audience of the *Child and Adolescent Psychiatric Clinics of North America*. For instance, a specific piece on child forensic ethics was not included in this collection, although elements of forensics are integral to and are included in the articles on psychotherapy, medical records, and professional communications. Similarly, although ethics in pediatric consultation-liaison psychiatry is not addressed in a typical fashion, the Sexsons' article on health care ethics committees is immensely relevant and important for child psychiatrists working in and interested in pediatric and general medical settings. Readers also are referred to the discussion of ethical issues in neuropsychiatric genetics by Fuentes and Martin-Arribas in the June 2007 issue of this *Clinics* series [1]. Perhaps the next issue on ethics can tackle medical errors, community child and adolescent psychiatry, infant psychiatry, ethical concerns that arise when working with autism spectrum disorders, and family therapy ethics—just to name a few other worthy topics.

I am most grateful to the contributors to this issue, especially for their enthusiasm and willingness to share their wisdom and expertise. I have come to a greater appreciation of the insights and anticipatory ethical guidance dispensed by the authors of the original issue on ethics in the *Child and Adolescent Psychiatric Clinics of North America* published nearly 13 years ago, many thanks to Drs. Schetky, Campbell, Etemad, George, Harrison, Koocher, Krener, Levine, McFarland, Overstreet, Quinn, and Tobin, who were vital to that effort [2]. And, as always, thanks to our extraordinary publisher at Elsevier, Sarah Barth, and to the outgoing Consulting Editor, Andrés Martin, MD, MPH and incoming Consulting Editor, Harsh K. Trivedi, MD.

Mary Lynn Dell, MD, MTS, ThM
Psychiatry and Behavioral Sciences
Emory University School of Medicine
492 Ponce de Leon Manor NE
Atlanta, GA 30307, USA

E-mail address: dellml@comcast.net

References

[1] Fuentes J, Martin-Arribas MC. Bioethical issues in neuropsychiatric genetic disorders. Child Adolesc Psychiatric Clin N Am 2007;16(3):649–61.
[2] Schetky DH. Ethics. Child Adolesc Psychiatric Clin N Am 1995;4(4).

ELSEVIER
SAUNDERS

Child Adolesc Psychiatric Clin N Am
17 (2008) xxi–xxii

CHILD AND
ADOLESCENT
PSYCHIATRIC CLINICS
OF NORTH AMERICA

Memoriam and Dedication

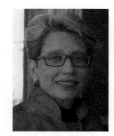

Henrietta L. Leonard, MD
(1954–2007)

> In dwelling, live close to the ground.
> In thinking, keep to the simple.
> In conflict, be fair and generous.
> In governing, don't try to control.
> In work, do what you enjoy.
> In family life, be completely present.
>
> —*Tao Te Ching*

Henrietta Leonard was kind, gracious, and amazingly personable. Her passion for science, medicine, and for life was infectious. Her ability to make others feel important was genuine. Yet, as one of her colleagues pointed out, "Henri's intelligence and accomplishments are exceeded only by her modesty." She always found time for her students and trainees, often well past their dates of graduation. She was meticulous in her work and provided clarity to the most intricate of issues. She balanced a full family life and a rich professional life. She played an important part in so many of our lives.

Beyond being an internationally acclaimed researcher, educator, editor, author, mentor, colleague, and friend, Henri was a central member of our academic family at Brown. She will be missed greatly and remembered fondly. Her legacy lives on in the hearts and minds of those who were fortunate to have known her. Her work lives on through the many patients whose lives she improved and the numerous trainees whom she nurtured and mentored.

1056-4993/08/$ - see front matter © 2008 Elsevier Inc. All rights reserved.
doi:10.1016/j.chc.2007.09.002   *childpsych.theclinics.com*

Henrietta was a staunch supporter of ethical conduct in pediatric research trials, including appropriate informed consent and assent procedures. We quite fittingly dedicate this issue on ethics to her.

Gregory K. Fritz
Jeffrey I. Hunt
Harsh K. Trivedi

ELSEVIER
SAUNDERS

Child Adolesc Psychiatric Clin N Am
17 (2008) 1–19

CHILD AND
ADOLESCENT
PSYCHIATRIC CLINICS
OF NORTH AMERICA

Theory Can Be Relevant: An Overview of Bioethics for the Practicing Child and Adolescent Psychiatrist

Mary Lynn Dell, MD, MTS, ThM[a,b,*],
Kathy Kinlaw, MDiv[c]

[a]Psychiatry and Behavioral Sciences, Emory University School of Medicine,
492 Ponce de Leon Manor NE, Atlanta, GA 30307, USA
[b]Clinical Ethics, Emory University School of Medicine, 1462 Clifton Road,
Suite 302, Atlanta, GA 30322, USA
[c]John and Susan Wieland Center for Ethics, Emory University, 1462 Clifton Road,
Suite 302, Atlanta, GA 30322, USA

Reflection on moral and philosophical aspects of medical practice, and the care of individuals suffering from physical and emotional ills, dates back at least to Hippocrates and the 5th century BCE [1,2]. Until a few decades ago, common belief was that a physician's general integrity, steeped in years of the best education available, then honed and refined through the experience of caring for ill individuals and their families, reliably led to attitudes and behaviors that prioritized the best interests of patients. American society and the profession of medicine had an unspoken consensus of what it meant to "do the right thing." However, the technological advances of the past 40 years, coupled with increased economic pressures and cultural, ethnic, and religious diversity, have led to the blurring of previously clear and unquestioned moral precepts in medical practice. Bioethics has become yet another discipline, with its own vocabulary, literature, and methodologies, in which child and adolescent psychiatrists must be fluent and current. This article provides an overview of basic concepts, various approaches to issues and schools of ethical thought, and a representative model for systematic analysis of ethical dilemmas in clinical practice.

Dr. Dell has received funding from the Templeton Foundation and the Louisville Institute.

* Corresponding author. 492 Ponce de Leon Manor, NE, Atlanta, GA 30307.
  E-mail address: dellml@comcast.net (M.L. Dell).

Fundamental concepts and definitions

Bioethics is filled with terms that are understood by many in a general way, but require definition when used in a technical sense. "Morality" refers to norms for behaviors that are accepted widely and form a consensus for sizeable groups, if not total societies. Morality includes not only rules, but beliefs, principles, and virtues that can be passed down through the generations. The terms "morality" and "ethics" are frequently used interchangeably. Ethics employs ways to think about and examine moral life [3,4]. According to Bernard Lo, ethics "connotes deliberation and explicit arguments to justify particular actions ... ethics focuses on the reasons why an action is considered right or wrong. It asks people to justify their positions and beliefs by rational arguments that can persuade others" [3].

Ethics can be divided further into "normative" ethics, or ethical theories that name and describe moral norms by which we abide, and "practical" or "applied" ethics, which deal with moral issues in particular contexts and professions [4]. "Medical" ethics, or "bioethics," then describes a discipline at the crossroads of life sciences and ethics. In a specific sense, it is an intellectual pursuit that has arisen from recent technological advances and their inherent moral challenges. Bioethics has extended beyond this backyard, however, into the domains of larger culture, law, media, public policy, theology, philosophy, the environment, and even history. It touches the most private, inner worlds of individual patients, affects their families and immediate friends, and extends into government and health policy. Lest the societal aspects of bioethics take on a larger-than-life persona intimidating to physicians in the trenches providing routine care, "clinical" ethics focuses on discerning the right thing to do in the present moment for the particular patient one is caring for at the time [5].

The history of bioethics: developments especially relevant to child and adolescent psychiatry

General medical ethics

Western medicine commonly traces the birth of medical ethics to the 4th century BCE and the Pythagoreans. Though Confucian writings from China and manuscripts from the Indian subcontinent bear similar ethical precepts, it is the oath of Hippocrates that has endured to the present day, inspired generations of students, and spawned numerous offshoots in the form of codes, oaths, covenants, and standards of conduct. Surprisingly, this oath was largely disregarded for centuries, finding favor in the Middle Ages because of its similarities to post-Constantinian Christianity. The second half of the oath includes many elements familiar to contemporary physicians, such as applying skills for the benefit of the sick to the best of ability and judgment, refusing to give harmful substances to patients, refraining from sexual relations with patients and household members, and respecting confidentiality [1,6].

The paternalism inherent to the Oath of Hippocrates and its concentration on benefits to individual patients proved to be fit companions for American practitioners and their evolving sense of professionalism through the 18th, 19th, and early 20th centuries. The majority of physicians in the United States in the 17th and 18th centuries were of British and French backgrounds and predominantly Christian. Christian ethics and virtues were essentially synonymous with good medical ethics and high standards of professionalism. Other qualities important to ethical practice, ranking just below Christianity, were those of male gentility: "proper birth, sufficient wealth, unblemished character, adequate learning, and civic service." However, by 1900, a minority of physicians were advocating for stricter attention to applied scientific knowledge, and that technically proficient skills were just as important, if not more so, than religious beliefs, virtue-based codes, and physician status in the larger community [7].

Indeed, with the emerging specialties of physiology, pathology, and microbiology came, by necessity, increased value upon objectivity and scientific medicine in patient-related care. In addition to technological advances, two other developments in organized medicine during the 20th century broadened the scope of bioethical concern and thought. These included the expanding role of hospitals and health care organizations, and the specialty and subspecialty movement in modern medicine. Diagnosis and treatment required specialized equipment and supplies too bulky and impractical for use in homes, so concentration of care in hospitals became more economical financially. Centralization of care in hospitals enabled better cooperation and coordination of care among burgeoning numbers of care providers, and by diminishing travel time, increased efficiency of physicians and nurses. As the medical fund of knowledge grew, focusing on particular organ systems and disease processes permitted physicians to not only continue rapid advances in care, but to build personal reputations and prestige. Indeed, just as much needed and appreciated technological advances in scientific aspects of medicine needed accompanying moral and ethical reflection, so too did the new accoutrements of medical professionalism: the elevated social and financial status of physicians and the risk of estrangement from the poor, working, and even middle-class, patients they served [8].

In the last 20 years, the discipline of bioethics has been influenced profoundly by imperatives to address health care financing, ethical concerns in human subjects research, genomics, and relationships with governmental agencies, pharmaceutical companies, and other private interest groups. The predominance of Protestant professional ethics has been tempered by other voices, including Catholic moral philosophy, Jewish and Muslim scholars, Eastern philosophers, secular humanists, legal experts, economists, politicians, and even patients and their families with no vested interests in dogma or protocol. Indeed, the broader background and context of medical ethics in which child and adolescent psychiatrists live and practice is expanding at an unimaginably rapid pace.

General psychiatric ethics

Until the 20th century, the history of psychiatric ethics largely paralleled that of general medical ethics in that the field was influenced significantly by contemporary Western philosophy and religious belief. Early Roman and later medieval understandings of psychiatric illness reflected early Christian convictions that mental illness resulted from sin, evil, witchcraft, and Satan. Those souls suffering from mental illness were judged to be mortal sinners or the offspring of such transgressors, or the victims of devilish activity to be associated with only at great risk to one's own eternal destiny. Of note, Eastern and Arabian medical practitioners had a much more sympathetic and enlightened approach to the mentally ill, but the more compassionate Eastern ways of care were largely unknown or unheeded by Western Europe at that time. However, pockets of humane care of the mentally ill arose in a few dedicated religious communities or orders, such as Geel, Belgium, and the Priory of St. Mary of Bethlehem (Bethlem) in London in the 13th century. As Europe's population increased, including the numbers of mentally ill needing housing and supervision, psychiatric hospitals became massive in size and quality again declined to levels of early medieval times. The mentally ill were sequestered in unsanitary, overcrowded asylums with criminals and others who needed to be separated from an enlightened society. Malnutrition, illness, abuse and neglect, and even death rates were extraordinarily high. Some of the "treatments" of the day were little more than sanctioned forms of abuse [9,10].

The French Revolution in Europe and the American Revolution in the United States signaled increased attention to the rights and humane treatment of the mentally ill. Philippe Pinel, superintendent of two large asylums in Paris at the end of the 1700s, is credited with removing chains, minimizing restraints, and communicating with patients to the fullest extent possible. In Philadelphia, the Pennsylvania Hospital under the leadership of Benjamin Rush pursued less physically constricting forms of restraint and less restrictive treatments and freedoms on hospital grounds, as tolerated by the patients. In New York, William Tuke and his grandson, Samuel Tuke, pioneered the Quaker-inspired "moral treatment" of psychiatric patients. While very paternalistic by modern standards, moral treatment promoted many benevolent practices, including exercise, conversation between patients and staff, art, reading, crafts, and table games. The idea was for caregivers to promote patients' abilities to help themselves, even if struggling with mental infirmity. Across the Atlantic at the Manchester Infirmary, Dr. Thomas Percival instituted a conduct code in 1803 for attending physicians dealing with the mentally ill that paralleled Quaker moral precepts and was related strongly to his Judeo-Christian beliefs. Percival's work was so respected as an advancement in professional ethical thought that it served as the basis for American Medical Association's first code of ethics at the time of that organization's founding in 1847 [9,10].

Dr. Worthington Hooker of Connecticut advanced ethical care of the mentally ill through *Physician and Patient; or, a practical view of the mutual duties, relations and interests of the medical profession and the community*, published in 1849. He advocated honesty with patients and treatment before they harmed themselves or others or ran afoul of the law. Until the developments in biological psychiatry in the mid-20th century, resulting in psychotropic medications and a more scientifically driven approach to the mentally ill, the practices of benevolent care of loosely regulated physicians and hospital superintendents, and segregating the insane from the rest of society in those residential facilities, were predominate in the United States and Western Europe [9,10].

Sadly, abuses in psychiatry have fueled many of the advances in psychiatric ethics. The largest abuses have come from the use of psychiatry by corrupt political and governmental authorities, such as those in Nazi Germany, Cuba, the Soviet Union, Northern Ireland, and China [11]. Other abuses have arisen from psychiatric institutions in conjunction with finances, such as abuses in Japan driven by the possibility of great monetary gains for private psychiatric hospitals, or unethical practices in the United States stemming from managed care and exploitation of third party payments [11,12]. Deinstitutionalism of psychiatric hospitals, large and highly publicized scandals in psychiatric research, and the personal abuses of power by individual clinicians regarding sexual and other boundary violations with patients—not to mention general bioethical issues that extend to psychiatry—all have spurred growing interest in psychiatric ethics [9,10,12].

Pediatric ethics

The belief that children should have access to sufficient food, clothing, shelter, parenting, education, and health care is largely a post-Enlightenment notion that has become stronger and more universally accepted in the late 19th and 20th centuries. Over the past century, children's health care has been advocated for primarily by leaders of the women's rights movement, some religious and charitable organizations, home nursing agencies, the emerging pediatric medical specialty, and later the legal profession, the social sciences, and various governmental agencies. Consensus grew that not only should children not be abused or neglected, but that they should expect preventive care and appropriate treatments for medical illnesses. From these developments came a very important impetus for ethical discourse-the fact that most decisions about medical care of children and allocation of resources for pediatric care and research are made by adults, not the target population of pediatric medicine and research [13].

Much of the pediatric ethics literature revolves around who has the power and responsibility for medical decision making involving minors. Most adults are presumed to have decision-making capacity and to be legally competent to make decisions regarding their own health care, but individuals under the age of eighteen years, by definition, are legally incompetent to consent to medical treatment and participation in research. Though some children, especially older adolescents, are capable cognitively of providing informed consent from a developmental perspective, they may not give legal consent in many situations, especially regarding life-threatening illnesses. Generally, parents or legal guardians are presumed to be appropriate medical decision makers for their children. Under the best interests standard, the parents or other surrogate considers not only the child's or adolescent's wishes, but also other factors relevant to the patient's health and welfare. When parents are available, they usually are presumed to know what is best for their child and will go to greater lengths than anyone else to advocate and obtain the best available care for their offspring. A closely related standard is that of substituted judgment, which refers to a surrogate decision maker acting as a patient would act if the identified patient were competent. The best interest standard clearly has greater relevance to pediatrics, as children by definition have never been competent and it is difficult to know completely what a noncompetent person would decide. In ideal situations involving pediatric care, shared decision making prevails. In shared decision making, parents, physicians, nurses, other health care professionals, and an older child or adolescent weigh the medical concerns, treatment options, and potential outcomes, and arrive at a consensus opinion about how to proceed. However, the final decisions fall legally and morally on parents or guardians of minor patients [13–15].

Child and adolescent psychiatry has also benefited from general pediatrics' refinement of informed consent and assent. The doctrine of informed consent directs physicians to provide explanations to parents or guardians of the illness, diagnostic procedures, and proposed treatment in common language, as well as the potential risks and benefits of the recommended treatments, alternative treatments, and no treatment at all. In addition, the caregiver is obligated to assess parental understanding of this information and the parental capacity to give consent. Though older children and adolescents cannot be regarded as autonomous decision makers, obtaining their assent for treatment facilitates healthy doctor-patient relationships and educates children about their illnesses, medications, procedures, and other treatments. The bioethics committee of the American Academy of Pediatrics has stated that assent should include developmentally appropriate explanations of a child's medical condition, tests, and treatments; an assessment of what the child understands regarding his or her care; and an indication from the minor patient about willingness to cooperate with recommended diagnostic and treatment procedures [16,17]. Obviously, these concepts are extremely relevant to subspecialties dealing with children and adolescents, especially child and adolescent psychiatry.

Finally, child psychiatrists are well advised to be aware of common ethical issues in general pediatric medicine, as many children, adolescents, and families dealing with acute and chronic medical problems and their associated stresses benefit from psychiatric care. Ethical dilemmas exist in neonatology, particularly regarding premature infants, congenital anomalies and genetic conditions, neurologic conditions, and feeding and hydration. Pediatric intensive care units deal with do-not-resuscitate orders, withdrawal of life-sustaining treatments, artificial respiration, ventilators, extubations, pain management, and end-of-life care. Adolescent issues include confidentiality, assent and informed consent, sexuality, contraception, substance use, and willingness to take medications and cooperate with recommended medical treatments. Details regarding adolescent confidentiality and parental consent to treatment, particularly involving sexual activity, contraception, substance use, and psychiatric evaluation and treatment vary from state to state. Physicians caring for adolescents are well advised to become familiar with the laws and policies in their jurisdictions and health care institutions [15,18–21].

Schools of bioethical thought

A complete review of the philosophical basis of modern bioethics is beyond the scope of this article. However, this section reviews some classic ethical frameworks and theories commonly used in medical ethics today.

The moral principles approach to bioethics

The principles approach to bioethics is largely associated with ethicists Tom Beauchamp and James Childress. These principles permeate classic ethical theories and are identifiable in common morality and professional ethical guidelines and codes. The four principles championed by Beauchamp and Childress include respect for autonomy, beneficence, nonmaleficence, and justice [22–25].

"Respect for autonomy" refers to respecting or honoring the decision-making capacities of independent, autonomous individuals. When patients have the mental abilities to understand, express preference and intent, and make voluntary decisions based on sufficient information, free from coercion or undue external influences or constraints, they are said to be autonomous for the purposes of medical decision making. In the last half of the 20th century, individual autonomy superseded the role of kindly paternalism in ethical medical practice, paralleling the ascendancy of autonomy and individualism in the American women's and civil rights movements [22,26,27].

"Beneficence" denotes the physician's duty to provide care that promotes the overall welfare of the patient, including balancing risks, benefits, and even costs. The alleviation of disease and the pain, suffering, and disability of illness and injury is the prime objective of a benevolent physician. Those physicians and patients for whom virtuous character traits in health care practitioners are important will tend to value beneficence more highly than those for whom scientific and technical fluency are paramount [23,27,28].

"Nonmaleficence" is the descendant of the Latin phrase *primum non nocere*, or "Above all, do no harm." It is the public face of the Hippocratic Oath. Many ethicists and many in contemporary society believe that nonmaleficence should be the primary consideration in patient care, trumping benevolence and patient autonomy. Much of the distrust of psychiatry stems from the previously mentioned abuses of psychiatric practice that have resulted in harms to individuals and even large groups of people, simply because they were different than the party in political power. When there are aspects of pain or other unpleasantness in a therapy or treatment intervention, these harms must be balanced and weighed against both immediate and longer-term benefits [24,27].

"Justice" is not a single principle per se, but a set of norms that guide treating individuals according to what is fair, due, or owed to them. Distributive justice has particular relevance to medical ethics as it informs the practical problem of allocation of health care resources. In a just health care system, access to services, medical products, medications, and trained professionals should be possible for all, with burdens of risks and costs distributed across society so as not to be prohibitive or burdensome for any in need of basic care and resources [25,27]. Justice can be considered on an individual basis, or microallocation, in which a child's family and care provider work together to determine adequate and appropriate care and how to best secure this according to market value and available resources, including financial, time, and professional costs. Macroallocation, involves justice associated with health care distribution for larger populations. Local, state, and national politics and economics are major determining forces [29,30].

Virtue ethics

Virtue ethics is an approach to ethical thinking in which the basic issues and judgments of ethical dilemmas concern and revolve around matters of character. The primacy of character rivals and often outweighs the overt rightness or wrongness of possible choices or action. Virtue ethicists might also go so far as to claim that without good or right character there cannot be right actions, behaviors, or conduct [31].

As one might predict, over the years there have been different opinions about which virtues are most important for physicians to possess, exercise, and nurture. The ethicist John Fletcher expounded a list of nine virtues clinicians should show forth, including: technical competence, objectivity and detachment, caring, clinical benevolence, subordination of self interest to patient care, reflective intelligence, humility, practical wisdom, and courage [32]. This list has been open to criticism by principlists and pure virtue ethicists for including elements of action (technical competence) and some principalist influences (clinical benevolence).

Virtue ethics has been promulgated on a more widespread basis by Pellegrino and Thomasma, both of whom are heavily steeped in natural law and Catholic moral philosophy. They note that modern bioethics has become a problem-solving vehicle, helping us confront dilemmas in the application of ethical principles to perplexing technological or diagnostic and treatment situations. Pellegrino and Thomasma defend their promotion of virtue ethics over what they dub "quandary ethics" in the following manner:

> ...quandary ethics is less successful in the more ancient branch of medical ethics—the ethics of character and the right and proper conduct of the physician as physician. Quandary ethics as it is now practiced places emphasis largely on the process of decision making, on the way to resolve clashes between prima facie principles such as autonomy, beneficence, and justice. It is less successful in recognizing that all choices—those made by the physician, the patient, patient surrogates, or the courts—ultimately must channel through physicians, patients, nurses, and other health professionals. ... the physician must exercise judgment on technical matters with implications for the good of the patient. No contract, no advance directives, no living will, no court order or ethics committee recommendation can cover all eventualities or anticipate those nuances or modulations of judgment that enter into the surgeon's incisions, the internist's prescriptions, or the psychiatrist's counsels [33].

The core set of virtues most helpful in ethical medical practice has shifted somewhat over the years, beginning with Socrates, Plato, and Aristotle, the Stoics, then through the Medieval Period, the Renaissance, and the Enlightenment to the present age of modern medicine [34]. Pellegrino, Thomasma, and other contemporary medical philosophers prioritize the following virtues, though not in hierarchical order: 1) fidelity to trust; 2) compassion; 3) phronesis, or practical wisdom; 4) justice; 5) fortitude; 6) temperance; 7) integrity; and 8) self-effacement. Other virtues include intellectual honesty, humility, and therapeutic parsimony [35]. Though in Western civilization these virtues grew from the Judeo-Christian tradition, virtue ethicists are quick to emphasize the universal development and recognition of these qualities throughout centuries of medical practice on multiple continents and in diverse cultures [36,37]. Perhaps a bit closer to home, as child psychiatrists in 2008 must navigate through the rapids of business, law, administration, education, neuroscience, technology, patient advocacy, pharmacology, psychotherapy, and public relations on a daily basis, virtue ethics may indeed be a helpful partner in psychiatric practice.

Feminist approaches to bioethics and the ethics of caring

In 1982, psychologist Carol Gilligan published her landmark book *In a Different Voice: Psychological Theory and Women's Development*, forever changing thought about gender differences in education, psychology, human development, theology, philosophy, ethics, and humanities in general. Gilligan and colleagues [38] proposed that males and females use a different lens through which to view, analyze, and address moral issues. Males tend to approach moral quandaries according to standards, rules, and hierarchies, whereas females approach similar matters and decision making in ways that strengthen and preserve interpersonal attachments and relationships. This approach to ethical and moral dilemmas, in no way restricted to the female sex, may serve to augment and enrich pre-existing problem-solving methods in bioethics.

Though the terms "feminist ethics" and "ethics of caring" share common features and often are used interchangeably, there are significant differences. Feminist ethics refers to a variety of schools of thought dedicated to reversing perceived and real male domination and female subordination. Subtypes include socialist, liberal, Marxist, radical, and psychoanalytic feminism, all with different approaches to address social ills affecting women in particular circumstances. Feminist bioethics is essentially the extension of feminist ethics and its methodologies to concerns confronting women in health care settings [39,40]. Feminist bioethics is concerned especially with issues of justice; availability of adequate health care for poor, oppressed, and marginalized populations; medical sequelae of abuse, neglect, and violence; political influences in medical care and its delivery; and community-based services for diseases especially prevalent in underserved groups [41,42]. Pure feminist bioethics extends the mission of leveling the playing field between the sexes to medical care, and may include rough and tumble remedies to these inequalities.

A feminine ethics of care emphasizes attention to the well being and nurturing of others, and employs empathy, compassion, and even sympathy, quite liberally. Care becomes a process worthy of attention in and of itself, with significance attached to the interactions between those giving and receiving care. An ethics of care includes not only the prescription of a psychotropic medication for a mood disorder, but also concerns itself with the concerns, feelings, and questions the individual patient may have about being diagnosed with that mood disorder. In cases in which a total cure may not be possible, physicians employing an ethics of care are able to shift into a palliative care mode without seeing themselves as having failed the patient because the most desired treatment outcome may not be possible. From the physician's perspective, there is overlap of the ethics of care with the principle and virtue of benevolence at its best. Like virtue ethics, the ethics of care is less likely than other schools to give clarity to specific strategies of problem solving in bioethical quandaries [38].

Casuistry

Casuistry is a method or approach to ethical issues that analyzes dilemmas on a case by case basis, enlisting general moral rules or principles as they are helpful in a particular instance. As early as the Greek Sophists, one can discern tension between absolute moral tenets, to be applied at all times to types or categories of moral perplexities, and the need for some flexibility when dealing with specific ethical quandaries. This has been true especially in major world faith traditions, particularly those with a book or body of sacred writings or teachings containing ethical, moral, and spiritual imperatives governing attitudes and behaviors. Such traditions begin with a certain precept or maxim, have these interpreted and passed on through layers of scholars with religious authority, preparing adherents of the faith to apply these moral values to particular situations in time, place, and circumstance. It is then understandable why casuistry, as a method of necessity, grew and thrived throughout early Western civilization and into medieval Christian Europe, and especially through much of Catholic moral thought. As the perceived need for absolute direction through principles and laws increased in the late 19th and 20th centuries, casuistry was viewed increasingly as inconsistent, not scientifically rigorous or reliably reproducible, and fell out of common favor and usage [43].

However, the emphasis of biomedical ethics on doing the right or best thing on a case by case basis has served to breathe new life into casuistry as an approach to ethical analysis. Prominent bioethicists Albert Jonsen and Stephen Toulmin published *The Abuse of Casuistry* in 1988, leading to renewed interest and respectability in this method, comparing it to the process of English common law. Jonsen and Toulmin defined modern casuistry as "the analysis of moral issues, using procedures of reasoning based on paradigms and analogies, leading to the formulation of expert opinion about the existence and stringency of particular moral obligations, framed in terms of rules and maxims that are general but not universal or invariable, since they hold good with certainty only in typical conditions of the agent and circumstances of the case" [43].

The advantages and contributions of casuistry are that it holds moral reflection close to individual cases, keeps the bedside ethical quandary at the forefront of care, facilitates the teaching and modeling of shared and practical wisdom patient care, and is user-friendly to a variety of other approaches of bioethical reflection and decision-making as they contribute to case-by-case analysis and problem solving. On the other hand, casuistry may thwart those physicians desiring clear, absolute guidelines about what to do in specific situations, and it can be ambiguous when it comes to clear explanations about why some principles or moral priorities are primary in one case but not in another case that, at least on the surface, seems quite similar in clinical fact and ethical circumstance [43].

The relationship between medical ethics and the law

More so than other illusive questions in bioethics education, medical ethics and the law is a relationship that perplexes and frustrates novices to bioethical thinking more than any other. Medical students, especially, have a tendency when confronted with an ethical quandary for which there is no totally satisfying remedy, to throw their hands up and exclaim, "So what does the law say I need to do about this?"

Bioethics and the legal system have a bidirectional relationship in which both have been affected profoundly by the other, but in any one case may be completely compatible regarding analysis and action plan, partially in agreement, or antagonistic and mutually exclusive. Medical, ethical, and legal thinking regarding pregnancy termination illustrate the variety of positions bioethics and the law can take on a particular topic, based on the details of a particular case. While the legal system at times has provided structure and guidance for issues with bioethical aspects, especially when rights and procedure are involved, it is also true that bioethics has informed legal analysis and proceedings involving life, death, and the care of minor children and those deemed incompetent and without medical decision making capacity. Indeed, bioethics and the law have blossomed into their own subspecialty areas in both parent disciplines [44].

Physicians do need to be aware of federal, state, and local laws, statutes, and codes with implications for medical practice, for these regulations and imperatives often reflect a consensus on ethical thought in larger society. However, as Bernard Lo points out in his textbook *Resolving Ethical Dilemmas: A Guide for Clinicians*, an introductory text often used in medical student education, law and ethics differ in their fundamental purposes. The law defines criminal, and thus minimally acceptable behavior, whereas bioethics strives to discern the best or optimal action or plan of care. The law may define statutory right or wrong behavior, whereas ethics encourages compassion and other virtuous attitudes and behaviors, even as the physician is behaving in a manner consistent with legal directives. In addition, clinicians can encounter ethical quandaries for which the law is silent. At other times, a physician compelled by ethical beliefs may be confronted with choices that are prohibited by law. Particularly in the specialty of psychiatry, in which cases may overlap considerably with criminal, juvenile, and family law, one must be familiar with the overlap, contradictions, and assistance legal thought can provide in instances of ethical dilemmas in clinical practice.

A helpful model for bioethical analysis

Dr. Albert R. Jonsen, a leading bioethics scholar largely responsible for the defense and renaissance of casuistry in medical ethics, in conjunction with colleagues Mark Siegler and William J. Winslade, have refined a practical model for ethical decision making in medical ethics (Box 1). Known as the "Four Topics" or "Four Quadrants Model," it provides not only physicians caring for patients, but also nurses, attorneys, clergy, allied health professionals, ethics committee members, hospital administrators, quality assurance reviewers, third-party payers, and others a systematic method

Box 1. Quadrants for case analysis

Medical indications
(Principles of beneficence and
  nonmaleficence)
What is the patient's medical
  problem? History? Diagnosis?
  Prognosis?
Is the problem acute? Chronic?
  Critical? Emergent? Reversible?
What are the goals of treatment?
What are the probabilities of
  success?
What are the plans in case of
  therapeutic failure?
How can patient be benefited
  and harm avoided?

Patient preferences
(Principle of respect for autonomy)
Is patient mentally capable and
  legally competent? Is there
  evidence of incapacity?
Patient's stated preference for
  treatment
Is patient informed of benefits or
  risks, do they understand and
  give consent?
If incapacitated, who is surrogate?
  What standards is surrogate
  using for decision making?
Do patient prior preferences exist
  (eg, advance directives)
Is patient unwilling or unable to
  cooperate with treatment? If so,
  why?
In sum, is patient's right to choose
  being respected to extent
  possible in ethics and law?

Quality of life features
(Beneficence, nonmaleficence,
  and respect for autonomy)
What are prospects, with or
  without treatment, for return
  to patient's normal life?
What physical, mental, and social
  deficits is the patient likely to
  experience with treatment?
Provider biases regarding
  quality of life?
Any point for patient when
  continued life undesirable?
Any plan or reason to forgo
  treatment?
Plans for comfort and
  palliation?

Contextual features
(Loyalty and fairness)
Are there family issues that might
  influence treatment decisions?
Are there provider issues that might
  influence treatment decisions?
Are there financial and economic
  factors?
Are there religious or cultural
  factors?
Are there limits of confidentiality?
Are there problems of allocation of
  resources?
How does the law affect treatment
  decisions?
Are there research or teaching
  issues?
Is there conflict of interest for
  providers or the institution?

Other key questions
1. What are the ethical dilemmas in the case? (Is there an ethical issue?)
2. What are the alternatives courses of action? What are the benefits and
   burdens of each? To whom?

Adapted from Jonsen, AR, Siegler, M, Winslade, WJ. Clinical Ethics: A Practical Approach
to Ethical Decisions in Clinical Medicine, 5th edition. New York: McGraw-Hill, 2006:1–11; with
permission.

of identifying and considering all aspects of an ethical issue or dilemma in a consistent, reliable fashion. Steeped in the tradition of casuistry, this model is compatible with principle ethics, virtue ethics, and other ethical schools, while simultaneously considering voices from religious, financial, legal, nursing, and family influences [45].

Topic one is "medical indications." In internal medicine and general pediatrics, this is often the most critical quadrant, though for all cases thorough consideration and understanding of the technical medical concerns is foundational to ethical analysis of any case. It includes diagnosis, prognosis, treatment options, side effects-essentially the clinical aspects of a case as they might be presented during medical rounds or a teaching conference. Guiding ethical principles are beneficence and nonmaleficence.

Topic two, "patient preferences," is informed by the principle of respect for patient autonomy. Does the patient have decision-making capacity and is he competent? Has she been given informed consent, and does she indeed understand the most important aspects of her illness and treatment? If the identified patient is a minor, has he been given information at a developmentally appropriate level and has he assented to the treatment plan? Has the patient expressed care preferences, either directly or through advanced directives? Is there a surrogate decision maker? Is the patient willing and able to cooperate with care? Is the team honoring the patient's right to choose, if at all possible?

Topic three, "quality of life," is informed by respect for autonomy, beneficence, and nonmaleficence. The team must understand what is important to the patient in daily living, how illness and treatments may affect his or her ability to be able to engage in work and play, whether there are aspects of the treatment or even the illness without treatment that are unacceptable to the patient, what biases caregivers may harbor in the analysis and actual care, and what the prospects are for adequate pain management or quality palliative care in the event of a terminal disease.

Topic four, "contextual features," is informed by ethical principles of loyalty and fairness. What are family, care provider, religious, spiritual, financial, legal, and cultural influences in this particular case? Are there distributive justice or resource allocation issues? What about confidentiality? Does any care provider or institution have a conflict of interest in regard to the identified patient, her family, or what she represents?

Case example

Joey is 17 year old Asian American male with inflammatory bowel disease, hospitalized on the general pediatric hospitalist service of a tertiary care children's hospital for treatment of infected and draining perianal fistulas. He was well known, even infamous, to all pediatric gastroenterology services in the region, for his nonadherence to care and physical aggression toward physicians and nurses was long-standing and well documented. He refused to take all medication, especially as an outpatient, because of cosmetic side effects associated with steroids and feelings of loss of control related to opiate pain medications. He had been discharged from multiple physician practices because of "noncompliance." The bulk of his medical care occurred during recurrent hospitalizations for intravenous (IV) antibiotics for infected fistulas and management for malnutrition caused by his bowel disease. Even when hospitalized, he refused IVs, adequate pain management, physical therapy, and whirlpool treatments. Nurses were afraid to care for him, for he had been physically aggressive toward a pregnant caregiver during a prior admission.

Joey's biological father is unknown, and he went to live with a maternal great aunt shortly after his mother died of a heroin overdose when he was 6 years old. The aunt has multiple health issues herself, and has been unable to have an effect on Joey's treatment adherence for the past few years. She has increasingly called police to force Joey to take his medications, but that has been less than effective over the past few months. Protective services has taken custody, but numerous foster homes have been as ineffective managing Joey as aunt has. When well enough, Joey does enjoy attending school, but even this does not seem to keep him motivated to cooperate with medical care. The school and aunt are convinced he is depressed, but he refuses to keep mental health appointments or try psychotropic medications because of the stigma associated with both. When Joey acts out and harms others, he is not kept by juvenile law enforcement authorities because of their inability to deal with his gastrointestinal disease and fear of a lawsuit. Thus, Joey bounces back and forth between foster homes and his aunt's home, based on the strategy of the current county caseworker, sometimes makes outpatient medical appointments in which he threatens or harms caregivers, does not adhere to treatment recommendations, does not attend school or psychiatry follow-up, receives no consequences for harming others, and receives essentially emergency medical care as an inpatient when he can no longer bear the pain and odor of his fistulas.

Past psychiatry consultants to the inpatient pediatric service have assessed Joey to be depressed, perhaps quietly paranoid as in a prodrome to schizophrenia, recommended perscription medications for imminent harmfulness to self or others, and helped document the need for one-to-one sitters for the safety of caregivers. Because of the strong emotions regarding Joey on the part of all caregivers and the difficult management issues involved, the new consultation liaison psychiatrist organized a care conference in which all disciplines, the aunt, and protective services caseworker could freely discuss their concerns and ideas at the same time and place. The psychiatrist facilitated this multidisciplinary meeting using the Four Topics Model to assure that all concerns were addressed.

Beginning with the "medical indications" quadrant, physicians reviewed the current status of the fistulas, nutrition, pain management, and depression, as well as treatment options and strategies. Physical therapy, nursing, and nutritionists were able to review their care as well. Though Joey had moderate to severe inflammatory bowel disease, the general consensus of all caregivers was that all problems could be adequately managed to the point of nominal pain, good nutrition, and the ability to attend school on a regular basis if Joey would keep outpatient medical appointments, take prescribed medications, and participate in physical therapy.

Next, the treatment team discussed "patient preferences." Joey's stated preference was not to be bothered with medical appointments and medications, regardless of how much pain he was in or how infected his wounds became. Though he was moderately depressed, he was not suicidal and had not harmed or threatened a caregiver during the last three hospitalizations. He refused outpatient psychiatric care and did not meet criteria for involuntary hospitalization. Although his legal decision-maker, his great maternal aunt, was competent and making decisions in his best interest, she was powerless to implement them. Joey, on the other hand, by definition incompetent because he was under the age of 18, was able to effectively refuse care because of aggressive behaviors, knowing that legal authorities would not jail him for violence because of his medical illness, and involuntary psychiatric facilities would also refuse admission for harmfulness to others because they, too, were unable to provide adequate medical care. This created the situation of a well-informed, but legally incompetent patient refusing care against the wishes of his legal guardian and medical team, and the medical, legal, and mental health systems unable or unwilling to cooperate on creative solutions.

In the "quality of life" quadrant, all disciplines and interested parties assembled agreed that Joey's current quality of life—in pain, bed-ridden with draining fistulas—was abysmal. However, this could easily be reversed and he could return to age-appropriate activities with merely adequate treatment.

The "contextual features" quadrant served the most helpful purpose of providing a structure for several sensitive issues to be discussed openly. Nurses and physical therapists were able to understand the cultural taboos of young women viewing an unclothed young man, even in the provision of necessary medical care. It was acknowledged that Joey's cultural predisposition was to not heed as authoritative the recommendations of his female physicians, nurses, physical therapists, protective service workers, psychiatrists, teachers, and even his aunt. Caregivers were able to safely express their desires to discharge him from care, even though no accepting physicians had been identified, because of their fears of injury and his abusive reactions toward them. Though no one present liked the fact that neither the legal nor psychiatric systems could force adherence to medical treatment, those physicians present were appreciative of being reminded that they could not refuse to care for Joey when he did come to medical attention, even if it was during acute inpatient encounters that might be avoided by regular outpatient follow-up. A hospital administrator was able to assure

Joey's aunt that he would not be denied by any part of that particular health care system.

In this particular case example, there were no overt changes in treatment plan. Joey's acute problems continued to be managed intensively until he was well enough to return to foster care; general pediatrics prescribed state-or-the-art care for inflammatory bowel disease that he was unlikely to follow; psychiatry recommended outpatient supportive psychotherapy and antidepressant that he refused; Joey's cultural and gender biases continued to sabotage care efforts; and his aggressive behaviors coupled with infected, draining fistulas continued to help him evade treatment or consequences in the mental health and legal systems. For some care providers, the main concerns in this case were purely medical, others worried about medicolegal ramifications if they refused to work with Joey, some believed the main problem was psychiatric; however, all agreed that numerous ethical concerns existed and were appreciative of the opportunity to address these. The use of the Four Topics Model in a one hour case conference was invaluable in reviewing the quality of care recommendations, medical and nonmedical considerations influencing treatment adherence, and in renewing commitment from the team of health care providers in the care of this very challenging young man. The team was able to define the services Joey needed when he was in their care, better understand their medical and moral obligations toward him, as well as renew their willingness to revisit the care plan as factors considered in the clinical ethics analysis changed.

Summary

Medical ethical theory and the history of bioethics, unlike some abstract or tangential domains of philosophical or theoretical ethics, are helpful for the understanding of not only the current state of bioethics, but also possible future trajectories of ethical medical practice that will affect physicians and patients alike. Child and adolescent psychiatrists need to be familiar with major ethical issues in general medicine, psychiatry, and pediatrics, in addition to those controversies that might be more specific to their subspecialty. Employing a systematic approach for the identification and analysis of ethical concerns, such as the Four Topics Model of Jonsen and colleagues, improves the child and adolescent psychiatrist's confidence that he or she not only is aware of ethical quandaries in practice, but is addressing these issues in a transparent, well-informed manner.

References

[1] Dyer AR, Miller MN. Ethics and psychiatry. In: Hales RE, Yudofsky SC, editors. Textbook of clinical psychiatry. 4th edition. Washington, DC: American Psychiatric Publishing, Inc.; 2003. p. 1629–49.

[2] Schetky DH. Ethics in the practice of child and adolescent psychiatry. In: Lewis M, editor. Child and adolescent psychiatry: a comprehensive textbook. 3rd edition. Philadelphia: Lippincott, Williams, and Wilkins; 2002. p. 1442–6.

[3] Lo B. An approach to ethical dilemmas. In: Lo B, editor. Resolving ethical dilemmas: a guide for clinicians. 3rd edition. Philadelphia: Lippincott, Williams, and Wilkins; 2005. p. 3–9.

[4] Beauchamp TL, Childress JF. Moral norms. In: Beauchamp TL, Childress JF, editors. Principles of biomedical ethics. 5th edition. New York: Oxford University Press; 2001. p. 1–25.

[5] Callahan D. Bioethics. In: Post SL, editor. Encyclopedia of bioethics, vol. 1. 3rd edition. New York: Macmillan Reference USA; 2004. p. 278–87.

[6] Veatch RM. Medical codes and oaths. In: Post SL, editor. Encyclopedia of bioethics, vol. 3. 3rd edition. New York: Macmillan Reference USA; 2004. p. 1488–504.

[7] Burns C. Medical ethics, history of the Americas: colonial North America and nineteenth-century United States. In: Post SL, editor. Encyclopedia of bioethics, vol. 3. 3rd edition. New York: Macmillan Reference USA; 2004. p. 1517–23.

[8] Jonsen AR, Jameton A. The United States in the twenty-first century. In: Post SL, editor. Encyclopedia of bioethics, vol. 3. 3rd edition. New York: Macmillan Reference USA; 2004. p. 1523–39.

[9] Musto DF. A historical perspective. In: Bloch S, Chodoff P, Green SA, editors. Psychiatric ethics. 3rd edition. Oxford: Oxford University Press; 1999. p. 7–23.

[10] Bloch S, Pargiter R. A history of psychiatric ethics. Psychiatr Clin North Am 2002;25: 509–24.

[11] Bloch S. Psychiatry, abuses of. In: Post SL, editor. Encyclopedia of bioethics, vol. 4. 3rd edition. New York: Macmillan Reference USA; 2004. p. 2172–8.

[12] Chodoff P. Misuse and abuse of psychiatry: an overview. In: Bloch S, Chodoff P, Green SA, editors. Psychiatric ethics. 3rd edition. Oxford: Oxford University Press; 1999. p. 49–66.

[13] Kopelman LM. Children: healthcare and research issues. In: Post SL, editor. Encyclopedia of bioethics, vol. 1. 3rd edition. New York: Macmillan Reference USA; 2004. p. 387–99.

[14] Ross LF. Children, families, and healthcare decision-making. New York: Oxford University Press; 1998.

[15] Lo B. Ethical issues in pediatrics. In: Lo B, editor. Resolving ethical dilemmas: a guide for clinicians. 3rd edition. Philadelphia: Lippincott, Williams, and Wilkins; 2005. p. 235–42.

[16] Committee on Bioethics of the American Academy of Pediatrics. Informed consent, parental permission, and assent in pediatric practice. Pediatrics 1995;95(2):314–7.

[17] Berger JE. Committee on Medical Liability of the American Academy of Pediatrics. Consent by proxy for nonurgent pediatric care. Pediatrics 2003;112(5):1186–95.

[18] Truog RD. Pediatrics, intensive care in. In: Post SL, editor. Encyclopedia of bioethics, vol. 4. 3rd edition. New York: Macmillan Reference USA; 2004. p. 2012–7.

[19] Kodish ED, Lyren A. In: Post SL, editor. Encyclopedia of bioethicsPediatrics, overview of ethical issues in, vol. 4. 3rd edition. New York: Macmillan Reference USA; 2004. p. 2017–9.

[20] Holder AR. Pediatrics, adolescents. In: Post SL, editor. Encyclopedia of bioethics, vol. 4. 3rd edition. New York: Macmillan Reference USA; 2004. p. 2004–12.

[21] Lantos JD, Moseley KL, Meadow W. Infants, medical aspects and issues in the care of. In: Post SL, editor. Encyclopedia of bioethics, vol. 3. 3rd edition. New York: Macmillan Reference USA; 2004. p. 1252–7.

[22] Beauchamp TL, Childress JF. Respect for autonomy. In: Beauchamp TL, Childress JF, editors. Principles of biomedical ethics. 5th edition. New York: Oxford University Press; 2001. p. 57–112.

[23] Beauchamp TL, Childress JF. Beneficence. In: Beauchamp TL, Childress JF, editors. Principles of biomedical ethics. 5th edition. New York: Oxford University Press; 2001. p. 165–224.

[24] Beauchamp TL, Childress JF. Nonmaleficence. In: Beauchamp TL, Childress JF, editors. Principles of biomedical ethics. 5th edition. New York: Oxford University Press; 2001. p. 113–64.

[25] Beauchamp TL, Childress JF. Justice. In: Beauchamp TL, Childress JF, editors. Principles of biomedical ethics. 5th edition. New York: Oxford University Press; 2001. p. 225–82.

[26] Miller BL. Autonomy. In: Post SL, editor. Encyclopedia of bioethics, vol. 1. 3rd edition. New York: Macmillan Reference USA; 2004. p. 246–51.

[27] Tong R. Nonfeminist approaches to bioethics. In: Feminist approaches to bioethics: theoretical reflections and practical applications. Boulder (CO): Westview Press; 1997. p. 53–74.

[28] Churchill LR. Beneficence. In: Post SL, editor. Encyclopedia of bioethics, vol. 1. 3rd edition. New York: Macmillan Reference USA; 2004. p. 269–73.

[29] Kilner JF. Healthcare resources, allocation of: macroallocation. In: Post SL, editor. Encyclopedia of bioethics, vol. 2. 3rd edition. New York: Macmillan Reference USA; 2004. p. 1098–107.

[30] Kilner JF. Healthcare resources, allocation of: microallocation. In: Post SL, editor. Encyclopedia of bioethics, vol. 2. 3rd edition. New York: Macmillan Reference USA; 2004. p. 1107–16.

[31] Statman D. Introduction to virtue ethics. In: Statman D, editor. Virtue ethics: a critical reader. Washington, DC: Georgetown University Press; 1997. p. 1–41.

[32] Fletcher JC, Quist N, Jonsen AR, editors. Ethics consultation in health care. Ann Arbor: Health Administration Press; 1989.

[33] Pellegrino ED, Thomasma DC. Virtue-based ethics: natural and theological. In: Pellegrino ED, Thomasma DC, editors. The Christian virtues in medical practice. Washington, DC: Georgetown University Press; 1996. p. 6–28.

[34] Pellegrino ED, Thomasma DC. Virtue theory. In: Pellegrino ED, Thomasma DC, editors. The virtues in medical practice. New York: Oxford University Press; 1993. p. 3–17.

[35] Pellegrino ED, Thomasma DC. The virtues in medical practice. New York: Oxford University Press; 1993.

[36] Pellegrino E, Mazzarella P, Corsi P. Introduction. In: Transcultural dimensions in medical ethics. Frederick (MD): University Publishing Group; 1992. p. 1–12.

[37] Murray RF. Minority perspectives on biomedical ethics. In: Pellegrino ED, Mazzarella P, Corsi P, editors. Transcultural dimensions in medical ethics. Frederick (MD): University Publishing Group, Inc; 1992. p. 35–42.

[38] Jecker NS. Contemporary ethics of care. In: Post SL, editor. Encyclopedia of bioethics, vol. 1. 3rd edition. New York: Macmillan Reference USA; 2004. p. 367–74.

[39] Tong R. Feminist approaches to bioethics. In: Feminist approaches to bioethics: theoretical reflections and practical applications. Boulder (CO): Westview Press; 1997. p. 75–98.

[40] Tong R. Feminist approaches to bioethics. In: Wolf SM, editor. Feminism and bioethics: beyond reproduction. New York: Oxford University Press; 1996. p. 67–94.

[41] Wolf SM. Introduction: gender and feminism in bioethics. In: Wolf SM, editor. Feminism and bioethics: beyond reproduction. New York: Oxford University Press; 1996. p. 3–43.

[42] Sherwin S. Feminism and bioethics. In: Wolf SM, editor. Feminism and bioethics: beyond reproduction. New York: Oxford University Press; 1996. p. 47–66.

[43] Jonsen AR, Toulmin S. The abuse of casuistry: a history of moral reasoning. Berkelet: University of California Press; 1988.

[44] Capron AM. Law and bioethics. In: Post SL, editor. Encyclopedia of bioethics, vol. 3. 3rd edition. New York: Macmillan Reference USA; 2004. p. 1369–75.

[45] Jonsen AR, Siegler M, Winslade WJ. Clinical ethics: a practical approach to ethical decisions in clinical medicine. 6th edition. New York: McGraw-Hill; 2002.

ELSEVIER
SAUNDERS

Child Adolesc Psychiatric Clin N Am
17 (2008) 21–35

CHILD AND
ADOLESCENT
PSYCHIATRIC CLINICS
OF NORTH AMERICA

Current Ethical Issues in Child and Adolescent Psychotherapy

Lee I. Ascherman, MD[a,b,*], Samuel Rubin, MD[a,b]

[a]Division of Child and Adolescent Psychiatry, The University of Alabama at Birmingham, 1700 7th Avenue South, Birmingham, AL 35294-0018, USA
[b]The Children's Hospital of Alabama, 1600 7th Avenue South, Birmingham, AL 35233, USA

The *Webster Unabridged Dictionary* [1] defines ethics as 1) "a system of moral principles," 2) "the rules of conduct recognized in respect to a particular class of human actions or a particular group...." These principles and rules are specified further by the American Psychiatric Association and particularized by the American Academy of Child and Adolescent Psychiatry. They serve to bind child and adolescent psychiatrists to a code that supports the professionalism and quality care that are necessary to gain the trust of children, families, and the society at large.

The treatment of children is based upon the precepts of first, to do no harm, second, to do what is in the best interest of the child, third, to protect the privacy of the child's communications, fourth, to respect the child as well as the family regardless of race, religion, socioeconomic status, education, or intellectual level, and fifth, to promote and support the highest level of development and autonomy in the child [2]. Additionally, we must resist pressures to control the child and coerce compliance at the cost of the individuality of our patient or compromise of the best treatment available.

The practice of psychotherapy, whether in the hospital or in the office, requires us to be able to establish rapport with the child or adolescent and with the parents or guardians. The establishment of a safe environment in which the patient can understand our respect for them and our interest in what they have to say is essential for the initiation of a process for evaluation and subsequent psychotherapy. Key to the patient's confidence in the safety of the therapeutic environment is their understanding that their words

---

* Corresponding author. Division of Child and Adolescent Psychiatry, The University of Alabama at Birmingham, 1700 7th Avenue South, Birmingham, AL 35294-0018.

E-mail address: lascherman@uabmc.edu (L.I. Ascherman).

will remain private. Protecting the child's privacy can be a complex and difficult challenge as we work with the parents to learn about their child's development in the context of family dynamics, with the school to evaluate the child's educational strengths and weaknesses, and with the justice system and other agencies to advocate for the child's need. The child and adolescent psychiatrist plays an essential role as the professional who integrates information and informs the child and the family of the options for treatment. Once treatment is recommended, third-party payors can encroach upon the family's and child's privacy with requests for data about the evaluation and the psychotherapy. This further challenges the child and adolescent psychiatrist to provide information that will justify support of treatment while preserving the confidences of the child and family.

Evolving ethical considerations

Some of the ethics-based rules that apply to the practice of child and adolescent psychiatry are clear and generally agreed upon [3]. For example, rules against sexual contact or harsh or abusive treatment are encoded as boundary violations. They are based on the recognition that such experiences traumatize, distorting and injuring the child's trust, self-esteem, and capacity for intimate relationships.

In other realms related to developments in biology and genetics, technology, and social changes, new ethical considerations emerge. Many areas relevant to the practice of psychotherapy are less clear than our basic "rules." For example, the use of the telephone for psychotherapy, audiovisual links for evaluation and treatment, and the use of the Internet and e-mail warrant careful attention and thoughtful consideration of issues relevant to privacy and efficacy.

Respecting boundaries

Psychotherapy with children and adolescents is an alone endeavor. Our experience of the patient's desires and aggressive impulses can induce us to action based on our own needs and conflicts. During any psychotherapy process, subtle instances can arise that pose risk for boundary problems. Work with preschool children offers many examples: the child who wants to sit on our lap or hug us. Sometimes children of this age may remove their shoes, raise their skirt, or want to take off their shirt. Others may want to invite us to their homes or have us attend a social or religious event. In all of these situations, the child and adolescent psychiatrist is challenged to refrain from actions that confuse boundaries and, instead, promote the child's expression of longings and impulses in words. Older children and adolescents may challenge boundaries by posing personal questions, such as those about marital status or whether we have children. Such questions indicate curiosity and are potential opportunities to understand the child further. Motivations for the questions can be explored without necessarily having to provide an answer to them.

Although there are no hard and fast rules, therapeutic neutrality can be a helpful guide for making our way with the child or adolescent in the psychotherapeutic process. This concept often is misunderstood. It does not mean that the child and adolescent psychiatrist does not care about the child or does not react with feelings to the evolving process. Rather, it refers to the therapist's need to remain "neutral" to the conflicts and desires of the child that strive for satisfaction with the therapist. Being "neutral" to these means that we neither encourage nor condemn them, but remain interested, wanting to understand their meaning for the child. This construct helps us to secure a position that protects the therapeutic space for the child and child and adolescent psychiatrist, inviting discussion rather than expression through action. It also is relevant to our work with parents or guardians as we strive to be aware of our reactions to them, using this awareness to inform our efforts to understand and help them.

The practice of psychotherapy with children and adolescents presents us with the responsibility to constantly monitor our own reactions to the patient and family and their reactions to us and to the treatment situation. Obviously, everything is not just transference and countertransference. There are outer reality issues and the child's real relationship with the child and adolescent psychiatrist that need to be considered; however, attunement to the patient's perceptions of us and our perceptions of him or her can greatly inform us about the child's conflicts. Sometimes, our reactions to a child, adolescent, or his or her family may be more about us than about them. Knowledge of the sources of our reactions and responses may free us to work more objectively and may restore a therapy process in jeopardy. When the child and adolescent psychiatrist remains puzzled by his or her reactions or the therapy process does not progress, consultation with a trusted colleague may be helpful. Occasionally, seeking treatment for oneself may be the best choice.

Autonomy of older children and adolescents

There is growing recognition by the judicial system of a minor's ability to contribute to decisions based on understanding and objectivity [4]. Whether recognized legally in any given jurisdiction or not, there remain clinical and ethical indications for children and adolescents to participate in decisions about treatment, including their psychotherapy. In addition to being respectful, the working alliance is strengthened when the child or adolescent feels that he or she has participated in an informed decision to pursue psychotherapy, rather than experience it as imposed by others.

Liability for dangerous patients, abandonment, and other current issues

Society's concerns about dangerousness have increased again in response to the recent tragic violence at Virginia Tech (Virginia Polytechnic Institute and State University in Blacksburg, Virginia). The dilemma between duty to the patient and duty to society was the subject of the Pace Law Review published in 1999–2000 entitled "Current Issues in the Psychiatrist–Patient Relationship: Outpatient Civil Commitment, Psychiatric Abandonment and the Duty to Continue Treatment of Potentially Dangerous Patients—Balancing Duties to Patients and the Public" [5]. This review contains extensive discussion of the difficulties predicting dangerous behavior. When working with patients with recognized risks for dangerousness, attentiveness and vigilance should increase when decisions to transfer or stop treatment are made. Although confidentiality and privacy must be considered, the child and adolescent psychiatrist also should be thoughtful and deliberate when contact with a patient with a potential for dangerousness is threatened to be weakened or lost. Erring on the side of safety for the patient, the patient's family, and the community is advised.

Protection of data about the child and family

The child and adolescent psychiatrist's responsibility to protect information about the child and his or her family dates to the Hippocratic oath. The duty to hold in confidence that which is revealed in the context of the doctor–patient relationship evolved in law as a responsibility incumbent upon the physician once the doctor–patient relationship, a fiduciary relationship, is established. The foundation of this responsibility lies in the Latin meaning of fiducia, "trust." A fiduciary is defined as "a person who stands in a special relation of trust, confidence or responsibility in his obligations to others" [6]. It is the physician who carries the responsibility to guard and protect the trust and confidence of his or her patient. Breach of the fiduciary relationship is a key legal condition for modern malpractice.

These principles also serve as the underpinnings of the psychotherapy relationship between the child and adolescent psychiatrist and patient. It is only with the establishment of trust and confidence that a therapeutic space can be created. Within this space, the child or adolescent can feel sufficiently safe to trust in his or her freedom to reveal what he or she thinks and feels without being judged, retaliated against, or violated by breach of his or her privacy.

Communication with parents and guardians

From its very beginnings, the profession of child and adolescent psychiatry has attempted to understand children in the context of their biologic heritage, family, community, and culture, exploring how these interact and influence the child's development. Variability in the relative influence of each of these forces from child to child has led to the development of a repertoire of interventions, including pharmacology, parent guidance, family therapy, individual therapy, and advocacy in schools and courts. A recommendation for individual psychotherapy usually reflects an appreciation that disturbance in the child's internal world (whether conceptualized as thoughts, feelings, or both) carries its own momentum, despite biologic and environmental interventions, and that these disturbances threaten to distort the trajectory of further development.

Those conducting psychotherapy with children and adolescents encounter unique challenges in their efforts to protect their patient's privacy. Child and adolescent psychiatrists rarely operate in a vacuum sealed from interaction with parents and guardians. When this does occur, it can reflect a parent's trust in the process and respect for their child's privacy or, more ominously, a lack of interest in his or her child's emotional life and an implicit delegation of responsibility for the child's well-being to the child and adolescent psychiatrist. In one situation, the child and adolescent psychiatrist may find him- or herself challenged to protect the privacy of the psychotherapeutic process from parents or guardians who are perceived as too intrusive. In another, he or she may appeal for greater involvement from parents who are perceived as too remote.

Regardless of where on this spectrum the child and adolescent psychiatrist finds him- or herself with a given patient, the ethical principles guiding one's conduct of communication with parents and guardians remain the same. Parents and guardians have rights to be informed about any treatment conducted for their child, including psychotherapy, and to be updated on their child's progress. In addition, a psychotherapy process with a child or adolescent that is too opaque to parents or guardians can elicit distrust sufficient to jeopardize the alliance and risk disruption of the process. The child and adolescent psychiatrist must balance the rights of parents or guardians and the clinical indications for some communication with them against the child's right for reasonable privacy and the clinical need for the child to be able to trust that he or she has sufficient privacy for the process to be effective. The child or adolescent who perceives one's therapist as too open a conduit of information to one's parents is likely to remove critical information from the process, rendering it compromised, if effective at all.

Upon recommending a psychotherapy process, the child and adolescent psychiatrist has the responsibility and opportunity to review with parents or guardians the structure of the psychotherapy frame and, importantly, its rationale. In addition to discussing schedule, duration of sessions, frequency, and estimated duration of treatment, issues relevant to the child's privacy should be addressed. Parents can be reassured that there is regard for their need to be informed about the process intermittently. The importance of such communication can be emphasized to parents who are inclined to be too remote. The frequency of sessions with parents or guardians is a clinical decision, integrating such variables as the age of the child, the severity of the child's problems, the severity of the parents' issues, the strength of the alliance with the parents and child, and the needs of the parents.

The challenges faced in balancing a child's need for reasonable privacy against the parents' need for reasonable information can be shared candidly with parents or guardians. Parents can be told that their child's confidence in the relative privacy of the process can be critical to its efficacy, but that their need for information also is respected to help them understand and parent their child. The parents also can be reassured that information suggesting imminent danger to their child or others would not be withheld from them. Empathy for the challenges of parenting, avoiding blame, direct acknowledgment of the child and adolescent psychiatrist's time-limited role with the child in contrast to the parents being there for the "long run," communication of hope that improvement in the child's relationship with his or her parents can be a consequence of the psychotherapy, and recognition that no parent can be a therapist to one's own child and remain an effective parent all serve to strengthen the alliance with parents and their comfort with their child's privacy.

The structure of the psychotherapeutic frame also should be reviewed with the child or adolescent. The rationale for periodic contact with parents or guardians can be discussed, highlighting that these contacts in no means abrogate the child and adolescent psychiatrist's responsibility to guard the child's privacy. The child or adolescent should be informed of the frequency of sessions with parents or guardians and should be invited to discuss what one would like communicated before such sessions. Together, the child and child and adolescent psychiatrist can anticipate what may arise in discussions with the parents. The child and adolescent psychiatrist also can provide the patient with an example of how one might frame an issue for the parents, inviting feedback as to whether this example is respectful of his or her privacy. Communication of broader themes that avoid details that the child would deem too personal is advised, eg, "Billy is working on how he can gain independence while still maintaining important ties to you as his parents." The child and adolescent psychiatrist also should offer to review with the child the session with his or her parent or guardian after it occurs. A summary impression of the session can be provided while maintaining reciprocal respect for the parent's or guardian's privacy.

One common challenge to any child's confidence in his or her privacy is a parent's appeal to have time with the child and adolescent psychiatrist at the beginning or end of the child's scheduled time. It is not unusual for a parent to want to report on what a child has done, with the implicit or explicit message that the child and adolescent psychiatrist address the issue in the upcoming session. Sometimes, the parent attempts to have this discussion in the waiting room. These types of communications challenge the confidence that a child or adolescent has in the autonomy of his or her process and privacy. It also disrespects the boundary of the child's time and therapeutic space. Fulfilling the parent's appeal for time at the beginning of the child's session, whether the child remains in the room or not, inevitably distorts the child's freedom to begin the session with his or her agenda, confusing for the child whether the child and adolescent psychiatrist is the guardian of the psychotherapeutic space or simply the agent of the parent. Meeting with a parent during the latter portion of the child's scheduled time or immediately after the session with the child can collude with the child's fantasy that the child and adolescent psychiatrist is reporting to the parent, constricting the child's confidence that one has privacy in sessions. Discussing issues with a parent in a waiting area is an obvious violation of the child's privacy.

Consideration of why a parent or guardian may press for a portion of a child's session can help to inform the child and adolescent psychiatrist's understanding of the child and parents. For example, a parent's appeal for contact during his or her child's scheduled session can reflect hunger for or envy of the attention being directed at one's child, anxiety about his or her child's privacy with the child and adolescent psychiatrist, or wishes for the child and adolescent psychiatrist to fulfill the role of a missing parent. The solution to the challenge of providing sufficient time to a parent or guardian without violating the therapeutic space established for the child is to structure a parent process separate from the child's time.

Written and verbal communication with parties outside of the family

Requests for information about a child or adolescent in psychotherapy can be abundant. The child and adolescent psychiatrist becomes the gatekeeper of information and guardian of his or her patient's privacy. In *Jaffe v Redmond* [7], The US Supreme Court upheld the patient's privilege with regard to the release of psychotherapy records, reinforcing the patient's right to privacy and the importance of the patient' s freedom to enter a psychotherapy relationship with confidence in the protection of one's privacy. With minors, that privilege becomes the right of parents or guardians unless state law gives that right to the minor before he or she reaches the age of majority; however, parents and guardians may not always appreciate the potential ramifications of releasing information. Even when legal authority to communicate written or verbal information to a third party is granted by a signed release of information, the responsibility of the child and adolescent psychiatrist to consider the ramifications of what is released to whom remains paramount.

The child and adolescent psychiatrist should respond to any request for release of information with consideration of its appropriateness and necessity and the potential impact of what is released on the child, the family, and the psychotherapy process. Child and adolescent psychiatrists are vulnerable to mistakenly think that they must respond to any request for information, absenting their discretion about what is shared with whom. This is particularly the case with requests for written reports, which often contain abundant information beyond the needs that generated the request. These reports also may contain information about family members.

When considering written or verbal communication to a third party, the child and adolescent psychiatrist should discuss the request with the child and the parents or guardian. If the child and adolescent psychiatrist has questions about the necessity of the release or concerns about the potential ramifications of such information, these should be communicated openly. If there is a decision to communicate with outside parties, careful consideration should be made as to what is said or sent, with streamlining of communication to the minimum necessary to achieve the goals of that request. Reports requested by schools, courts, or hospitals should be reviewed carefully, scrutinizing whether the content is congruent with the needs of the request and whether the reports contain information about the child or others that is beyond what is needed. The child and adolescent psychiatrist always should consider the long-term fate of what is released, including whether the setting receiving the material will be able to guard the privacy of these records in ways appropriate for their content. When records communicate more than is needed for the purpose of the request, the child and adolescent psychiatrist can compose a summary letter that includes the information needed and no more. Although less convenient than sending already prepared documents, the duty to protect a patient's privacy always should outweigh such convenience.

Psychotherapy records also should be segregated from the main medical record. Rarely, if ever, should there be a reason to release process. Child and adolescent psychiatrists practicing in settings with centralized records in a medical records office should guard against portals that could allow anyone other than the treating child and adolescent psychiatrist to make decisions as to what is copied and released.

The child or adolescent and their parents or guardians should be involved in discussions about whether to release information and what information should be released. What will not be released should be highlighted, emphasizing that the child and adolescent psychiatrist, as guardian of the psychotherapy process, will not communicate details about the child or family that are not relevant to the needs of the request. Requests for communication with others that are initiated by the child and adolescent psychiatrist also should be discussed with parents or guardians and patients. Ideally, discussions with the child or adolescent should occur separately from discussions with parents or guardians, so that each has maximum freedom to speak openly. Please refer to the article by Recupero elsewhere in this issue for a related discussion of medical communications, including attention to medicolegal considerations.

Ethical and clinical considerations with e-mail and telephone communication

Many of the pertinent issues that child and adolescent psychiatrists face with the availability of electronic communication are discussed by Kassaw and Gabbard [8] in their 2002 review of the topic. While noting specific situations in which e-mail communication might have a constructive potential, they highlight three areas of ethical concern: "1) problems inherent in the mechanics of E-mail, 2) privacy and confidentiality issues, and 3) the loss of essential elements of the therapeutic action associated with the psychiatrist-patient relationship." All of these issues are relevant to psychotherapy with children and adolescents.

Limitations to the ability to ensure the security of information communicated electronically pose risks to privacy, despite the "illusion of security" that passwords promote. Technological vulnerabilities, together with human error (ie, inadvertent access to files or visibility of screens), provide sufficient rationale for caution against maintaining detailed electronic material related to psychotherapy. Recent incidents gaining national attention involving the theft or loss of electronic information only reinforce the need to avoid electronic preservation of such personal material as that which would exist in a psychotherapeutic exchange.

Conducting psychotherapy through electronic communication also is problematic. E-mail communication in exchange for direct communication in the office deprives the child and adolescent psychiatrist of critical information related to facial expression, body language, and voice tone. Emotion is drained from word text, spontaneity is lost, and the potential to edit communication is maximized. Reciprocally, the patient is deprived of the voice tone, facial expression, and body language of the child and adolescent psychiatrist, essential elements of communication that have a strong influence on the therapeutic relationship, process, and course. Cyber communication also may collude with the child's or adolescent's avoidance of direct communication about particularly important issues, including those related to safety. Electronic communication easily promotes a quality of remoteness in a relationship, contrary to the method and aims of the psychotherapeutic process.

The establishment of e-mail exchange as a forum for communication also distorts the traditional therapeutic space. A reliable time and place for contact and therapeutic work is exchanged for more amorphous cyberspace. Direct contact and visibility is replaced by invisibility. Even scheduled electronic communication concentrated to a reliable time can degenerate easily to more erratic communication that parcels information and dilutes therapeutic intensity. In addition, the fantasy that the child and adolescent psychiatrist as psychotherapist is available on demand is reinforced by irregular communications and responses. The child and adolescent psychiatrist also places him- or herself at risk for missing important messages about safety when precedent is established for e-mail as a sanctioned form of communication. Critical information often is diluted with other messages and affectively may be cold by the time the therapist electronically receives the information or responds. Please refer to the article by Recupero elsewhere in this issue for additional discussion regarding electronic communications.

For similar reasons, the use of the telephone as a regular alternative to direct face-to-face sessions also is discouraged. The loss of the visibility of the patient to the therapist and the therapist to the patient can seriously limit communication and understanding. Issues of key importance are more likely to be avoided. This avoidance may be less apparent to the therapist because of the absence of visual cues. Patient and therapist also can become more vulnerable to competing visual stimulation that detracts from attention to the therapeutic relationship and process.

Hospital psychiatry and the psychotherapeutic relationship

The child and adolescent psychiatrist conducting a psychotherapy process with a patient who is hospitalized faces unique challenges in balancing one's ethical obligation to maintain the privacy of the psychotherapy relationship with the need for open communication in the hospital setting. This is true whether the child and adolescent psychiatrist conducting the psychotherapy also is conducting the hospital treatment or whether hospital treatment has been referred to a colleague. In the latter scenario, it is easier to maintain an identity as psychotherapist, but some liaison to members of the inpatient team will still be likely.

Hospitalization should not mandate loss of privacy in the psychotherapy relationship. Principles for communicating with parents can serve as a guide for what material is communicated to the larger inpatient team. The child and adolescent psychiatrist as psychotherapist can use one's knowledge of the child to enhance the treatment team's understanding of the child without providing more information than is essential. What might be said to the treatment team should be discussed first with the child. As with outpatient treatment, the child and adolescent psychiatrist conducting the psychotherapy should clarify early in one's contact with the hospitalized patient that the therapist cannot hold information directly relevant to the child's safety or the safety of others. If such issues arise, it is best to explore them sufficiently so that, preferably, the child brings this information to the treatment team.

The challenges of practice in a "small community"

The challenge to maintain therapeutic boundaries with patients and their family members is greatest within smaller communities in which paths outside the therapeutic relationship are much more likely to cross [9]. Although the "small community" often is thought of as the small town or more isolated rural area, small communities also are common within larger metropolitan areas. They exist in neighborhoods, school districts, ethnic and religious subcultures, professional groups, work places, and common socioeconomic circles. In addition to the greater challenges maintaining boundaries and avoiding conflicts of interest within such communities, it also is harder for the psychotherapist to remain relatively anonymous. Far more information about the psychotherapist may enter and influence the psychotherapeutic space, often without the immediate knowledge of the therapist. As a consequence, the patient and the child and adolescent psychiatrist can feel constraints to the freedom that should be inherent to the psychotherapy process.

Overlapping relationships within small communities should be avoided whenever possible. Care should occur when referrals are made that carry potential for conflicts of interest or compromised anonymity. Despite the awkwardness of declining such referrals, it always is best to refer to a colleague when problems are anticipated. In communities so small that an alternative is not available, the child and adolescent psychiatrist who accepts such a patient must maintain additional vigilance to guard the psychotherapeutic space. Discussing these issues with the child and parents at the onset of treatment is recommended. This will help to reinforce the therapeutic frame and avoid misunderstandings about limiting contacts outside the treatment relationship. The child and adolescent psychiatrist also must anticipate that by entering a treatment relationship with that child and parent, social relationships with them will not be possible in the future.

Public encounters

Public encounters with patients pose challenges to privacy and confidentiality and to the child and adolescent psychiatrist's anonymity. Although often unpredictable, some public encounters can be anticipated and avoided. When a child and adolescent psychiatrist is aware that a child or parent may be at an event that he or she attends, one may choose to avoid the event or discuss the potential encounter with him or her ahead of time. In communities in which interface is likely to happen at some time or another, the child and adolescent psychiatrist may anticipate this with one's patient, allowing for some preparation for when it occurs.

Acknowledgment of a relationship with a patient in a public setting can be experienced as a violation of the patient's privacy and confidentiality. A lack of acknowledgment can be experienced as a snub. In general, it is best for the child and adolescent psychiatrist to explain to one's patient and his or her parents that, in the case of encounter outside of the office, one will err in the direction of not acknowledging them unless they initiate an acknowledgment. In the latter case, the child and adolescent psychiatrist should keep in mind that an acknowledgment initiated by a patient or parent, even one that seems overtly extraverted, may result from anxiety rather than any real indifference to their privacy. Given that the child and adolescent psychiatrist is the guardian of the patient's confidentiality, it is best to respond with a socially appropriate response without encouraging much discussion or introduction of others. In subsequent clinical contact, it is useful to explore the patient's reactions to the encounter, especially if he or she does not bring it up.

Privacy versus secrecy

The *American Heritage Dictionary of the English Language* [6] defines privacy as "the condition of being secluded or isolated from the view of, or from contact with, others." Secrecy is defined as "the quality or condition of being secret or hidden, concealment" [6]. Although there is some overlap in the definitions and common connotations of privacy and secrecy, the terms are not identical for the purposes of understanding the psychotherapeutic relationship. Although information shared within the therapeutic space contains information that can be perceived as secret, its therapeutic purpose is to promote freedom within this space to not hide, rather than to hide, from others for some covert purpose. The US Supreme Court ruling of *Jaffe v Redmond* [7], affirming the patient's privilege for releasing the content of psychotherapy, emphasizes the patient's right to privacy and freedom to seek treatment by trusting in that right. The Court wrote, "If the privilege were rejected, confidential conversation between psychotherapists and their patients would surely be chilled..."

Despite the psychotherapist's understanding of the distinction between privacy and secrecy, children and adolescents, parents, and hospital teams are vulnerable to misconstrue protection of the patient's privacy as a collusion of secrecy. For the child or adolescent to use the psychotherapeutic space freely and optimally, and for the parents or guardians to maintain sufficient trust in the therapist and process, it is crucial to clarify the distinction between privacy and secrecy at the beginning of the treatment relationship and at subsequent junctions when there is evidence that such misunderstandings of this distinction reemerge.

Countertransference

Moore and Fine's *Psychoanalytic Terms and Concepts* [10] includes in its discussion of the term "countertransference" "...feelings and attitudes toward a patient... derived from earlier situations in the analyst's life that have been displaced onto the patient...Others include all ...emotional reactions to the patient, conscious and unconscious, especially those that interfere with... understanding and technique. This broad purview might better be designated *counterreaction*."

The construct of countertransference is related intimately to neutrality, defined by Moore and Fine [10] as "...keeping the countertransference in check, avoiding the imposition of one's own values on the patient, and taking the patient's capacities rather than one's own desires as a guide...The concept also defines the recommended emotional attitude of the analyst - one of professional commitment or helpful benign understanding that avoids extremes of detachment or overinvolvement."

The relevance of countertransference and neutrality to the ethics of conducting psychotherapy lies in the critical importance of the child and adolescent psychiatrist's attention to his or her emotional reactions to one's patient and one's patient's parents or guardians. Although such reactions are unavoidable and may provide useful information toward understanding patients, it is incumbent upon the treating child and adolescent psychiatrist to exercise vigilance as to how one's reactions might influence one's conduct of the psychotherapy process. When the child and adolescent psychiatrist is aware of an intensity of feelings toward a given child or adolescent or that such feelings have influenced one's behavior toward one's patient or one's patient's parents in ways that deviate from one's usual practice, greater self-scrutiny is warranted. Such deviations in intensity of feelings or behavior also serve as serious warning signs for a potential for boundary violations, placing child and therapist at risk. When this occurs, it is critical to avoid the predictably strong temptation to rationalize what is unfolding. Consultation with supervisors or colleagues is critical to avoid any enactment that is detrimental to all. Common warning signs in the behavior of the therapist include recurrent lateness to sessions, extensions of sessions, touching of patients, gifts to the patient, and contact with the patient outside of scheduled sessions, especially outside of the office setting.

The influence of the child and adolescent psychiatrist's values on one's attitude toward one's patients or one's patient's parents or guardian also warrants vigilance. Child and adolescent psychiatrists will encounter patients and families holding a variety of cultural, religious, and political beliefs that may differ from their own. Respect for their beliefs is essential. In addition, children and adolescents often communicate internal conflict about their beliefs and values. When this occurs, the child and adolescent psychiatrist should refrain from the temptation to interject one's values as a means to assist the child with his or her conflicts. Rather, one should remain respectful of one's patient's dilemma, helping him or her to arrive at his or her own acceptable solutions, even when those solutions may not be consistent with one's own beliefs and values.

More than one therapist

In most cases, it is problematic for a child or adolescent to be engaged in concurrent psychotherapy processes. At a minimum, the patient is at risk for perceiving conflicting and potentially confusing messages from his or her therapists. In addition, in response to perceptions of each therapist, the patient is vulnerable to omitting key aspects of him- or herself from both of the psychotherapy processes. For example, the therapist attempting to address more central issues may be at risk for being devalued, whereas the therapist farther from these issues becomes idealized. Both therapists, in turn, develop incomplete and potentially distorted views of the patient.

A few treatment situations may allow for concurrent psychotherapy processes. When these are undertaken, vigilance to the potential risks must occur. Some hospital programs provide inpatient therapists other than the child or adolescent psychiatrist treating the patient outside the hospital. When such arrangements exist, sanctioned communication between these therapists is essential so that the therapists' efforts are coordinated and coherent to the patient and family. In general, the inpatient therapist's focus should be on those issues most immediately relevant to the events precipitating hospitalization. Ideally, the outpatient psychotherapist can enhance the inpatient therapist's understanding of the child or adolescent without disclosing nonessential information that the patient has shared in confidence.

Patients who have eating disorders and substance abuse disorders may work with more than one psychotherapist when the roles of each are distinguished clearly. In this situation, the role of one child and adolescent psychiatrist is to focus almost exclusively on the problematic behavior, providing monitoring and support, whereas the other provides a more open-ended, judicious exploratory process as a means to support the patient's overall growth and development, including the navigation of stressors that place one at higher risk for relapse. Here again, ongoing communication between therapists is essential to promote coherence for the patient and family and to minimize the potential drifts toward idealization and devaluation that can occur.

In some clinical settings, one clinician works with the child or adolescent while another works with the parents or guardians. This model protects the integrity of the child's time, especially when the parents or guardians have significant, ongoing needs of their own; however, it does little to enhance parents' or guardians' trust in their child's psychotherapy process unless there is constructive communication with them about that process. This can be done by the clinician working with them, by the clinician working with their child, or by both. Both clinicians should maintain awareness that they are vulnerable to distorted views of the child and parents influenced by what they hear or experience in their respective processes. Ongoing communication between the clinicians helps to protect against this. Each clinician will be challenged to communicate enough to the other to help inform his or her understanding, without disclosing details that violate the child's or parent's reasonable privacy.

Summary

Core ethical principles for the conduct of psychotherapy with children and adolescents transcend times, trends, and jurisdictions. Advances in technology, variations in state law, and the evolution of federal law should stimulate consideration of how these ethical principles apply to new situations; however, the guiding compass remains the psychotherapist's obligation to create and protect the integrity of the psychotherapeutic space to provide the child or adolescent the freedom to identify, examine, explore, and hopefully resolve the issues that bring one to treatment. Boundaries, privacy, confidentiality, and the patient's autonomy are components of this space. Together, they reflect a basic respect for the patient central to professional conduct and essential to any effective treatment process.

References

[1] Random House Webster's unabridged dictionary. 2nd edition. New York: Random House; 2001.
[2] Schetky DH. Preface. Child Adolesc Psychiatr Clin N Am 1995;4(4):XIII–XXIV.
[3] Schetky DH. Boundaries in child and adolescent psychiatry. Child Adolesc Psychiatr Clin N Am 1995;4(4):769–78.
[4] Redding RE. Children's competence to provide informed consent for mental health treatment. Wash Lee Law Rev 1993;50:569–753.
[5] Sentiman LC, Kaufman G, Merton V, et al. Current issues in the psychiatrist-patient relationship: outpatient civil commitment, psychiatric abandonment and the duty to continue treatment of potentially dangerous patients-balancing duties to patients and the public. Pace Law Rev 2000;20:231–62.
[6] Morris W. The American heritage dictionary of the English language. 1st edition. New York: American Heritage Publishing Co., Inc.; 1969.
[7] Jaffe v. Redmond, 518 U.S. 1 (1996).
[8] Kassaw K, Gabbard GO. The ethics of e-mail communication in psychiatry. Psychiatr Clin North Am 2002;25:665–74.
[9] Simon RI, Williams IC. Maintaining treatment boundaries in small communities and rural areas. Psychiatr Serv 1999;50(11):1440–6.
[10] Moore BE, Fine BD, editors. Psychoanalytic terms and concepts. New Haven (CT): The American Psychoanalytic Association and Yale University Press; 1990.

ELSEVIER
SAUNDERS

Child Adolesc Psychiatric Clin N Am
17 (2008) 37–51

CHILD AND
ADOLESCENT
PSYCHIATRIC CLINICS
OF NORTH AMERICA

Ethics of Medical Records and Professional Communications

Patricia R. Recupero, JD, MD[a,b]

[a]The Warren Alpert Medical School of Brown University, 345 Blackstone Boulevard,
Providence, RI 02906, USA
[b]Butler Hospital, 345 Blackstone Boulevard, Providence, RI 02906, USA

Child and adolescent psychiatrists typically produce two types of written communication about the patient: internal records, such as medical records and psychotherapy notes, and external communications, such as correspondence or consultation with other caregivers, schools, or courts and individuals in the legal community. Internal records are designed to document the patient's treatment and condition and are maintained primarily to support the psychiatrist's recall of essential aspects of the patient's history. They also may be maintained for review, or to support reimbursement, by third parties, as well as to communicate with other caregivers who may access the record in the care of the patient. Although internal records are created primarily for the use of the treating psychiatrist and, possibly, third parties involved in the patient's care, they are subject to lawful subpoena in litigation (eg, custody disputes, dependency proceedings, malpractice lawsuits, and other legal proceedings). External communications, such as letters to pediatricians or reports to schools, are written specifically for the use of third parties. Ethical considerations (eg, honesty, patient autonomy, confidentiality, and professionalism) apply to internal records and external communications, but considerations may differ depending on the context in which a particular document was created. Because there is a lack of published literature concerning the ethical implications of records and documents in child and adolescent psychiatry, this article draws heavily on the forensic literature and lessons that may be learned from the law.

Communications

Child and adolescent psychiatrists may work as consultants or as treatment providers. Consultants frequently interface and collaborate with other

---

E-mail address: patricia_recupero@brown.edu

professionals in the child's life, and information sharing may be necessary. Concerns about confidentiality of the information exchanged are of special importance. For example, a consultant who is asked to evaluate a child for special educational needs usually would not have a need to disclose to the school the child's reports of sibling rivalry issues.

Treatment providers also may be requested to help with consultations, particularly in educational settings, where such consultations may be clinically appropriate for the child [1]. Hospital and residential stays for children have been decreasing, increasing the burden placed on schools to manage more psychiatrically ill students and increasing the need for psychiatrist school consultants [2]. Under the Individuals with Disabilities Education Act (IDEA), children with disabilities, including "emotional disturbances," are afforded legal protections to ensure that they receive an adequate education [3]. Children covered by the IDEA are entitled to individualized education plans (IEPs), and IEP teams frequently require the assistance of mental health professionals to help determine what constitutes an "emotional disturbance" and whether it is covered by the IDEA [4,5]. In school consultations, disclosure should be restricted to the minimally necessary amount required for the purpose. For example, the disclosure of the diagnosis, medication, and specific school services recommended usually would suffice.

Some child psychiatrists also conduct forensic evaluations and provide assistance with competency evaluations, juvenile justice system issues, and opinions in custody disputes, to mention a few. Although the ethical aspects of forensic child and adolescent psychiatry are beyond the scope of this article, readers may find Ratner's [6] analysis in an earlier issue of the *Child and Adolescent Psychiatric Clinics of North America* informative. The dilemma of being the treating clinician and the evaluator at the same time may be particularly difficult for a child to understand and may have a detrimental effect on the therapeutic relationship [7].

Treatment providers frequently are required to perform consultant functions in the course of their work. Because trust is the cornerstone of a successful therapeutic alliance, treatment providers should plan to devote extra attention to working with the patient to be sure that true informed consent is given by the parent or guardian [8]. Also, the child should have an understanding of the purpose and extent of the disclosure. Ideally, where appropriate, the child should see the clinician as acting as his/her agent in making the disclosure.

Thoroughness and honesty

For records to be complete, thorough documentation should commence at the outset of the treatment or consultation. Balancing "thoroughness" with confidentiality is not always easy. Records should reflect what one has done, but not necessarily every detail that one has learned during the course of evaluation and treatment. Keeping in mind that records may be subpoenaed or even released at a patient's request, the prudent clinician would not record inappropriate material, such as details of a child's envious description of a sibling. Notation of "significant sibling rivalry issues explored" should suffice.

When first sitting down to talk with the patient, family members, school officials, or others, it may be helpful to repeat and articulate problems that prompted the request for a consultation or treatment. Agendas may differ among the various persons involved in the case (eg, child, parents, teachers, legal agencies) [9]; therefore, it may be necessary to help those involved to reach a common understanding of the problem. The consensus may be incorporated into the psychiatrist's subsequent case formulation. After an understanding of the problem has been reached, one may help to articulate the goals of treatment and to specify these in the record. It may be necessary to revisit the case formulation and treatment goals later in the patient's treatment as new information becomes available.

In all records and professional communications, truthfulness is paramount. As Diane Schetky, MD, explained:

> Patients or parents may request that diagnoses or codes be altered out of concerns about confidentiality or so they can receive better reimbursement. The psychiatrist may be tempted to exaggerate the patient's condition to have needed services approved or to obtain higher reimbursement rates. There may be the temptation to alter dates of service, as when Medicaid will not pay for a parent visit on the same day the child is seen, regardless of how far they have traveled... Regardless of one's motives, these practices are fraudulent, and, as such, are subject to criminal prosecution. The psychiatrist who engages in fraud may also be subject to ethical investigations and sanctions [10].

Incorrect or misleading information in a patient's record, or in communications with third parties, may result in substandard care and, possibly, harm to the patient. Patients or families concerned about stigma may request that psychiatric diagnoses or clues (eg, prescribed psychotropic medicines) not be recorded. Psychiatrists must help families to understand that failing to record such information may result in harm to the child. For example, a pediatrician needs to be aware that a child is on an anticonvulsant or mood stabilizer, such as carbamazepine, because of the medical risks associated with the medication as well as drug–drug interactions.

A thorough medical record requires the documentation of the reasoning and authorization leading to disclosures of confidential or sensitive information. Such records should be in legible writing, detailed, and signed and dated by the patient or parent legally able to authorize the disclosure.

Collaboration and cooperation

A major distinguishing aspect of child and adolescent psychiatry, as opposed to other specialties in psychiatry, is the necessity of collaborative and cooperative work. The importance of collaboration begins with the initial evaluation of a child or adolescent. Collateral information, such as pediatric examinations and parent or teacher observations about the child's behavior, often aids significantly in formulating an accurate diagnosis. Ongoing communication with other care providers often is necessary throughout a period of treatment or consultation, and cooperating with family and other caregivers in the child's life helps to tailor the treatment to the needs of the individual patient [11]. Furthermore, failing to take other caregivers into consideration can have a severely detrimental effect on the course of treatment. In *Argus v Scheppegrell* [12], a physician was held liable for continuing to prescribe addictive substances to a young woman whose mother had called to advise the physician that her daughter had developed an addiction; the girl died from an overdose of the prescription drugs.

Involving the patient's family is important to providing effective, ethical care. When communicating with families, it is helpful to involve them as much as possible in the treatment plan. Providing education and learning from patients and their families are equally important aspects of the ethical practice of child and adolescent psychiatry. To strengthen an alliance with skeptical or resistant parents, the psychiatrist may provide them with copies of medical literature supporting treatment recommendations, refer to resources (eg, American Academy of Child and Adolescent Psychiatry [AACAP]), and provide patient- and family-oriented brochures [13]. One should not merely give the referral or document; one should follow up to ensure that the information provided was understood and that the issue was addressed adequately. Recording in the patient's chart some follow-up statement, such as "Patient inquired as to the meaning of agitation in the booklet and how it applied to him" is an excellent practice. It supports informed consent as having taken place and that the clinician and the patient have a working relationship.

Autonomy and dignity

Although "minors' autonomy" is a potentially contradictory phrase, the ethical principle of patient autonomy applies to the practice of child and adolescent psychiatry. In records and communications, as with other aspects of psychiatric practice, care must be taken to avoid undermining the patient's sense of autonomy and dignity. In child and adolescent psychiatry, autonomy and dignity are linked closely to questions regarding the patient's competence and capacity to consent to, or refuse, treatment or disclosures of confidential information. Such concerns often are an important part of the patient's record or the psychiatrist's communications about the patient.

A sophisticated understanding of these issues will aid in improving treatment and in avoiding ethical problems with records and documents. Although the patient cannot dictate what is put into his record, he may be able to understand that a record will be kept as in any other doctor's office and that he might ask the clinician to exclude certain material, if appropriate.

Competence and decision-making capacity often are relevant in consultation settings as well; they may figure into child custody proceedings or juvenile dependency hearings, and they are integral to situations in which the requirement of parental consent would be detrimental to the child. Therefore, it is appropriate to discuss with the child, especially a mature minor, how the patient would like the clinician to report findings related to a custody proceeding or similar situation.

Among the more ethically important parts of a patient's record is the informed consent process and documentation, whether involving consent for treatment or consent for disclosure of confidential information or release of records [10]. In most cases involving minors, the child's parents must give informed consent, and the child should be afforded an opportunity to assent to the treatment or disclosure in question. Consent may not be required for emergencies (homicidality or suicidality), but attempts to obtain consent in such situations, or justification for why it was not obtained, should be recorded [14]. When parents disagree about the child's treatment or disclosures, the custodial parent (if the parents are divorced) has the legal right to consent. If it is unclear which parent has custodial rights, consulting with an attorney may be necessary [14]. Retaining a copy of the custody document in the child's chart may be helpful.

When parents give consent, it is nonetheless recommended that psychiatrists include children in the decision-making process. Even where they are not legally able to give informed consent, minor patients may give their assent to treatment or disclosures. If the ultimate decision-making power rests with the clinician or parents, and the child's wishes cannot be respected, the child should be aware of this and should be allowed an opportunity to be heard and treated with respect.

Information provided to children should be appropriate to their development and maturity. Providing the minor patient with the choice to assent or to provide informed consent may enhance the therapeutic alliance and may offer the child a unique opportunity to exercise his or her legal rights, reasoning skills, maturity, and decision-making capacity [15]. Whether given by the parent or by the patient, consent and assent must be thorough, informed, and documented in the patient's chart, and copies may be provided to the family as well.

Even if hospitalization or commitment is required, a minor may still be deemed otherwise competent: "As with adults, commitment to a mental health facility should not render [legally] incompetent an adolescent who is otherwise decisionally capable" [16]. Psychiatrists should exercise caution in their choice of words and phrasing with respect to a minor patient's competence, capacity, or lack thereof. Written opinions regarding a patient's competence or decision-making capacity may "follow" the patient in other settings and have lasting effects on the patient's legal rights. For example, if the patient later becomes involved in a custody dispute between his parents, the court may subpoena his mental health records, and an attorney for a parent may attempt to disqualify the child from testifying by calling his competence into question. Evaluations and opinions regarding competency or capacity should, in most cases, be specific to the situation at hand. If a minor is deemed incompetent because of judgment rendered faulty by a severe mood disorder, the records should state that the cause of the impaired judgment is the (treatable) mood disorder. In such a case, treatment may render the patient competent to consent if the patient's development and the relevant laws allow for the minor's consent.

If, after consulting state law and reviewing legal advice, the physician determines that the minor should be allowed to consent to treatment without involving parents, documenting one's reasoning and evidence of the minor's level of competence may minimize related legal risks and help to protect the patient's autonomy. Before the minor's consent is accepted, a determination of maturity is necessary. This may involve a full assessment of the minor's capacities, as well as his or her understanding of treatment and consequences; as an expert in child development, it is appropriate for the psychiatrist to conduct this evaluation [15,17]. A finding of competence generally requires three elements: thorough understanding of the relevant information; capacity (skills in communicating, reasoning, deliberation regarding risks and consequences); and freedom from undue influence, fear, guilt, or coercion [18]. There are no guidelines for conducting competency evaluations with minors, and research in this area has been scant [19].

Nonetheless, mature adolescents who clearly have the mental functioning required to give an informed consent may be legally incompetent to do so. The law sends conflicting messages to children and adolescents. As noted by a legal scholar, a 14-year-old can be tried as an adult in criminal proceedings but cannot legally consent to medical treatment; a 15-year-old runaway may consent to treatment, but a more mature 15-year-old living with his parents cannot [16]. Child and adolescent psychiatrists are in a unique position to help foster a child's sense of autonomy and dignity, even when the law, or other authority figures in the child's life, do not. Whenever the law permits and the child's competence is evident, the psychiatrist should endeavor to respect the patient's decisions. When disagreements arise as to the best interests of the child, and parties disagree, it may be necessary to consult with legal experts.

Respecting patients' dignity often calls for censorship of some communications, even where there is consent for disclosure. Much of this censorship may be summarized by the warning to "avoid unnecessary details," particularly when incorporating patient report into records, including psychotherapy notes. The psychiatrist should be aware that parents and children may request to view records. In some states, the clinician is allowed to edit or re-dact portions of a record in the event that parents request to view the record; however, in most states, parents are legally entitled to view the entire record [13], possibly including psychotherapy notes. Furthermore, children also are legally entitled to full access to the entire record upon reaching the age of majority. Therefore, when writing records or communications, it may be helpful to keep potential future readers in mind. Consider omitting any un-necessary details that would be harmful for parents or children to read, as well as details that parents or children would not want disclosed to one an-other. Protecting such confidences protects the patient's and family's dignity and serves the ethical principle of nonmaleficence, sometimes referred to as "first, do no harm (*primum non nocere*)." This "censorship" typically in-volves substituting general language for specific quotations (eg, "child ex-presses anger toward father" instead of "child yelled 'I hate him [father]!'"; "parents frustrated with child's behavior" instead of "parents re-port 'He's driving us crazy!'"). Additional omissions may involve sensitive personal information (eg, "explored sexual thoughts" instead of "patient re-ports sexual fantasies involving his teacher").

Confidentiality

In child and adolescent psychiatry, protecting a patient's confidentiality is among the most important, and the most difficult, ethical concerns that may arise. The legal principle of psychotherapist–patient privilege [20] is related closely to the ethical notion of confidentiality, but privilege is defined more narrowly, and a psychiatrist's ethical duty to protect a patient's confidenti-ality may exceed one's legal obligations; however, clinicians do hold a legal duty to protect the confidentiality of their patients, and, in some cases, that of patients' family members as well. In the event of an unauthorized breach of confidentiality, the patient or family may decide to sue for breach of con-fidentiality, malpractice, or even invasion of the patient's privacy and other torts [21]. Even in the absence of a lawsuit, the psychiatrist might be subject to ethical sanctions, such as suspension or loss of license, for egregious breaches of a patient's confidentiality.

Some of the most difficult ethical decision making in child and adolescent psychiatry involves questions of confidentiality and privacy when there is conflict between family members, or conflict between a child and his or her parents. When parents are divorced or separated, it is of the utmost im-portance that the psychiatrist not divulge confidential information to the noncustodial parent without explicit consent from the custodial parent, and, ideally, assent from the minor patient as well [13]. Some states have laws about whether minors can protect confidential information from dis-closure to parents [14], and some specifically require the adolescent patient's consent before releasing medical records with sensitive topics, such as abortion or sexually transmitted diseases (STDs), to parents [22]. When these laws do not apply, however, parents are able to access their child's records against the child's wishes.

Regarding disclosures to individuals outside the family, parents or legal guardians typically have the legal right to waive the child's privacy rights [23]; however, in *Abrams v Jones* [24], the Texas Supreme Court upheld a mental health professional's right to refuse to disclose information from the child's mental health record when disclosure of such information would not be in the child's best interests, even when the information would be relevant to proceedings in a custody dispute. Special care is due when conducting family sessions or family therapy. In *Mrozinski v Pogue* [25], a custody dispute, a child's therapist disclosed information from family sessions to the noncustodial parent's attorney that the custodial parent believed to be confidential. The therapist relied on the 14-year-old patient's authorization and affirmed that the custodial parent was not a patient during family treatment sessions. The court ruled that psychiatrists can be held liable for unauthorized disclosure of private information about the child's family members. In emphasizing this point, the court in *Mrozinski v Pogue* wrote: "The strongest public policy considerations militate against allowing a psychiatrist to encourage a person to participate in joint therapy, to obtain his trust and extract all his confidences and place him in the most vulnerable position, and then abandon him on the trash heap of lost privilege" [25].

The patient and family should be informed, at the beginning of a treatment or consultation, as to the limits and exceptions to confidentiality [8]. Such limits and exceptions include emergencies and dangerous behavior (eg, suicidality or homicidality) [26]; mandatory reporting of child abuse; risk for imminent harm to others (the duty to warn or to protect) [27]; legal settings, including divorce and custody disputes; and criminal proceedings. To ethically protect the patient's confidentiality, however, patients may need some explanation as to what each of these limits or exceptions means. For example, the grounds for reporting "child abuse" differ by state, and the definition of abuse may include physical abuse, sexual abuse, neglect, and, in some cases, emotional maltreatment [14]. If Jane Doe, aged 15, is dating John Roe, aged 19, she may not be aware that if they become sexually active, the state may classify their behavior as child abuse, triggering mandatory reporting. In states where "emotional maltreatment" is defined as child abuse, patients may need clarification regarding when an argument is not just an argument.

In a variety of legal settings, a valid subpoena may compel testimony, deposition, or disclosure of records [28,29]. In juvenile courts in particular, protections for minors' privacy and confidentiality seem to be eroding in recent years [23]. Additionally, children have little say in what aspects, or how much, of their mental health record is disclosed in dependency proceedings [23]; in such cases, the court acts *in loco parentis* and, thus, consents to the release of the records. Furthermore, children should be aware that information disclosed to third parties could be disclosed to others. For example, in some school districts, school nurses and officials are required to notify parents when a student is pregnant [22].

Confidentiality concerns may arise when therapy focuses on sensitive issues [9], such as the patient's drug abuse, delinquent behavior, sexual identity or sexual activity and STD testing, past child abuse, pregnancy and abortion or adoption, and personal beliefs (eg, racist beliefs). For some patients, the mere fact of having been treated by a mental health professional may be associated with stigma. Confidentiality concerns related to sensitive topics should trigger extreme care on the part of the clinician, given the potentially disastrous consequences of a disclosure or breach of confidentiality. Legal scholar Katner [23] recounted a case in which an adolescent girl attempted suicide following her therapist's disclosure of the girl's HIV status; although it was not specified to whom the therapist made the disclosure or how the news had spread, the girl's teacher, and, later, her classmates, learned of her HIV status. Unauthorized disclosures of sensitive information may permanently mar the child's or adolescent's ability to trust mental health professionals and others. Conversely, failing to disclose information when disclosure is necessary to protect the patient's safety may be equally unethical. Such decisions may be difficult, but the psychiatrist must weigh potential outcomes to protect the patient's best interests.

There are additional steps that one may take to protect minor patients' confidentiality. Restricting staff access to confidential records and psychotherapy notes reduces the chances of disclosure without the psychiatrist's oversight. When an attorney for a father in a custody dispute served an improper subpoena and the mother's physician (without the patient's authorization) released medical records containing information about her mental health treatment to the father's attorney, the patient was entitled to sue the physician for breach of confidentiality [30]. In school consultations, children and others who meet with the psychiatrist should be informed as to how the information might be used or shared, as well as what information may be included in nonmedical records, such as student or employee files [2]. The Association of Child and Adolescent Psychiatric Nurses states that "[c]hildren have the right to have their records kept private and to be told about the conditions under which information about them will be disclosed without their permission" [31]. Forewarning patients and families about limitations and exceptions to confidentiality protects their autonomy and reduces the likelihood that a necessary breach will be traumatic and provoke legal action. Such advance warning should be done in writing and documented in the patient's chart. Printed material, such as a patient's rights document or a Health Insurance Portability and Accountability Act privacy notice, may be beneficial; however, a discussion about the contents of such material that is memorialized in the chart is helpful.

When disclosure of confidential information is necessary, consider involving the patient in decisions about what information to release, to the extent possible [23]. If the child is involved in the decision and consents to the

disclosure, there may be less harm to the child's ability to trust authority figures and others, and the child may have a stronger sense of autonomy and
dignity. Furthermore, as Schetky [10] explained, not all authorized disclosures are ethically appropriate: "Even when there is consent for release of
information, the psychiatrist must delicately balance how much information
a school needs to know about a child's turbulent family life to help a child
while respecting the family's wish for privacy." The psychiatrist, in deciding
what material to disclose, should keep the child's best interests in mind as
a guiding point for such ethical decisions.

Objectivity and neutrality

Child and adolescent psychiatrists should strive to remain as objective
and neutral as possible when dealing with families and others in the child's
life. Such a task is not simple, particularly in the event of family conflict or
custody disputes. When possible, treating clinicians should try to avoid becoming involved in legal disputes involving the patient or family, particularly custody battles. Typically, in custody disputes, "… both parents
believe that their litigation position is in the child's best interest" [32]. In
such disputes, one frequently hears allegations about one parent that may
or may not be true; recording such suspicions or allegations in professional
communications or records may have lasting implications, even for allegations that have a foundation of truth.

Allegations of child abuse are common in high-conflict divorce cases, but
they frequently are dismissed by investigative clinicians as being the result of
spite between parents or not being sufficiently serious to warrant protective
state custody [33]. If abuse is suspected, reports may warrant investigation
into the likelihood of truth or falsity of the claim or suspicion. One court,
considering a lawsuit against a therapist for a wrongful child abuse report
filed during a custody dispute, held that "a mental health care provider
owes a duty to any person, who is the subject of any public report or other
adverse recommendation by that provider, to use due care in formulating
any opinion upon which such a report or recommendation is based" [34].
Families have succeeded in lawsuits against clinicians who accept reports
of sexual abuse without questioning "red flags" suggesting that the allegations may be false [35], and families also have succeeded in lawsuits for damage suffered as a result of "recovered" but false "memories" of childhood
abuse [36,37]. Research shows that children are suggestible; in the absence
of information to support a child's claim, and without further investigation,
psychiatrists should be wary of recording or repeating serious allegations in
a chart or communication if there is a reasonable chance that the claim may
be inaccurate [28]. One might record simply that a third party reported
something, rather than presenting such reports as factual information.

Perhaps one of the most challenging ethical demands for the child and
adolescent psychiatrist is remaining neutral. In the course of treating or

evaluating a child, one often hears information that provokes strong reactions and triggers judgments; however, having a good relationship with the child's parents often is a necessary requirement to continue to provide treatment or consultation [11], because alienated parents may choose to cease bringing their child for appointments or to seek the services of a different clinician. In medical records and professional communications, the child and adolescent psychiatrist should strive to avoid blaming and accusatory or inflammatory language. Parents whose child needs the help of a psychiatrist frequently are defensive and insecure about their parenting skills and family relationships, and psychiatrists should be prepared to respond in a reassuring, supportive manner that keeps lines of communication open [26]. One should carefully monitor countertransference reactions during case formulation and when writing notes or other communications that may become part of the medical record. Despite knowledge of the numerous factors (including genes and environment) that may interact when a child presents with problematic behavior, psychiatrists frequently attribute blame to parents, even when such blame is not appropriate or is not helpful to the treatment; clinicians who more often identify the parents as the problem may unconsciously behave in ways that betray their belief, alienating parents and creating obstacles to successful treatment [38]. Conversely, another pitfall to avoid is the temptation to side automatically with a child's parents. Parents often view the therapist as an authority figure who can help to advance their agenda [9], and whether in the record or in an authorized disclosure, the psychiatrist should be careful not to place the parents' interests above the best interests of the child.

Electronic communications

Although a full discussion of the ethical implications of electronic communications is beyond the scope of this article, technological improvements often bring new ethical dilemmas, several of which bear noting, albeit briefly. As noted by Terry and Francis [39], electronic medical records and electronic health records carry numerous benefits and drawbacks. Among the benefits of such records are the ease of information exchange and coordination of care; automated scanning for drug interactions; portability of the records; thoroughness, particularly when records are shared among providers; the possibility of patient involvement in maintaining the record; automatic reminders for medication refills and appointments; and numerous others. Frequently cited drawbacks include risks to patient privacy, confidentiality, and data security; potentially large impacts from errors; and the potential for employment or insurance discrimination related to long-standing conditions recorded in the patient's record.

The Internet has played a critical role in the intellectual and social development of today's children and adolescents. The Pew Internet and American Life Project conducted research showing the growing importance of social networking (eg, Web sites such as MySpace) in the lives of adolescents [40]. Child and adolescent psychiatrists should understand the importance of these media in the lives of their patients, but respecting personal boundaries remains important. For some patients, there may be a therapeutic benefit in the child's mind of being able to meet the clinician in cyberspace, but such communications may carry extreme confidentiality risks. Being familiar with MySpace may help the clinician to relate to his patients, but creating a MySpace profile and adding one's patients to the public list of "featured friends" may not be ethically appropriate. Posting public comments to a patient's blog or online journal may transgress important boundaries.

In some cases, e-mail communication with patients, parents, or third parties may be appropriate. One benefit to e-mail communication is the relative ease of retaining thorough and legible documentation of what was, and what was not, communicated [41]. Fortunately, an evolving body of literature provides guidance on navigating the complicated legal and ethical issues involved in electronic communications [42,43]. When e-mail or chat conversations delve into clinical matters, a practice known as e-therapy, additional ethical concerns may arise [43–46]. Professional Web sites offer unique opportunities for networking and outreach among child and adolescent psychiatrists. Olson and Kutner [47] offered psychiatrists several helpful tips and suggestions for communications with the news media and with the public through news media. Additional resources address ethical and legal concerns specific to psychiatry Web sites [48,49].

Professional activities

In addition to maintaining medical records and communicating with parents, teachers, and other figures in the child's life, the practice of child and adolescent psychiatry frequently involves other types of professional communications, including research and professional or political correspondence. To serve the best interests of patients, professional ethics may call for communication with third-party payers and insurance providers, as well as political activism or advocacy work, particularly when the psychiatrist is made aware of policies or procedures that may be harmful to patients and their families [8]. Activities such as letter writing, submitting newspaper editorials, and communicating with officials about psychiatry-related business or politics are part of one's professional communications, and ethical standards do apply. In the United Kingdom, a child psychiatrist was suspended for "serious professional misconduct" when he mailed to primary care physicians and patients copies of letters that he had written, questioning the competence of other psychiatrists and criticizing them for disagreeing with his views [50]. In some letters, he hinted that the psychiatrists in question may have been medically negligent and may be unfit to practice. Psychiatrists, as professionals, are held to a higher ethical standard than that of the man on the street. Consequently, there may be grave consequences or sanctions for ethically inappropriate communications.

As with communications to family members and school officials, the psychiatrist should try to avoid the use of jargon and unnecessary details about a particular case. Journalists may request opinions on stories that capture news headlines, but to maintain professionalism, psychiatrists should refrain from speculating on diagnoses and details of a particular case, particularly if they have not evaluated the individual in question. If the psychiatrist has evaluated the individual, then the usual rules about confidentiality and privilege apply, and information should not be divulged to the media unnecessarily. Furthermore, no matter how interesting a patient's case may seem, psychiatrists should strive to avoid exploiting a patient's story for personal or professional gain. The psychiatrist owes an ethical duty to the child or adolescent to place the patient's best interests above the psychiatrist's interest in building one's curriculum vitae. In communications with others about the practice of psychiatry, professionalism is essential.

Summary

Although space constraints prevent a thorough discussion of the relevant ethical issues in medical records and professional communications, readers are advised to consult existing ethical guidelines and regulations from the American Medical Association [51], the American Psychiatric Association [52,53], and the AACAP [8]. The Health Insurance Portability and Accountability Act of 1996 specifies that some content from medical records can be disclosed without a patient's consent, but only the "minimum necessary," and "psychotherapy notes" have stricter privacy protection [54]. State laws may provide even stricter ethical protections. Liability insurance carriers and professional affiliations can be excellent sources for guidance on ethical matters. Additional lessons may be learned by following legal news and screening recent cases for ethical implications. When presented with an ethical problem or a difficult decision, the child and adolescent psychiatrist should not rely solely on his or her own judgment, nor rely too heavily on the recommendations of interested parties, such as parents. To resolve difficult ethical dilemmas, one may consult with ethics experts and seek feedback and support from colleagues who are able to give reasoned, unbiased opinions.

References

[1] American Academy of Child and Adolescent Psychiatry. Practice parameter for the assessment and treatment of children and adolescents with bipolar disorder. J Am Acad Child Adolesc Psychiatry 2007;46(1):107–25.

[2] Bostic JQ, Bagnell A. Psychiatric school consultation: an organizing framework and empowering techniques. Child Adolesc Psychiatr Clin N Am 2001;10(1):1–12.

[3] Glick DB. Statutory spotlight: Individuals with Disabilities Education Act 2004. 9 U.C. Davis J. Juv. L. & Pol'y 439; 2005.

[4] Mount KA. Children's mental health disabilities and discipline: protecting children's rights while maintaining safe schools. 3 Barry L. Rev 103;2002.

[5] Ash P. Children and adolescents. In: Simon RI, Gold LH, editors. The American Psychiatric Publishing textbook of forensic psychiatry. Arlington (VA): American Psychiatric Publishing, Inc; 2004. p. 449–70.

[6] Ratner RA. Ethics in child and adolescent forensic psychiatry. Child Adolesc Psychiatr Clin N Am 2002;11:887–904.

[7] Strasburger LH, Gutheil TG, Brodsky A. On wearing two hats: role conflict in serving as both psychotherapist and expert witness. Am J Psychiatry 1997;154(4):448–56.

[8] American Academy of Child and Adolescent Psychiatry. Code of ethics. Available at: http://www.aacap.org/galleries/AboutUs/CodeOfEthics.PDF. Accessed April 17, 2007.

[9] Koocher GP. Ethical issues in psychotherapy with adolescents. J Clin Psychol 2003;59(11):1247–56.

[10] Schetky DH. Ethics in the practice of child and adolescent psychiatry. In: Lewis M, editor. Child and adolescent psychiatry: a comprehensive textbook. 3rd edition. Philadelphia: Lippincott Williams & Wilkins; 2002. p. 1442–6.

[11] American Academy of Child and Adolescent Psychiatry. Practice parameter for the assessment and treatment of children and adolescents with oppositional defiant disorder. J Am Acad Child Adolesc Psychiatry 2007;46(1):126–41.

[12] Argus v Scheppegrell, 472 So.2d 573, (La. 1985).

[13] Vernick AE. Forensic aspects of everyday practice: legal issues that every practitioner must know. Child Adolesc Psychiatr Clin N Am 2002;11:905–28.

[14] Fortunati FG Jr, Zonana HV. Legal considerations in the child psychiatric emergency department. Child Adolesc Psychiatr Clin N Am 2003;12:745–61.

[15] Redding RE. Children's competence to provide informed consent for mental health treatment. 50 Wash. & Lee L. Rev 1993;695.

[16] Hartman RG. Adolescent autonomy: clarifying an ageless conundrum. 51 Hastings L.J. 1265;2000.

[17] Kuther TL. Medical decision-making and minors: issues of consent and assent. Adolescence 2003;38(150):343–58.

[18] Kenny NP. A teenager's refusal of assent for treatment. Med Ethics 2002;9(3):3.

[19] Tan JOA, Fegert JM. Capacity and competence in child and adolescent psychiatry. Health Care Anal 2004;12(4):285–94.

[20] Jaffee v Redmond, 518 U.S. 1 (1996).

[21] Zelin JE. Physician's tort liability for unauthorized disclosure of confidential information about patient. 48 A.L.R. 4th 668, 2004.

[22] Prober M. Please don't tell my parents: the validity of school policies mandating parental notification of a student's pregnancy. 71 Brooklyn L. Rev 2005;557.

[23] Katner DR. Confidentiality and juvenile mental health records in dependency proceedings. 12 Wm. & Mary Bill of Rts. J. 511;2004.

[24] Abrams v Jones, 35 S.W.3d 620 (Tex. 2000).

[25] Mrozinski v Pogue, 423 S.E.2d 405 (Ga. App. 1992).

[26] Bird HR. Presentation of findings and recommendations. In: Wiener JM, Dulcan MK, editors. Textbook of child and adolescent psychiatry. 3rd edition. Washington D.C: American Psychiatric Publishing, Inc; 2004. p. 215–8.

[27] Tarasoff v Regents of the University of California, 551 P.2d 334 (1976).

[28] Sikorski JB, Kuo AD. Forensic psychiatry. In: Wiener JM, Dulcan MK, editors. Textbook of child and adolescent psychiatry. 3rd edition. Washington D.C: American Psychiatric Publishing, Inc; 2004. p. 903–27.

[29] Nelken ML. The limits of privilege: the developing scope of federal psychotherapist-patient privilege law. Review of Litigation 2000;20:1–43.

[30] Crescenzo v Crane, 796 A.2d 283 (N.J. Super. Ct. App. Div. 2002).

[31] ACAPN (Division of ISPN) position statement on the rights of children in treatment settings. J Child Adolesc Psychiatr Nurs 2000;13(4):183–4.

[32] Paulsen JW. Family law: parent and child. 54 SMU L. Rev 1417; 2001.

[33] Johnston JR. Building multidisciplinary professional partnerships with the court on behalf of high-conflict divorcing families and their children: who needs what kind of help? 22 U. Ark. Little Rock L. Rev. 453; 2000.

[34] Montoya v. Bebensee, 761 P.2d 285,289 (Co. App. 1988).

[35] Althaus v. Cohen, 710 A.2d 1147 (1998 Penna Super) rev in part, remanded by 562 Penna 547, 756 A.2d 1166 (Penna 2000).

[36] Kisch WJ. From the couch to the bench: how should the legal system respond to recovered memories of childhood sexual abuse? 5 Am.U.J. Gender & Law 207;1996.

[37] Ramona v. Superior Court of Los Angeles County, No. B111565, 57 Cal. App. 4th 107 (Cal. Ct. App. 1997).

[38] Johnson HC, Cournoyer DE, Fisher GA, et al. Children's emotional and behavioral disorders: attributions of parental responsibility by professionals. Am J Orthopsychiatry 2000; 70(3):327–39.

[39] Terry NP, Francis LP. Ensuring the privacy and confidentiality of electronic health records. 2007 U Ill. L. Rev. 681.

[40] Lenhart A, Madden M. Teens, privacy, and online social networks: how teens manage their online identities in the age of MySpace. Pew Internet & American Life Project, April 18, 2007. Available at: http://www.pewinternet.org/pdfs/PIP_Teens_Privacy_SNS_Report_Final.pdf. Accessed April 26, 2007.

[41] Ash P. Malpractice in child and adolescent psychiatry. Child Adolesc Psychiatric Clin N Am 2002;11:869–85.

[42] Recupero PR. E-mail and the psychiatrist-patient relationship. J Am Acad Psychiatry Law 2005;33:465–75.

[43] American Psychiatric Association Council on Psychiatry and the Law. Frequently asked questions (FAQ): e-mail in psychiatry. Available at: http://www.psych.org/psych_pract/ clin_issues/cybermedfaq.cfm. Accessed April 26, 2007.

[44] Recupero PR, Rainey SE. Forensic aspects of e-therapy. J Psychiatric Practice 2005;11(6): 405–10.

[45] Recupero PR, Rainey SE. Informed consent to e-therapy. Am J Psychother 2005;59(4):319–31.

[46] American Psychiatric Association Council on Psychiatry and the Law. Frequently asked questions (FAQ): e-therapy. Arlington, VA: American Psychiatric Association; 2006. Available at: http://www.psych.org/psych_pract/clin_issues/etherapyfaqs.cfm. Accessed April 26, 2007.

[47] Olson CK, Kutner LA. Media outreach for child psychiatrists. Child Adolesc Psychiatric Clin N Am 2005;14:613–22.

[48] Recupero PR. Legal concerns for psychiatrists who maintain web sites. Psychiatr Serv 2006; 57(4):450–2.

[49] American Psychiatric Association Council on Psychiatry and the Law. Frequently asked questions (FAQ): medical practice websites. Available at: http://www.psych.org/ psych_pract/clin_issues/medpracticewebfaq.cfm. Accessed April 26, 2007.

[50] Dyer O. Psychiatrist suspended for undermining patients' trust in treatment. BMJ 2004;328: 1516.

[51] American Medical Association. Principles of medical ethics. Adopted June 17, 2001. Available at: http://www.ama-assn.org/ama/pub/category/2512.html. Accessed April 26, 2007.

[52] American Psychiatric Association. Principles of medical ethics with annotations especially applicable to psychiatry. Washington D.C: American Psychiatric Association; 2001.

[53] American Psychiatric Association. Opinions of the ethics committee on the principles of medical ethics with annotations especially applicable to psychiatry. Washington D.C: American Psychiatric Association; 2001.

[54] 45 C.F.R. §164.508 (a) (2).

ELSEVIER
SAUNDERS

Child Adolesc Psychiatric Clin N Am
17 (2008) 53–66

CHILD AND
ADOLESCENT
PSYCHIATRIC CLINICS
OF NORTH AMERICA

A Doubtful Guest: Managed Care and Mental Health

Edie Rosenberg, MBA, David Ray DeMaso, MD*

Department of Psychiatry, Children's Hospital Boston, 300 Longwood Avenue, Boston, MA 02115, USA

> "*It joined them at breakfast and presently ate*
> *All the syrup and toast, and a part of a plate.*"
> –Edward Gorey

Like the title character in *The Doubtful Guest*, managed care appeared uninvited on the health care scene more than 2 decades ago and shows no sign of going away any time soon [1]. Engineered by health plans and employers who were upset with rising premium costs, it has since been embraced in the public sector as well. It has changed the way that mental health providers practice and even the way that they think. Central features of managed care include the establishment of selected provider networks, preauthorization of covered services that meet payer-defined standards of medical necessity, use management and review, and a shift away from traditional fee-for-service financing to shared-risk arrangements that include capitated or prepaid contracts and retention of a portion of provider payments until after performance goals are met. In behavioral health services, much of the growth in managed care occurred belatedly, during the 1990s, and appeared increasingly in the form of separate organizations that were charged with managing mental health and substance abuse benefits "carved out" from medical benefits.

Although the ultimate goal of managed care was to contain costs and optimize the use of resources available for a defined group, it held the promise of additional benefits. Chief among these was improving health care quality through the establishment of standards of care, reducing variability across providers, and holding providers accountable for outcomes. Another was the notion that if insurers could control expenditures for the insured,

* Corresponding author.

E-mail address: david.demaso@childrens.harvard.edu (D.R. DeMaso).

some of the saved resources could be applied to extending coverage to the increasing numbers of Americans who had no health coverage at all [2].

It is safe to say that most mental health providers have been reluctant witnesses to and participants in the successes and failures of the managed care promise. This article examines the ways in which mental health services have been particularly affected by managed care and describes how to address some of the ethical conflicts that have always existed, but have been immeasurably transformed by managed care. We also suggest that there can be no real improvement for mental health providers in the ethical minefield of managed care until they stop focusing on how distressed they are about it and start dealing with the larger, systemic issues in psychiatry and American health care that brought them to the minefield in the first place.

Managed care as the great evil?

The angst engendered in many mental health providers at the mere mention of managed care is not hard to understand. Mental health treatment is inherently private and requires trust to be effective. In no other medical specialty is the doctor–patient relationship so tied to outcome. Managed care symbolizes an intrusive third party, a challenge to the provider's autonomy. Information may need to be shared with a reviewer, altering the notion of confidentiality and introducing concerns about how the information will be used. Additional hours must be spent on administrative tasks. The method of treatment may be dictated, with decisions about "medical necessity" and coverage resulting in altered treatment plans and possible discontinuation of care. Income is threatened or reduced. Instead of focusing solely on the needs of an individual patient and family, the provider is suddenly put in the position of being a double agent, asked to act on behalf of the patient and the health care system in which the patient is enrolled. Conflicts of interest, including those resulting from certain forms of financial payment and incentives based on performance, are inevitable.

Still, the vehemence with which some mental health providers describe the threat posed by managed care is noteworthy and shows no sign of abating. Some have even characterized the relationship between psychotherapist and managed care organization as "traumatic bonding," a connection forced on providers by the need for economic survival that can result in transformation akin to that seen between hostage and captor in the "Stockholm syndrome" [3]. Reading about the alleged evils of managed care, one is hard-pressed to remember some of the evils of the fee-for-service system that preceded it, most notable among them the incentive to overtreat and the harm caused by unnecessary procedures that resulted. There also was little incentive to engage in prevention or health promotion activities.

From the point of view of an individual patient or provider, however, there is no question that the fee-for-service system was the golden age, or, as Reinhardt [4] aptly put it, "the fairy tale that health care is a free lunch." There was free choice of providers, claims were paid without argument or negotiated discounts, and the amount and type of care were decided solely by the provider with the consent of the patient. Equally important is that employer costs for this uncontrolled system were largely invisible to consumers, because of the way that deductions appeared on paychecks and because there was little cost sharing at the time that health care was received [4]. In this context of seemingly limitless resources, it is no wonder that patients and providers alike responded poorly to the limit setting and reduction of choice that were imposed by managed care.

There are additional reasons why, amid all of the upheaval and concern about managed care among the medical community at large, it would be reasonable to assume that mental health care would be particularly impacted by it. These include factors affecting the behavior of managed-care plans (increased opportunities for cost shifting to state programs or family members and the availability of clinicians other than physicians to provide care); factors affecting patients (the stigma associated with mental illness and the characteristics of the illness itself making patients less likely or able to advocate for themselves); and factors affecting clinicians (the criteria used to review psychiatric care are less clear or predictable than in other specialties) [5]. Psychiatrists are more than twice as likely as primary care physicians or other medical specialists to report intensive prior authorization requirements and three times as likely to face frequent denials [5]. They report that their staff spent less time appealing review decisions than other physicians, but that seems to be because psychiatrists themselves are devoting more time to the appeals process; they also report being less successful than other physicians in resolving disputes [5].

In a survey of physicians' beliefs about the impact of managed care on their practices, psychiatrists seem to be more concerned than are other physicians about their ability to make clinical decisions in the best interest of their patients without the possibility of reducing their income [6]. They also are less likely to agree that it is possible to maintain continuing relationships with patients over time that promote the delivery of high-quality care. Their concerns about patient continuity and the impact of managed care on the patient–provider relationship might have to do with a shift in behavioral managed care toward nonphysicians providing psychotherapy and reliance on psychiatrists for medication management [6].

Are these subjective assessments of the impact of managed care on practice to be believed? Certainly they should be viewed with caution. One of the most frequent complaints about managed care is that it creates pressure on physicians to increase productivity, to see more patients in less time. Physicians report that office visits have gotten shorter and that it is increasingly difficult to spend adequate time with patients. Between 1989 and 1998, however, two large data sets showed that the average duration of visits for primary and specialty medical care actually increased for prepaid and nonprepaid visits [7]. It could be that physicians perceive that visits are shorter because their case mix is more complex and the visits feel rushed or because of the amount of time they are spending on administrative tasks, but the reality is that medical visits are not shorter [7].

In contrast, a separate study of trends in the composition and duration of visits to psychiatrists, using one of the data sets above, found that between 1985 and 1995, visits in office-based psychiatry became shorter, less often included psychotherapy, and more often included a medication prescription [8]. It is fair to say that psychiatry has been disproportionately affected by some of the changes wrought by managed care. This is principally due to the special nature of the treating relationship in psychiatry and its exquisite sensitivity to the effects of cost-containment methods used by managed care organizations, the limited reimbursement levels, and the lack of parity in coverage with medical benefits.

Physicians, as a group, have been concerned about reduced fees under managed care and their effect on income; however, physician incomes, with the exception of a dip in 1994, increased throughout the 1990s [9]. A study of psychiatrists' salaries, however, revealed lower, flatter salary patterns than those for physicians in all other specialties [10]. Although compensation to psychiatrists has increased in the past 5 years, on an annual basis, the increase has failed to keep pace with inflation [11]. Even if reimbursement levels for psychiatrists were on par with those for other specialties, psychiatrists would still be alone in having the added difficulty of trying to integrate care when patients' mental health benefits are carved out.

Ethics and managed care

Given the unique position in which mental health providers have found themselves since the advent of managed care, it is no surprise that many of them continue to believe that "ethical managed care" is an oxymoron. Ethical dilemmas are conflicts about competing values. In the fee-for-service world, the responsibility of the physician was to focus solely on the needs of an individual patient. Having a third party intrude on the doctor–patient relationship to impact treatment is an affront to the autonomy of the therapeutic dyad and represents the introduction of one or more competing values. Does the doctor care about the 47 million uninsured Americans? Probably. Does he think that their situation has anything to do with the patient in his office? Not likely. The larger context of using resources to maximize "the greatest good for the greatest number" is not relevant to his treatment plan. In addition, our doctor is a smart man and not quite so magnanimous. He knows that whether or not his patient gets 3 or 33 or 333 sessions authorized by the reviewer has an impact on the profitability of the managed care company, not on the uninsured millions (some of whom he continues to treat at greatly reduced fees after they lost their jobs and were dropped from the rolls of the managed care company).

The mental health provider and the managed care reviewer are not having the same conversation; they are not engaging the same ethical dilemmas. This is why the exchange is so untenable and why even to participate in it is contrary to everything in the doctor's training. If the doctor is being honest with himself, however, he knows that, on some level—even as he rejects the managed care reviewer's unsubstantiated standards of care and definitions of medical necessity—the reason why he is in this position is, in part, because he and his colleagues have not substantiated any standards of care either. There is more ambiguity about norms of treatment and their efficacy in psychiatry than in other areas of medicine, making the review process more challenging for clinicians [5]. The definitions of psychotherapy are too numerous to count, and it is not clear how many sessions of what kind are needed to effect a given treatment outcome.

It is tempting for the mental health provider to say anything that he needs to say to the managed care reviewer, even lie, to obtain authorization for the treatment that he "knows" is best for his patient. In 1995, the American Academy of Child and Adolescent Psychiatry's (AACAP) professional code of ethics was modified to include annotations with special reference to evolving health care delivery and reimbursement systems. The code now specifically states that "child and adolescent psychiatrists must not misrepresent problems, services, or diagnoses to circumvent limitations of their patients' coverage" [12]. This, in itself, is extraordinary, a tacit recognition of the ongoing moral conflict experienced by psychiatrists in the world of managed care.

A study of physicians' attitudes and beliefs revealed that many physicians sanction the use of deception to obtain care when denied authorization by a third-party payer [13]. Physician support for deception was higher when presented with hypothetical situations with greater clinical severity and immediate patient risk. It also was higher in areas of the country with higher managed care market penetration. Of note, internists who were the subjects of the study were much more likely to sanction falsely documenting suicidal ideation for a patient seeking treatment for a recurrent history of profound depression with past suicide attempts than they were to claim someone had a deviated septum to obtain cosmetic rhinoplasty; however, psychiatric referral ranked below falsely claiming someone had a suspicious breast lump to get a screening mammogram [13].

Another study found that alternate diagnostic coding strategies were a common part of practice for physicians evaluating children with mental health conditions [14]. The most frequent reason cited was diagnostic uncertainty and the difficulty of describing mild, borderline, or subthreshold conditions in developing children. Less frequently mentioned reasons were to obtain needed patient services and physician reimbursement. There also was undercoding related to the desire to avoid labeling and stigmatization and concerns about confidentiality and parental acceptance. The survey revealed the physicians' belief that insurance and managed care organizations have created a system that fosters the use of alternate diagnoses, and that coding issues occur more frequently with behavioral disorders compared with other medical conditions [14].

It is true that physicians are hindered in their efforts to code procedures and diagnoses accurately if they want their patients to be able to access their insurance benefits, because the plans do not accept many of the codes, despite the transaction and code sets standards mandated by the Health Insurance Portability and Accountability Act (HIPAA). It is not surprising that physicians believe that coding issues occur more frequently with behavioral disorders, because of the uncertainty in the field and because the existence of carve-out plans makes it difficult for physicians to use coding systems consistently across specialties. A pediatrician, for example, would not be on the provider panel for a patient's behavioral carve-out plan, so he typically could not use mental health codes and get reimbursed. This has important implications for innovative efforts to expand the involvement of pediatricians in the provision of psychopharmacology services to address access issues created by the critical shortage of child and adolescent psychiatrists.

Practical considerations: confidentiality

If opting out were a choice, most mental health providers would "just say no" to managed care. Because only a small percentage of providers can limit their practice to private, self-pay patients, it is useful to consider strategies for ethical survival when dealing with managed care organizations in everyday practice. Sharing patient information in the age of managed care is almost always first on any list of issues of concern. The principles are the same as they were before managed care, with allowances to accommodate the more recent HIPAA regulations, and there always have been instances when information disclosure is required by law. Getting informed consent to disclose information can raise different issues in treatment, however, when the disclosure is for administrative purposes (eg, getting authorizations for treatment or claims paid) than when it is for clinical purposes (eg, speaking with a child's teacher or pediatrician).

HIPAA regulations specify that written authorization from a patient or guardian is required to use or disclose private health information for purposes other than to provide patient care, receive payment for services, or to support health care operations. The disclosure must be guided by the recipient's reasonable need to know the information, which is the "minimum necessary" standard [15]. There are also sometimes applicable state laws that regulate information disclosure, which could be more stringent than HIPAA requires, and there are numerous HIPAA requirements beyond obtaining consent to release private health information (eg, the need to track certain disclosures and provide a list of them to the patient when requested).

Because of the sensitivity of the information divulged in treatment, mental health providers generally have maintained a higher standard than the law requires, obtaining permission for the release of information even when it is related specifically to patient care. Similarly, although insurance companies and managed care organizations are covered entities under HIPAA—and so subject to the same use and disclosure regulations as the provider—ethical considerations would require a psychiatrist to obtain the patient's consent to release information to a plan or reviewer, even if the disclosure is for the purpose of getting a claim paid.

In some practice settings, patients sign a blanket consent to release information accompanying the assignment of benefits to a provider or facility. This is insufficient, as is relying on any consent a patient may have signed when he enrolled in the managed care plan. To be HIPAA-compliant, an authorization to request or release information should state who is authorized to do so, describe the information to be requested or released, list any restrictions or exclusions, list the purpose of requesting or releasing it, specify from/to whom it may be requested or released, have an end date, and specify the patient's right to revoke the release at any time.

More to the point, obtaining consent to release information, like obtaining informed consent to do a procedure or research study, is not about the signature. It is about ensuring that the patient understands the information on the piece of paper and what it means. A signature does not replace a detailed discussion with the patient about what information will be shared with the managed care organization to make sure that the patient is aware of the way his health coverage works and the possibility that the treatment plan could be altered as a result of the review. It also affords the opportunity for the patient to specify any restrictions on sharing information, which a mental health provider should honor, even if it precipitates a separate discussion about how treatment can proceed if the patient's benefits cannot be accessed.

It also is important to distinguish between procedures established to comply with laws and business decisions adopted within the context of one's practice. One can be bound by law to share information with a noncustodial parent about a minor child's treatment, for example, but the business decision one might make in this instance would be to warn the custodial parent about the release and discuss its implications, even though this is not legally mandated. In general, conflicts of interest can be mitigated by transparent disclosure.

If a provider is going to be transparent, however, it might be preferable to deal first, outside the therapy, with any negative feelings he harbors toward the managed care organization for putting him in the position of needing to have the discussion in the first place. One study suggested that if prospective patients know that their therapists have negative perceptions of managed care, their own expectations about therapy changed. They were more likely to believe that managed care would have a negative impact on treatment and were less likely to pursue treatment or use insurance benefits, expect to benefit from treatment, expect to form a strong working relationship, and trust that the therapist would work in their best interest [16].

Practical considerations: coding and billing

Diagnosis and procedure codes should be straightforward. A mental health provider uses one to describe the illness or injury he thinks requires treatment and the other to describe the treatment he performs. In practice, however, they can generate great uncertainty and frequently are at the center of ethical quagmires related to meeting the treatment authorization, medical necessity, or coverage criteria of managed care plans. It is tempting to view coding as merely an administrative headache required to get claims paid. But before there was billing, there was a need to classify what physicians observed and what they did about it, a need for a common language so they could compare notes and evaluate results. The reason why we should care about the accuracy of coding and the adoption of uniform standards is that there is no way to make advances in medicine without agreement about what we are seeing and measuring.

That said, it gets murky when coding is the basis on which health care claims are paid, and there is no agreement among insurance plans and managed care organizations about which codes will be accepted. Some coding decisions are not ambiguous. There is no controversy in deciding whether to use the code for "family therapy with patient present" or the one for "family therapy without patient present." Although family therapy often is not reimbursed with the latter code, it is clearly unacceptable to say that the patient was there when he was not. The situation also is uncomplicated if a child and adolescent psychiatrist sees the parent of his patient alone for half of a psychotherapy hour and the content of the session is exclusively about the child; this still would be individual psychotherapy billed under the child.

Less clear, however, is how a psychiatrist should decide whether to use evaluation and management codes (99xxx) or the diagnostic interview and psychotherapy codes (908xx). Both are plausible, and, presumably, the answer depends on which codes the patient's health plan will cover. Similarly, the psychiatrist will be sure not to put a V-code diagnosis in *Diagnostic and Statistical Manual of Mental Disorders, Fourth Edition Revised* (*DSM-IV-R*) as the primary diagnosis on a claim form, because the service will not be covered by the patient's insurance. The pediatrician may avoid *DSM* or *International Statistical Classification* mental health diagnoses altogether because they will be denied by the patient's medical carrier, and he is out-of-network for the patient's behavioral health carve-out plan.

Even with all of the ambiguity, certain principles apply. A physician has to represent accurately what he is treating and how; the correct codes must be used to be paid legally for a service. The physician's documentation has to support the codes used; if something is not documented, it did not happen. He must distinguish between time-based codes and those that are not time dependent and know that even when he is using an evaluation and management code that is based on the extent of the history and examination performed and the complexity of medical decision making, he should use total time to determine the appropriate code to use if counseling and coordination of care represent more than 50% of his time. How to calculate time depends on where he is. Only his face-to-face patient time counts in an outpatient setting, but all of the floor time spent on a patient's case counts in an inpatient setting, not just time spent at the beside talking directly to the patient.

The bad news is that coding is complicated, and it changes all of the time. The good news—other than that it is worse for surgeons—is that AACAP has an excellent Current Procedural Terminology (CPT) training module that is updated every year. This should be required reading for every psychiatrist. The larger issue is that coding and billing procedures should be transparent, like other aspects of doing business with managed care plans. A patient should not be surprised by anything that appears on an explanation of benefits sent by his health plan. Some patients, especially in large practice settings where the billing may be viewed as removed from the therapeutic relationship, do not want to engage in conversation about business details. The growth of behavioral health carve-out plans has meant that the patient generally is not involved in obtaining authorization for treatment, the primary care physician often is no longer the gatekeeper for these services, and the mental health provider deals directly with the managed care organization. Sometimes even the existence of a separate organization managing mental health benefits is a surprise to the patient.

Whether or not the patient wants to discuss coding, billing, and other business arrangements, there are at least two reasons why it is imperative for the mental health provider to do so. The first is that a patient's managed care organization may limit services or impose review requirements that actually interfere with the care. The second is that, from a broader perspective, patients need to understand the nature of their benefits and how their health plan works to be able to make choices, advocate for themselves, and be informed consumers in an era of major upheaval in health care. It always was part of the treatment agreement to negotiate a fee arrangement; managed care simply has broadened the discussion enormously and amplified the potential ethical concerns. To avoid misunderstandings that could, in and of themselves, affect the treatment, a mental health provider should discuss with his patient the diagnosis and treatment plan, how the managed care organization authorizes and reviews services, what information will be provided to the plan, any limits in treatment of which he is aware, the amount of reimbursement provided and the amount for which the patient is responsible, and what will happen in the event that services are not covered. Any financial arrangements between the provider and the plan that could create a conflict of interest also should be discussed [17].

One additional benefit to an open discussion of financial arrangements with patients is that it reduces the temptation to engage in "creative" coding and billing practices. Advocating for patients within established professional guidelines and boundaries is one thing; misrepresentation to circumvent plan rules is another. Physicians should be mindful of the new antifraud measures that were part of the Deficit Reduction Act of 2005, signed into law in 2006 [18]. In addition to increasing federal investigation, prosecution initiatives, and enforcement of rules and regulations in the Medicaid arena, it included provisions requiring some providers to adopt specific policies about compliance with false claims laws. These laws allow individuals to bring suit against providers submitting false claims, provide protection for "whistle-blowers," and allow for such individuals to share in recoveries made. Although government enforcement focuses on Medicaid and Medicare, billing rules and laws against false billing apply to nongovernmental payers as well. Most importantly, the standard of intent under the false claims laws does not require actual awareness of the falsity of a claim. Deliberate ignorance or reckless disregard of the truth or falsity of a claim or any statement made in connection with the claim also is a violation.

Future considerations: beyond managed care

Many mental health providers have been so focused on their frustrations in dealing with managed care and the great harm that they believe is being done to their patients that they have not viewed it in its larger context. When the focus is purely on the individual patient, managed care is the evil enemy, corporate profiteers co-opting a public good (health care) for private gain. Viewed another way, as a reflection of our choices in allocating resources, managed care is *us*. Or, as Sabin [19] put it, managed care is "our society's effort to craft a private-sector solution to the public-policy problem of health care limits and fair resource allocation while pretending that the problem does not exist. Put bluntly, managed care is…rationing in drag."

We could have taken another route and, like much of the rest of the developed world, adopted a national system of universal health care coverage. This would have required an acknowledgment that resources are not infinite and explicit decisions about what would and would not be covered. But this is not the American way. So what we got instead was a market-driven response to the uncontrollable costs of the 1980s—managed care—that was advertised as being able to reduce costs and still provide all necessary services [19]. Because consumers do not mind reducing costs in the abstract but are averse to having their own care curtailed in any way, the backlash against managed care that resulted was large and entirely predictable [20].

In response to the backlash, there has been a flood of legislation putting restrictions on managed care organizations and establishing various patients' rights [2]. The focus of media coverage often is a particular patient denied a particular treatment by a particular managed care plan, with much gnashing of teeth and a follow-up story in which it is noted that the treatment was approved. Instead of engaging in rational discussions about what minimum standard of care should be available to all, we are debating health care reform case by case.

Missing in the reaction is any acknowledgment that limits have always existed; they were not invented by managed care organizations. In the fee-for-service era, out-of-pocket costs in the form of deductibles and coinsurance tended to be higher for consumers. Consumers influenced the use of resources by choosing when to seek care and from whom, and they shared in the costs accordingly. Under managed care, consumers do not choose the limits placed by their health plans to control costs, and the lack of choice comes at a time when they have more information about treatment options and new technologies [21]. The issue for many consumers seems to be choice, not limits per se. A study of consumer attitudes about managed care showed that consumers were markedly unhappier with the performance of their health plan when they did not choose the plan, and consumers without choice had more negative opinions about insurers and managed care in general. Therefore, what seems to matter is not just the type of health plan a person has, but whether he has a choice in the matter [22].

The transition to health care plans with reduced personal choice and increased cost-containment controlled by third parties has led to increased distress and unique ethical challenges. But it would be a mistake to limit the discussion to how to behave ethically in a treatment relationship in the world of managed care. Resolving these dilemmas is important, but unless the larger ethical issues in health care are addressed, it is insufficient. Managed care *is* rationing, but only one form of it. If we restrict ourselves to advocating for the patients in our offices, we have ceded the debate about system priorities. Why should we care? We should care because the current system has completely excluded 15% of our friends and neighbors, for whom "competing values" translates into no health care at all, and because it is in our interest to do so. If we can engage in rational planning about medical necessity and resource allocation, making evidence-based informed choices, then perhaps we can avoid having the same argument with one managed care reviewer after another, day after day after day. This has happened in Oregon, where key stakeholders, including the public, systematically and democratically defined health care priorities [23]. Although the actual performance of the Oregon plan has been mixed, it is a start.

Mental health providers need to be proactive in creating standards so that they can then advocate for their use. To inform the standards, obviously, more data are needed on what providers do and on what works and what does not. Providers should be excited about working with

managed behavioral health care organizations to get outcomes data, not re-
senting the initiatives that they bring to the table. They should do this because "pay-for-performance" mechanisms are increasingly common and
because mental health providers need to be able to measure the quality of
the services that they provide to participate effectively in the larger
discussion.

In the past decade, there has been significant consolidation among managed behavioral health organizations, so that only a few organizations now
enroll most covered lives. Although carve-outs present challenges to providing integrated care, they are large repositories of data that can be used to
measure service use, outcomes, cost, and quality. Carve-outs have been successful in lowering costs and maintaining or even improving access, but
quality of care has been harder to measure [24]. There also is evidence
that managed care strategies tend to "democratize" the provision of services, with reductions in care comparable across groups with varying intensity of illness. More people are getting care, but there is less variation in the
care that they are receiving; therefore, the sickest patients might not be well
served [25].

It is easy to understand why mental health providers have largely rejected
the validity of controls placed on their practices by managed care organizations. To remain fixed in this place, however, is shortsighted and is not, in
the long run, helpful to patients. Managed care, in one form or another,
is here to stay. Providers should be spending time collecting data that will
demonstrate which interventions provide optimal benefit with the most efficient use of resources. They also should be studying the effect of various
managed care practices on treatment and outcomes. If they are creative,
providers will think about the larger context, about prevention and the social, economic, and environmental factors beyond our interventions that
contribute to improved patient functioning. Perhaps this knowledge can
be used to exploit the flexibility that carve-outs afford. If mental health providers can demonstrate that providing preventive intervention services in
schools is cost-effective, for example, perhaps they can contract with a behavioral carve-out company to pay a set amount for a clinician's time in
a school instead of billing a greater amount for outpatient services on
a fee-for-service basis.

Innovative approaches to prevention and treatment will require creative
new administrative and business practices. The mental health provider in the
school, for example, will need to record prevention or collateral contact encounters without necessarily having formulated or recorded a diagnosis or
having performed a procedure listed in the CPT manual. Most managed
care organizations still have claims payment systems based on counting
face-to-face authorized visits, even if contracts include financial terms that
involve shared risk and are not exclusively fee-for-service. Mental health
providers currently have billing systems that require the registration and
capture of individual patient encounters.

Innovative approaches also will require changes in training programs. School-based services or preventive interventions, for example, require different skill sets than those currently taught in most programs. Seminars on competing values in the allocation of health care resources and on patient advocacy in its broadest, public policy context should be required. Trainees get a lot of experience filling out forms to get sessions authorized and justifying the need for an inpatient stay, but do they get a chance to examine and evaluate different criteria for determining medical necessity? It would be a remarkable exercise to have a group of trainees and faculty from different medical specialties meet regularly for a year to produce their own "Oregon plan" and debate its merits.

In recent years, the tenor of the public debate on health care in this country has shifted from reforming managed care to reforming the health care system as a whole. There is increased focus on quality and increased recognition that choices have to be made, because resources are not infinite. Mental health providers should take note and move beyond blaming managed care to promoting changes in practice. Advocating for the patient in treatment continues to be critically important, but so is advocating at the state house. Ultimately, the only way to move the debate forward and effect meaningful change in the health care system is to combine knowledge with advocacy and proactively define the standards that are needed to make the necessary choices.

References

[1] Gorey E. The doubtful guest. New York: Harcourt; 1998.
[2] Stone D. Managed care and the second great transformation. J Health Polit Policy Law 1999;24:1213–8.
[3] Weisgerber K. The traumatic bond between psychotherapists and managed care. In: Weisgerber K, editor. The traumatic bond between the psychotherapist and managed care. Northvale (NJ): Jason Aronson Inc; 1999. p. 3–36.
[4] Reinhardt UE. The predictable managed care *kvetch* on the rocky road from adolescence to adulthood. J Health Polit Policy Law 1999;24:897–910.
[5] Schlesinger M, Wynia M, Cummins D. Some distinctive features of the impact of managed care on psychiatry. Harv Rev Psychiatry 2000;8:216–30.
[6] Sturm R, Ringel J. The role of managed care and financing in medical practices: how does psychiatry differ from other medical fields? Soc Psychiatry Psychiatr Epidemiol 2003;38: 427–35.
[7] Mechanic D, McAlpine D, Rosenthal M. Are patients' office visits with physicians getting shorter? N Engl J Med 2001;344:198–204.
[8] Olfson M, Marcus SC, Pincus HA. Trends in office-based psychiatric practice. Am J Psychiatry 1999;156:451–7.
[9] Luft H. Why are physicians so upset about managed care? J Health Polit Policy Law 1999;24: 957–66.
[10] Dial T, Haviland M, Pincus H. Faculty salaries in psychiatry and all faculty departments, 1980–2001. Psychiatr Serv 2005;56:142.
[11] Kanapaux W. Compensation levels hold steady, but future uncertain. Available at: http:// psychiatrictimes.com/showArticle.jhtml?articleID = 175802456. Accessed September 6, 2007.

[12] American Academy of Child and Adolescent Psychiatry. Annotations to AACAP ethical code with special reference to evolving health care delivery and reimbursement systems. 1995. Available at: http://www.aacap.org/galleries/AboutUs/CodeOfEthics.PDF

[13] Freeman V, Rathore S, Weinfurt K, et al. Lying for patients: physician deception of third-party payers. Arch Intern Med 1999;159:2263–70.

[14] Rushton J, Felt B, Roberts M. Coding of pediatric behavioral and mental disorders. Pediatrics 2002;110:e8.

[15] Felt-Lisk S, Humensky J. Appendix G. American Psychiatric Association minimum necessary guidelines for third-party payers for psychiatric treatment. Privacy issues in mental health and substance abuse treatment: information sharing between providers and managed care organizations: final report. Available at: http://aspe.hhs.gov/datacncl/reports/MHPrivacy/appendix-g.htm.

[16] Pomerantz A. What if prospective clients knew how managed care impacts psychologists' practice and ethics? An exploratory study. Ethics Behav 2000;10:159–71.

[17] Acuff C, Bennett B, Bricklin P, et al. Considerations for ethical practice in managed care. Prof Psychol Res Pr 1999;30:563–75.

[18] Deficit Reduction Act of 2005, Pub. L. No. 109-171, 120 Stat. 4 (Feb. 8, 2006).

[19] Sabin J. Managed care and health care reform: comedy, tragedy, and lessons. Psychiatr Serv 2000;51:1392–6.

[20] Mechanic D. The managed care backlash: perceptions and rhetoric in health care policy and the potential for health care reform. Milbank Q 2001;79:35–54.

[21] Thorpe KE. Managed care as victim or villain? J Health Polit Policy Law 1999;24:949–56.

[22] Gawande AA, Blendon RJ, Brodie M, et al. Does dissatisfaction with health plans stem from having no choices? Health Aff 1998;17:184–94.

[23] Sabin J, Daniels N. Setting behavioral health priorities: good news and crucial lessons from the Oregon health plan. Psychiatr Serv 1997;48:883–9.

[24] Frank RG, Garfield RL. Managed behavioral health care carve-outs: past performance and future prospects. Annu Rev Public Health 2007;28:303–20.

[25] Mechanic D, McAlpine D. Mission unfulfilled: potholes on the road to mental health parity. Health Aff 1999;18:7–21.

ELSEVIER
SAUNDERS

Child Adolesc Psychiatric Clin N Am
17 (2008) 67–92

CHILD AND
ADOLESCENT
PSYCHIATRIC CLINICS
OF NORTH AMERICA

New Media and an Ethics Analysis Model for Child and Adolescent Psychiatry

Norman E. Alessi, MD[a],*, Vincent A. Alessi[b]

[a]University of Michigan School of Medicine, Department of Psychiatry,
825 Victors Way, Suite 310, Ann Arbor, MI 48108, USA
[b]Oberlin College, 101 North Professor Street, Oberlin, OH 44074, USA

Members of the child and adolescent psychiatric community frequently find themselves asked to discuss issues about media, specifically regarding its effects on their patients. Fueled by almost limitless advances, media is an area in which we often are asked to make ethical decisions; parents ask if their children should watch television, and if so, how much; if they should allow their children to use the Internet; if they should provide them video game systems, and if so, what types of games should be allowed; if their child has Asperger syndrome, will the use of the Internet interfere with the child's social development; should their adolescent be allowed to have a MySpace account; and if their adolescent is depressed, will their access to MySpace sites lead to a greater risk of self-injurious behavior? The understanding of how these questions should be answered requires more than just familiarization with old forms of media, but also an education in the recently introduced media modalities that have revolutionized the way information is transferred and communications are made.

The ethics of media as they relate to child and adolescent psychiatry is an area of great significance due to the increasingly fundamental role that media plays in both our lives and those of children and adolescents. Despite the important role of media in day-to-day life, the realm of the ethics of media has remained largely unexplored. This area of thought is intractable due to the rapid development of new forms of media—which are qualitatively distinct from those which preceded them—and the less-than-rapid progression of current understanding as informed by empirical research,

---

* Corresponding author.
E-mail address: nalessi@umich.edu (N.E. Alessi).

1056-4993/08/$ - see front matter © 2008 Elsevier Inc. All rights reserved.
doi:10.1016/j.chc.2007.08.002   *childpsych.theclinics.com*

given the comparatively slow pace at which it progresses. Furthermore, the ethics of media—new media in particular—is an uncharted area, because the production and subsequent use of new forms of media results in new dimensions of experience and effects in general that are impossible to understand through an analytical framework based on data gathered from old forms of media. We propose a model that will serve as a foundation for the clinician's development of an ethical framework regarding questions about new forms of media as they pertain to child and adolescent psychiatry.

This article is divided into two parts: (1) a description of media, in particular the myriad forms of newer media; and (2) a proposed model for ethical considerations about media modalities as they pertain to child and adolescent psychiatry. Hopefully through understanding what it is about media that has changed to warrant its delineation into "old media" and "new media," combined with a model that allows for the appreciation of the ethical ramifications of these forms of media, the psychiatric community's analysis of issues regarding the interaction between new media and the child and adolescent will be enhanced.

Current media thought

The term *media* is most frequently used to refer to the medium through which information as *content* is transmitted in a communication between a sender and a receiver, though it has also come to refer specifically to the content of a given communication. As evinced by the lack of reference to the differences between forms of media or communication mediums in the medical literature, content analysis, or policy creation, it would appear that many health professionals accept this sweeping generalization of media as sufficient in spite of its patent ambiguity. Even though there exists a general consensus among media theorists that the term *media*, when used as a catch-all term for "means of communication," is a gross oversimplification that can often lead to confusion and misunderstanding. Many clinicians, including child and adolescent psychiatrists, have yet to evolve their use of the term; yet to continue to use yesterday's concepts to work out today's problems can only lead to insufficient solutions and frustration. Therefore, it is important that we first define what it is that we are dealing with (eg, media) before speaking of how to conceptualize its ethical implications.

Contrary to how it is generally understood, media is not merely content-devoid of an association with its mechanism of distribution, nor is it only a delivery system for content. The actual catalyst of a message's effect on a receiver/user is the content it carries, but it is largely determined by the medium through which it is transmitted. That is, the effect of any given information is dependent on how it is transmitted, received, and interpreted: the effect of a given form of media, insofar as how it allows for the transfer of information, is distinct from and almost always far greater in effect than the information it may contain [1]. Consequently, a thorough understanding of the medium is at least as crucial to an accurate understanding of the effect of a communication as is an understanding of the content.

At no other time is an appreciation for the scope and the power of media's potential impact more important. The combined use and immersion in the many modalities of media has enmeshed our lives and the children and adolescents we care for into a *mediascape*, a world inseparable from the media that connects us to the world [2]. An exclusive reliance on content analysis, though adequate in the past, is no longer sufficient for either gaining an appreciation of the clinical impact of media or conceptualizing its ethical implications.

Evolution of media

We live in a world network of national and international communication so complete and complex that it permeates almost every facet of our everyday lives; however, this situation is fairly new. Often this modern web of communication is thought of as being media in general and is therefore considered a relatively recent innovation. However, media in general has existed for thousands of years, progressing through various forms as the necessities of the times have demanded, technologies of the day have allowed, and an individual's momentary means could provide. It is relatively recent that provision of various forms of media such as mail, pictures, written works, music, and plays are no longer a luxury of a society's affluent few. Beginning in the mid-nineteenth century and accelerating during the beginning of the twentieth century, many forms of media became more available and readily accessible. Newspapers, magazines, and the radio where available to almost everyone through fixed delivery systems, allowing for what was a wide distribution at the time, but in such a way that severely constrained the degree of freedom an individual had in shaping their personal experience. As a result of this unidirectional distribution, the resulting media experience of the user was that of a passive observer. Such forms of media fall within the category of old media, which refers not just to content or a medium's associated technologies, but to the experience the media is limited to supplying the user; the experience of flipping through the leafs of a letter or pamphlet is very different from exploring the pages of a Web site.

The world was changed significantly with the discovery and increased exposure to forms of media such as television, film, and the telephone. We had progressed from using media in which there was a static and fixed linear representation of information (eg, the pages in a book) to forms that allowed their audience a limited degree of choice (eg, multiple channels on the television or radio). The media has evolved into modalities which allow for interactive and nonlinear presentation of content that can be actively shaped by the preferences of the user, such as the World Wide Web and the Internet, smart phones, podcasts, teleconferencing, Wikipedia, and networked virtual worlds [3].

What is new media?

Though in recent years there has been a great deal of interest in new media, there is currently no universal definition for new media. This lack of an agreed-upon definition is due to the unrelenting change of the modalities that comprise new media, due to the constant introduction of new technologies and the novel dimensions of experiences they provide. Consequently, a static definition of new media is not possible. The Internet has evolved into the World Wide Web, from homepages to Web sites, and from interactive Web pages to blogs to social networks; similarly, the telephone has evolved from the land line to the cell phone to the smart phone. Each evolutionary step forward adds to the complexity of understanding the definition of new media.

There have been multiple definitions of new media that have come from diverse areas of thought, each giving explanations that are distinct from one another, though also being individually incomplete; each focuses on only one or two qualities of new media to the exclusion of others. This would not necessarily be a bad thing, provided that all of these definitions were read at the same time. The following three examples demonstrate how new media definitions generally look at one or two circumstantially pertinent qualities, rather than attempting a thorough explanation which then is specifically applied:

- New media are interdisciplinary works using recently developed electronic media. This includes works that take advantage of what is possible with recent developments in software and with hardware devices (monitors, projections, printouts, three-dimensional fabrications, and so forth) that employ that software [4].
- New media is a generic term for the many different forms of electronic communication that are made possible through the use of computer technology. The term is in relation to old media forms (eg, print newspapers and magazines) that are static representations of text and graphics. Use of the term *new media* implies that the data communication is happening between desktop and laptop computers and handhelds, such as personal digital assistants, and the media from which they obtain data, such as compact discs and floppy disks [5].
- Fifty-seven percent of American teenagers create content for the Internet—from text to pictures, music, and video. In this new media culture, people no longer passively "consume" media (and thus advertising, its main revenue source) but actively participate in them, which usually means creating content, in whatever form and on whatever scale. This does not have to mean that "people write their own newspaper: "It could be as simple as rating the restaurants they went to or the movie they saw," or as sophisticated as shooting a home video [6].

In the first example, Delahunt emphasizes the role technology plays in the increase of communication, defining new media as the digital collaboration allowed by new technologies. Similar to the first, the second definition relies on a strong reference to computer technologies, focusing on the resulting intercommunication and digital media convergence. Distinctive from the previous two, the last example emphasizes the user's participation in forming their own media experience by using technology for the purpose of interacting and exchanging information with others. It keys into the idea that new media is not how and what is handed down to a passive audience, but how user input can craft the experience. New media can exist in many forms, more so than old media. New media can involve technology, software, and social and interpersonal experience, yet it is not solely any of these, but all of them and much more.

It should be apparent that new media is a complex area that involves sophisticated delivery models and new types of human interfaces, content, and experience. The latest forms of new media continue to push the boundaries of what is considered possible and challenge the limits of their own definition. It is understandable that the first two descriptions we looked at were focused on hardware. It was through technologic advances that unrestrained innovation created new media of today and later allowed for rapid price reduction, making almost any technology widely available within years, if not months, of its discovery. The constant advance of technology has given rise to the unique experiences that distinguish new media from old media, and it is the continuation of this process that guarantees that new media will continue to redefine itself.

Any set definition of new media can only be temporarily accurate at best. Instead of trying to provide a definition, we instead will provide an eight-level model that considers multiple dimensions of a modality and offers an all-inclusive representation (Fig. 1). Moving from modes of transmission and types of technologies to individual and social levels of impact, the layers become gradually smaller from top to bottom so as to represent how each level possesses less and less ability to change the actual form of the modality itself: networks and hardware play the largest role in determining the modality, whereas individual experience, social impact, and interactive experience have a far less direct effect on the actual form of the modality. The eight levels and their representative components follow.

Communication and network technology

Including cable, satellite, wireless, and other technologies of infrastructure, this layer refers to the basic contentless link between an audience/user and the media modality; the string that holds together the paper cups of the old children's telephone and the vast web of cables extending through most countries would both fall into this domain [7]. The organization and basic structure of this system of connections only applies to those modalities that are networked such as the Internet, in such cases providing the fundamental limitations within which all other dimensions are constrained.

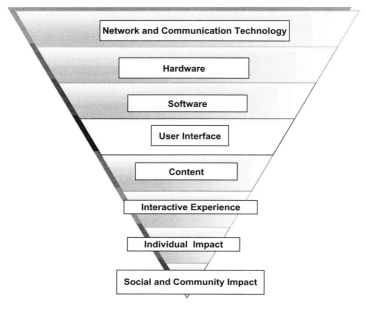

Fig. 1. Multilevel new media model.

However, in free-standing modalities such as video games, which are not necessarily networked, there are no such constraints—though a user no longer interacts with multiple other users, which carries its own set of hazards.

Hardware

This level includes televisions, handheld devices, video game systems, cell phones, and computer processing units. Such devices allow and mediate access to the information/content either received externally, such as from a network, or stored internally within the hardware itself in the form of a hard drive, CD, and so forth. Hardware is the most visible aspect of media, because it is the physical object that allows a person to interact with content. It is most frequently discussed in public forums and is often most likely to be compared with older technologies.

Software

The term *software* generally refers to the programs that manage, decode, and decipher content into a form accessible to the user/audience. Software adds the intelligence to hardware by receiving, processing, and presenting the information it receives. In nonlinear systems of information presentation (ie, new media), information managed by the software includes the input of the user as well as data from the hardware itself.

User interface

User interface refers to any entity through which content can engage the user/audience. The means by which this is accomplished are included in this layer; one example is the Web browser application that interprets the flow of computer code through the Internet into meaningful information. However, in some forms of media the interface is either a part of the hardware (eg, the keypad in an arcade game) or the content itself (eg, in a first-person shooter video game), which is modulated by the user's input alone. Often invisible to those who do not use new media, interfaces such as a video game character or an avatar (both representing a user), Internet browsers, Web pages, and even certain smart phone layouts are all examples of the kind of user interfaces that often fail to be seen by those who only use old media.

Content

The information that is rendered by the interface to the user, forming the basic substance of the message, could be the words of a piece of writing, the image of a user's videogame character killing an enemy, the moving pictures of a pornographic clip, or the sounds from a smartphone. Content may be the most evident component of any given media experience, and consequently is referred to most often. However, the effect of content is constrained by the infrastructure, hardware, software, and interface through which it is transmitted, with the media being far more important in the creation of the interactive experience. In a way, content is the substrate through which the effect of a medium can be felt by the user.

Interactive experience

Interactive experience refers to the actual general reaction of a user to the content they perceive. This may consist of many overlapping areas of phenomenologic sensations.

Individual impact

The unique response a person has to the elicitation of differing sensations provoked through the interactive experience is referred to as *individual impact*. Two adolescents can experience a MySpace site with reference to suicide quite differently depending on their state of mind.

Social and community impact

The larger implications of new media arise from similar and complimentary personal experiences occurring en masse. The ability to facilitate the cohesion of entire demographics of individuals is one of new media's greatest and, to some, most concerning strengths. Two examples are MySpace and YouTube, social networking applications that are changing the social expectations of today's youth.

At the heart of new media is the transformation of the production, transmission, and presentation of information from analog hard copy to digital binary. As new media becomes increasingly digitized, it also becomes increasingly integrated into computer technologies in general, becoming more and more broadly disseminated as computers and communication networks. Before the arrival of new media, one might have read a book or have gone to a library for references; now, however much of this work may be performed online. Though college classes were once exclusively experienced within a lecture hall or classroom, increasingly, the average student will now receive their daily dose of collegiate pedagogue through an e-lecture, with syllabus and associated reading found on a school Web site and delivered via podcast. At the end of the day, youth may visit their MySpace or Facebook site to see who has visited their personal Web page, check their messages, respond to e-mails, and perhaps spend some time in an online world such as that provided by the highly successful Second Life or World of War Craft, where they may have accumulated enough rare game items that they may sell them to other players in the real world.

Beyond appreciating what composes new media case by case, the concepts that arise from the combination of multiple modalities functioning simultaneously is pertinent to a better understanding of their effects in general. Though there are many ideas whose creation are attributed to the evolution of media, there are three important concepts associated with new media and the functionality made possible by its underlying technologies: convergence, connectivity, and immersion.

Convergence

Convergence is the coming together of multiple technologies facilitating the discovery, creation, reuse, transmission, and sharing of information. This is strongly influenced by the flow of media across multiple modalities as allowed between and among multiple media industries. Digital technology implies a convergence of all media forms; in the words of Henry Jenkins, "In the world of media convergence, every important story gets told, every brand gets sold, and every consumer gets courted across multiple media platforms" [8]. For example, MTV has recently introduced an online world in which users have virtual characters who inhabit a composite virtual world formed of the worlds of MTV's sitcoms and dramas. Realistic down to every detail, users can even interact with the virtual characters of their favorite shows.

Connectivity

As a result of the convergence of multiple media modalities, the amount of information a person can receive and send increases. Everyone is familiar with seeing either their teen, or others, with their cell phone, communicating via voice, text, pictures or video; at home they may instant message their friends, or go to their MySpace Web site and add to their online content; they may even have a blog they manage and share with "friends." More broadly speaking, the incredible connectivity allowed by the Internet has given rise to online collections of hypertext-linked Web pages called *wikis* (*wiki wiki* means "rapidly" in the native language of Hawaii), which allow all users to freely access, add, and edit information in real time [9].

Immersion

Immersion is the ability for an individual to become immersed in a "virtual reality" that can have many forms, from video games such as Halo to three-dimensional online worlds, Second Life, Club Penguin (a virtual world designed specifically for grade school children), or the combination of individual experiences a given media modality provides during the course of a day (ie, the sum of time spent on computers, cell phones, video games, and so forth). We exclude books, mail, and phones, and old media in general on the basis of limited immersive experience offered to the passive observer resulting in a lack of the user's ability to ascend to interactive audience. Convergence also overlaps with this concept: as more and more media encapsulate the world experience of an individual, their mediascape experience can undermine their relationship with certain aspects of reality.

These three concepts reflect how the evolution of technology has resulted in new modes of communication and experience that are revolutionizing media. However, these concepts make an analysis of the impact of media particularly difficult. Whereas there are reports that document the number of households that use the Internet and the average age of those who access the Web, there has been no research on topics related to these three concepts, despite their visibility and importance. However, this should come as no surprise given that there are no metrics that would allow accurate quantitative analysis or qualitative understanding of their significance. It is in part due to these limitations that the development of ethical guidelines in the area of new media is particularly difficult.

Differentiating old media from new media

A review of the literature concerning media and psychiatry demonstrates that the core issues often involve old media questions. This is not to say that "old media as new media" cannot occur and have impact, but there is a difference. For those who were exposed to old media predominantly before the development of new media, the difference may not be readily evident nor seem that important [10,11]. This is most apparent when one believes that getting their journals online is new media. It is old media in the sense that you can read each posting as a journal article; but it is not in that it can also be treated as new media. You can read this month's issue online as well as all quoted references associated with each article online; in addition,

you can access several blogs that deal with a particular article's topic and
even contact the author via e-mail with questions. Twenty years ago, these
tasks would have taken several days, if not weeks; now they can be done in
a fraction of that time. Fig. 2 provides a general breakdown of media into
old media and new media along the lines addressed in Fig. 1.

Why is it important to discern between old media and new media?

In a clinical setting, it is necessary to identify what forms of media represent linear and/or limited forms of information presentation (ie, old media)
and what forms of nonlinear information presentation (ie, new media) to
which an individual is being exposed. Using the conceptual definition and
criteria provided here, the individual modalities that shape a patient's

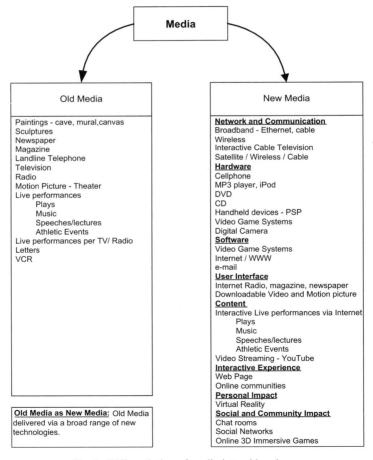

Fig. 2. Differentiation of media into old and new.

mediascape experience can be generally assigned to one of three classifications listed below.

Old media

In old media, one can read the news in a newspaper or magazine. Articles are linear and free-standing. To read further, one has to either go the library or review old copies one might own or borrow from friends.

Old media as new media

In old media as new media, one can approach reading the news on the Internet as if it were an old media newspaper or magazine. It can be linear and formatted to appear as if it were a "newspaper" or magazine. One can ignore links embedded in the text that would hyperlink a reader to another reference, magazine, newspaper article, associated video, sound files, graphics, e-mail to an author. Just because one uses the Internet does not necessarily mean that it becomes a new media delivery system.

New media

To appreciate the effect of new media, one has to understand the experience is more than reading several documents, seeing associated videos, or listening to numerous sound files. The metaphor of experience is one of entering a portal of limitless information in multiple forms that can be accessed via multiple devices at all times. Therefore, one can read an article or review a number of pertinent associated and historical documents, videos, lectures, and sound files. E-mails can be sent to an author, or their blog or vlog might be accessed to see if there is continued discussion. A number of Push technologies may be engaged to provide continued information about the article or author-related articles. An article serves as a portal to a vast domain of data, information, and knowledge.

New media is about an alteration in experience, not just content. The combination of cell phones with text messaging, wireless Internet that can be accessed from almost anywhere, video games accessible from both home and mobile platforms, and all other types of media delivery systems add up to a continuous experience of information, instead of intermittent exposure where convenient. Because the new media experience of today is very different compared with that of the past, we must apprise the issues it creates through its possible effects on the developing child and adolescent.

No demographic is at a greater risk for the problems associated with new media than the child and adolescent demographic. This is not only because children and adolescents are more vulnerable to violence and poor role modeling on television—it also has to do with how the average child and adolescent grows up with the technologies of new media surrounding them, seamlessly integrated into their world experience. This familiarity with the interaction and immersion of new media means that children and adolescents typically have a far greater ability to allow themselves to become consumed by the virtual experience created by the regular engagement of multimedia modalities. Their conception of reality, often filled with forms of media such as video games, television, computers, and the Internet is in many ways devoid of any nontechnological grounding that could put the information they receive into perspective. Consequently, the young more readily suspend disbelief (if there can be said to be any) in the relative falsity of media experience, treating it as much more than a means of communication (as their parents might) but rather as a multifaceted virtual world through which many of the lessons normally taught through life experiences are learned instead through media. For these reasons and more, the need to incorporate the broader effect of media on children into clinical practice is greater than in any other age group.

Media ethics

Traditionally, the term *media ethics* is used to refer to the field of applied morality that describes the principles of acceptable conduct and standards surrounding the execution of media in general (eg, the practice of journalism, broadcast media, censorship, and production of print and electronic content). Though professionals in these fields seem to also find themselves having to struggle to maintain a set of new media-savvy ethical guidelines, their ethical concerns are generally limited to those issues relevant to a production-oriented setting, ignoring such things as the areas of convergence, a concept that is very important when trying to understand the formative force of media on the autonomy for users. The concerns addressed herein are not directed at the process of production and distribution of media per se but instead target the ethical implications of new media as they arise within child and adolescent psychiatry. Currently, no clear ethical standard or system of analysis exists to confront the concerns of the user side of the media experience, much less an analytical framework that takes into consideration the demographic of its audience in a way that is relevant to child and adolescent psychiatric communities, especially given a patient's psychopathology.

Although media ethics in the traditional sense includes considerations of community standards, journalistic integrity, censorship, and bias, discussions of media ethics must not only address a broader range of topics such as video games, social networks, online virtual worlds, and collaborative online sites, they must do so with a perspective that is not so concerned with the production of media, but is instead focused on the effect of media on children and adolescents—both those diagnosed with psychiatric disorders and those not—and the responsibilities of the psychiatric community that arise thereof.

As in many areas, there is no universal ethical framework for the analysis of new media, nor is there a moral code to be followed, although many simple examples exist that might lead clinicians to believe they have made the correct recommendation and may lead parents to believe they have done the "right" thing. What are believed to be moral decisions must not be confused with ethical analysis. Morality is a system to define and judge right and wrong, whereas ethics is the study of that system, constituting how you decide when you must make a choice between two conflicting things that are right and/or two things that are wrong. For example, whether a child should be allowed to watch television or use the Internet is an ethical issue, for it is not a simple question of yes or no for many parents, but a question of how much and how long—yet other parents may believe there should be no media exposure. Few parents, however, would question whether a child should be allowed to view pornography. Ethical analysis requires attention to evidence, skill with valid debate, and patience with complexity; the pursuit of this process requires both time and dedication. It seems that one of the most dangerous prospects of any system of morality or ethical analysis is the ease with which one can rationalize the unreasonable. In a similar spirit, Edward R. Murrow is said to have once complained, "What is called thinking is often merely a rearranging of our prejudices." It is crucial, for any of the following to be of value, to have a critical eye while not sacrificing an open mind.

Because our questions involve a clinical health setting, one could argue that we are dealing with biomedical ethics; yet because we are involving the principles that underlie the professional role that child and adolescent psychiatrists play in making decisions about media, one could argue that we are also dealing with professional ethics. Because both of these fields are crucial to understanding the ethical implications of new media in general, a representative model must by default consider questions from professional, bioethical, and even traditional media ethics to be considered relevant to child and adolescent psychiatry. To our knowledge, this has not been clearly stated in the literature, nor has it been accepted by any medical or psychiatric professional society.

Given the tremendous scope of new media and its potential for unlimited growth, it would be preposterous to believe that the ethical issues that surround such a subject can be adequately answered through the construction of rules and dictums to be applied rotely. What is necessary is an ethical system of analysis that is not built upon a rigid set of tenets and assumptions, but is instead capable of including whatever forms of media emerge as technology continues to evolve and reflects our ever-increasingly sophisticated model of human development and associated psychopathology. The sort of analytical scaffold provided is designed to facilitate ethical analysis in both old and new areas of media, yielding a degree of continuity and insight far greater than prior models, and to support the creation of potential strategies on a case-by-case basis with attention to detail and an understanding of the media under consideration. For example, one can ask whether children should be exposed to violence via a certain media. This model incorporates how violence in a newspaper article, violence in a TV news broadcast, and violence in a three-dimensional immersive game are all quite different in many ways. The ethics of the broadcast, its content, and potential impact can be analyzed to determine whether it should be watched and what the impact of watching versus not watching might be. One can also ask if the violence needed to be shown or why was it decided to be shown. The complexity is greater in the three-dimensional game, leading one to have a much more difficult time coming to a clear ethical conclusion. But in neither case might there be a simple dictum or moral code that would or could reasonably cover all media and violence unless a framework is used.

Old media ethics as moral dictums

The development of new information technologies and their availability to all youth has prompted an escalation in the questions concerning the potential effects of "media" on children and adolescents. The amount of available content alone would seem to warrant placing limitations on access to various forms of media, especially those containing excessive or explicit violence, sexual content, or any other type of content that might, generally speaking, have serious and persistent consequences. Though produced by new media interactions, such ethical decisions are almost always based on old media ethics, which is fundamentally rooted in a causal model that assumes there is progressive impact associated with progressively more advanced forms of media and an inverse relationship associated with age (Fig. 3). From this model, media impact is assumed to become greater as we move from letter-print to image to moving images (video and movies), having less effect the older the person. Though this way of thinking is sometimes appropriate, it is often applied to too many situations, resulting in limitation of media exposure in a way that is excessive and/or unfair.

This causal model provides the basis of ethical analysis concerning old media and the moral guidelines that have been proposed involving children and adolescents. For example, as of 2007, many professional organizations have issued warnings concerning the dangers of violent games: the joint statement made by the American Academy of Pediatrics, American Academy of Child & Adolescent Psychiatry, American Psychological Association, American Medical Association, American Academy of Family Physicians, American Psychiatric Association states that "Numerous studies

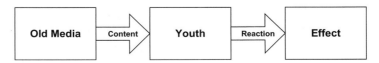

Fig. 3. Old media ethics analytic model.

conducted by leading figures within our medical and public health organizations—our own members—point overwhelmingly to a causal connection between media violence and aggressive behavior in some children. The conclusion of the public health community, based on over 30 years of research, is that viewing entertainment violence can lead to increases in aggressive attitudes, values and behavior, particularly in children" [12]. It is clear that there is a general professional consensus that exposure to media, or at least certain kinds of old media content, must be done with caution if at all. There have been many studies that address the potential impact of violence in films and TV on the expression of violence and provide significant correlations to justify these edicts. Yet these edicts do not provide a platform for new media ethical analysis, only a moral dictum based on empirical research, a system that we have previously established to be ineffectual for the use of fully understanding new media as it evolves.

New media ethical analysis: a model for decision making, not dictum creation

Whereas old media ethical analysis in child and adolescent psychiatry has to do with issues concerning content such as images of violence or nudity or aural presentation of vulgar words and concepts, the ethical analysis of new media has to be concerned with a greater range of modalities as well as the broader range of questions that arise from these. As illustrated in Fig. 4, it is easy to think that all that is needed is to modify the linear ethical model used to evaluate old media so it includes additional parameters which more finely characterize a media modality's actual effect (eg, user interface, interactive experience, and the social and community impact). Though this model

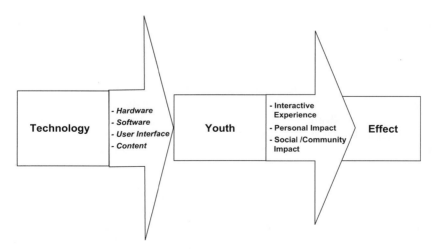

Fig. 4. New media ethics analytic model.

represents a vast improvement from using old media logic alone, it still falls short of acceptable: any system of analysis of new media cannot simply be a unidirectional system of media experience accumulation, which explicitly regards the individual as passive and ignores the fact that they play an active role in the formation of the media they receive and send, a key difference between previous linear systems of analysis. As shown in Figs. 3 and 4, new media ethics has to account for the agency that it provides to its users, which translates into a certain degree of responsibility over the content to which a user is exposed. It is with this agency and consequent responsibility that the ethical implications of new media become clearest: altering a form of old media before was not cause for major concern, because that form of old media was simply an object that was passively enjoyed, quite separate from the individual—whereas now, some new media can be considered as an extension of the user themselves.

Changing access to a single mode of old media was simply an ethical matter only insofar as its effects; there is nothing intrinsically wrong with changing a form of old media per se. On the other hand, altering and some-times even sharing in certain forms of new media is an act of inherent ethical interest: due to new media's interactivity, you are in fact altering an exten-sion of the individual themselves, not just on the level of the objects from which they choose, but with their very capacity of choice—an effect that is exacerbated when networks are included. Inflexible moral dictums may work to an acceptable degree in old media systems of reasoning, but due to the new dimensions of consideration brought forth by new media, we must take a much more considerate approach to our decisions regarding it. Because analysis is at the core of ethics, not the inescapable demands of moral law, it is important to use a technique that facilitates analysis. The examples that were given involve media ethics, not for a biomedical ethical model, but those that are consistent with production. With this in mind, we offer our own model, which we believe to be directly applicable to child and adolescent psychiatry.

The following analytical progression (Fig. 5 and Table 1) is designed to help increase the understanding of the ethical ramifications of new media and facilitate clinical decision making, while not interjecting any pre-established laws or inflexible guidelines. This analytic model reflects in part the general strategy put forth by Potter [13], involving the delineation of the ethical question, followed by potential outcomes, principles that might be applied as well as an assessment of the loyalties involved. From this, either action or further consideration is pursued [13,14].

Step one: define the question, define the media, define the impact

Given that this is a case-by-case analytical model, it is obvious that we must begin with the ethical question at hand. The first issue concerns the identification of the type of media in question, and the second concerns whether the question concerns the impact on a child, adolescent, or provider

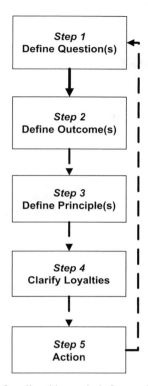

Fig. 5. System of media ethics analysis for psychiatry (SMEAP).

or involves a media issue alone. If there is any ambiguity about what type of media is involved in a given situation, it may be helpful to reference the first half of this article and consult the conceptual definition of new media that was provided. Once the modality and its potential effects are understood, it should be determined what effects are relevant to the child or adolescent and the circumstances surrounding them—the general levels of impact on the individual, their friends/network buddies, family, community, and specific culture.

Step two: define outcomes

Before determining what ethical principles are relevant in a specific case, we must discern what potential outcomes might arise if the processes (ie, the "use" of the modality) continues, and what outcomes might arise if it stops. The impact areas are divided into three areas involving the child or adolescent, the provider, and the media issues themselves. The presence of mental illness and how it might be worsened and the developmental issues that might arise at different ages are suggested as areas for consideration. For the provider, the potential for professional negligence is most important,

Table 1
System of media Ethics Analysis for Psychiatry (SMEAP)

Step	Definitions	Dimensions for consideration
1	Define questions	Media
		Old or new; media not delineated by content alone
		Child or adolescent
		Age of the child
		Developmental difficulties
		Presence of mental illness
		Practitioner's role
		Are there questions of responsibility or negligence?
		Traditional media issues
		Broad range: from acquisition to production to first amendment rights
2	Define outcomes	Child or adolescent
		Worsening or development of behavioral difficulties
		If mental illness present, assess potential impact on its stability and severity
		Developmental issues
		Early development: 12 months to 6 years of age
		Impact on bonding?
		Separation anxiety?
		Impact on executive functioning?
		Stranger anxiety?
		Separation individuation?
		Elementary school: 7–11 years of age
		Impact on the development of interpersonal skills?
		Group skills?
		Academic skills?
		Concentration and organization?
		Cohesiveness of the family?
		Middle school: 12–14 years of age
		Group identity?
		Self-esteem?
		Body image?
		Substance abuse?
		Sexual activity?
		High school: 15–19 years of age
		Social skill development?
		Substance abuse?
		Social values?
		Academic performance?
		Practitioner's role
		Does the media issue place the practitioner at risk if not dealt with? If so, what might be the impact if not dealt with?
		Traditional media issue
		To adequately deal with this issue, refer to the article under media ethics

(*continued on next page*)

Table 1 (*continued*)

Step	Definitions	Dimensions for consideration
3	Define principles	Use guidelines of professional organizations if available AACAP, AAP If the question does not appear to be dealt with by existing guidelines discuss with peers, review literature or access counsel from professional organizations
4	Clarify loyalties	Must be defined based on a consideration of the case and the patient and their abilities Patient, parents or guardians, school, law enforcement, human services
5	Action	If possible, take action that appears to reflect the summation of the factors that you have identified If it is not possible to take action, repeat the cycle with an attempt to determine the factors that had not been identified in the first analysis

and when considering media issues, the specifics of the question must be considered from that perspective.

Step three: define principles

For most clinical bioethical situations, the principles used would be those stated for either the American Academy of Child and Adolescent Psychiatry and/or the American Academy of Pediatrics [15]. This area is most important insofar as it informs an individual of how the foreseeable outcomes align with their own profession's general code of conduct; though it is unlikely that they will deviate from common sense, it is a point that is important to clearly establish nonetheless. Of greater concern are those situations that might arise not related directly to the principles of their professional organization. In that case, a practitioner might either speak with peers or with their professional organization itself to seek guidance.

Step four: clarify loyalties

Who are the parties involved and who is the child and adolescent psychiatrist representing? The answer to these questions will then serve to guide the psychiatrist in understanding who it is that he/she represents, and therefore whose interest they are serving. In many cases, there will be several interested parties who think that the child or adolescent is the one that needs to be helped or constrained and that the psychiatrist should follow their requests.

Step five: action

Determine the best course of action based on the information gained through the previous steps. If there is no apparent justifiable decision, it may be helpful to reconsider the answers you provided to previous questions and repeat the cycle. The information collected may not be simple enough to result in a simple action. One would expect that to be the case given the potential complexity of the summation of the media and its areas of impact. Yet the guidelines, if followed, will help to illuminate a broader range of factors than if just dealing with the situation in an offhand manner with little consideration other than reliance on dictums as suggested earlier.

The following two cases provide opportunities to demonstrate application of the analytic model.

Case 1

The mother of an adolescent girl e-mails you to tell you that she has been to her daughter's MySpace webpage and her daughter has of late been describing promiscuous behavior with a number of boys. The mother wants you to get her daughter to remove the material, stop using MySpace, and stop acting out. Mom also discusses how on the site the daughter talks about not taking her medications and lying about this. The mother gives you her daughter's MySpace user name so that you can read it for yourself.

Define problem

Can you acknowledge that you know of the posting to the girl? Can you tell her who told you? Can you read it without telling her? Is her mother or your reading it a violation of confidentiality? Does she understand what is and is not public?

Impact area

The daughter has told you recently that guys treat her as if she were a "slut." Do you discuss with her how these postings undermine her self-esteem and worsen her depression? Does discussion of the situation undermine her relationship with her family? Will her acting out worsen if the postings are discussed?

Define principles

Define principles using the AACAP code of ethics:

Principles I, II, V: Acknowledges and respects individual differences, placing them before personal bias. (Having the MySpace site is not the problem, its content and how she has used it is the problem.)

Principle VII: Addresses the right of parents and professionals to be informed. (It was appropriate for the mother to inform the clinician of the site and her concerns.)

Principle VIII: Addresses the rights of an adolescent to make decisions on their own behalf. (Given that anyone can start a MySpace account without permission of their parents and post whatever content they choose, it is difficult for a parent or a clinician to mandate the content—or for that matter, their involvement. Therefore, the clinician must respectfully act to both support and help evaluate the decisions of the youth.)

Principle XI: The role of the clinician in establishing an understanding with the youth of confidentiality and its limits. (The clinician in this situation should divulge how they came to learn of the site and other information, but they should then discuss whether their decisions and discussion can be shared with her parents.)

Clarify loyalties

The adolescent is the identified patient and she needs assistance. Given her age and the nature of her difficulties, it is important to maintain this relationship.

Action

Because the adolescent girl is your patient, it is important that you be forthright and honest. You have to discuss with her the e-mail from her mother. Because MySpace is accessible to anyone with a user name and anyone can obtain a user name, it is open to anyone and therefore not private, as a diary might be. After reading it, you discuss with her the implications of the postings, how people regard her, and how this affects her self-esteem. You convince her that the material in question should be removed, but she wants to keep her site. She admits the lying and wants help with her future postings and lying.

Case 2

A mother contacts your office saying that her 6-year-old son has started to act odd over the last several months. He has become more aggressive, hitting other kids and even the teacher at school. He had been designated "emotionally impaired" by the school. She mentions that this seems to have worsened after playing his 15-year-old brother's video game. You learn that the mother was aware of his video game use but had not thought anything of it due to her own online gambling habit.

Define problem

What type of games does the child play? First-person shooter, immersive, online? What role does his brother play in his access to these games? What responsibilities does his older brother have in the care of his younger brother? Is this abusive behavior on his older brother's part? Is this contributing to the delinquency of a minor, and should charges be brought against him? Does the mother's online gambling minimize her insight to the point that it jeopardizes the child's well being? If so, what is the clinician's responsibility to the child and his brother to address this? Does the mother's behavior constitute neglect and should the clinician act accordingly?

Impact area

Does the child have an associated diagnosis that would place him at greater risk than other kids? What areas are showing impact? Interpersonal relatedness? Modulation of affective expression? Poor sublimation of anger and other affects? Distortions of social cognition? To what degree have these been worsened by the exposure to games?

Define principles

Define principles using the AACAP code of ethics:

Principle: I: Statement of major commitment to children and families and professional competence. (The problem extends beyond making a DSM-IV diagnosis and the prescription of a medication. Clearly, much has to be learned about the brother and the mother, possibly resulting in an intervention involving the entire family.)

Principle II: Addresses the commitment to "do no harm" and reduce the potential harmful interactions of others. (The pertinent questions involve the degree to which the brother and mother are consciously, unconsciously, or unknowingly allowing the child to be traumatized by his exposure to violent video game material.)

Clarify loyalties

The child is the identified patient, yet his brother and his mother both have difficulties as well. The child's best interest has to be maintained above all else, including separation from his family if all else fails.

Action

First, the type of media involved has to be explored and characterized. This may take additional time on the part of the clinician to determine the nature of the game and the extent of the child's involvement. In the assessment of the child, attention must be given to the content of his aggression and if possible his communication about the games. If necessary, his brother should be interviewed about the games, their access by his brother, and his mother's supervision of him. The mother should be interviewed to determine the extent of her online gambling and the extent to which she neglects her child during play. Is this a gambling addiction? Does she have the ability to parent her child? Clarification is needed.

Recommendations

1. Make the responsibility of considering media ethical concerns part of the Code of Ethics for the American Academy of Child and Adolescent Psychiatry. The American Academy of Pediatrics has two policies that deal with media: "Media Violence" and "Media Education" [16,17]. Both state the significance of the role of the pediatrician in dealing with this issue at multiple levels, including individual, family, and community. However, both of these policies are over 5 years old and

are based solely on research of old media not reflective of the technologies and potential concerns of the day. Such a code should be a part of the code of ethics for the American Medical Association and the American Psychiatric Association as well, yet its immediate relevance is most apparent in child and adolescent psychiatry given the vulnerabilities of our populations and the potential risks media poses.

2. When discussing media ethics, differentiate between professional, biomedical, and media ethics. Is this an issue of what a professional should do, what the responsibilities are of the media producers, or the potential effects of a media on a child and adolescent and what might be acceptable as it relates to that patient?

3. Attempt to clarify whether you are referring to old media, old media as new media, or new media. Ethical issues will arise in each setting but it is important not to underestimate the impact of the new media and its influencing factors by reviewing past literatures.

4. When discussing new media ethical concerns, attempt to evaluate and discern the potential impact of associated technologies as opposed to content alone. New media will almost always involve new technologies that transform the experience. Therefore, the focus of the analysis must reflect an understanding of the media and its resulting experience.

5. Consider the significance in your patient and any disorders they may have. Rarely is there any reference to the media needs and requirements of our populations or the particular impact they may have on our populations. Are the effects of old or new media greater on psychiatric populations than normal children? Are they more likely to have negative effects? Are they more likely to have positive effects? If so, does that have clinical ramifications for the child and/or his or her family? If they have a pervasive developmental disorder, spending a great deal of time in Second Life or Club Penguin may be far more fulfilling than the isolation they may experience in their real world. The virtual world experience can potentially be used to transition to the real world. The essential question is: "Will they help or harm my patient?"

6. Clinicians should discuss with their child and adolescent patients how they spend their time. Furthermore, they should determine how much time their patients are spending using a technology that involves them in an alternative or "virtual reality." If the clinician is unfamiliar with the technology, they should not only ask about the time and experience but ask their patient to show them where and what they are doing—or, if there is little time during their sessions, investigate for themselves the nature of the experience. It is not enough to merely assess the media according to the child's or parent's description. They would not have the sophistication to readily evaluate the areas potentially involved, nor their implications.

7. Apply the ethical framework provided in cases in which there is a lack of ethical clarity. Spend the time to understand the problem, consider potential recommendations, and, if necessary, discuss with peers.

Summary

The moral dictums pertaining to media today are not the result of ethical analysis and do not reflect the complex issues that surround new media. Much of what is referred to in the literature and is discussed by professional organizations as media is in fact old media or old media as new media. Continued reference to these as the major sources of connectivity is a fallacy. New media and its potential effects must be understood as being more than content alone but reflective of the technologies that compose them and the experiences that arise thereof.

In our review of potential ethics analysis models and tools, none was able to adequately deal with the ethical issues and concerns that arise within the clinical relationships of child and adolescent psychiatry. Our proposed stepwise model is inclusive of the three potential areas subsumed under the category of *media ethics* and allows the delineation of specific topic areas, their impact, principles and value, and loyalties that may have bearing on a specific situation.

Hopefully, these observations and recommendations will lead to the beginning of further thought in this area and improved care of the children and adolescents in which these issues are present.

To aid the reader, the Appendix provides a list of suggested Internet sites that deal with several issues that we have explored here, including media, virtual reality, ethics, and media ethics.

Appendix

Internet sites of interest

Media

- http://www.digitalcenter.org/pages/current_report.asp?intGlobalId=19 (The Center for the Digital Future at the USC Annenberg School)
- http://www.childrenssoftware.com/default.html (Children's Technology Review)
- http://www.eff.org/ (Electronic Frontier Foundation)
- http://www.epic.org/ (Electronic Privacy Information Center)
- http://newmedia.iupui.edu/ (Indiana School of Informatics)
- http://www.leasttern.com/Tech/ethics_safety.html (Internet Law, Ethics and Safety)
- http://wiki.media-culture.org.au/index.php/Internet_as_a_new_media_references (M/Cyclopedia of Media)
- http://www.artlex.com/ArtLex/n/newmedia.html (New Media)
- http://www.cyberjournalist.net/news/000,147.php (Online News Association)
- http://www.stateofthemedia.org/2007/ (State of the News Media 2007)

- http://news.com.com/8301-10,784_3-9,713,568-7.html?tag=recentPosts (Tech News Blogs)
- http://www.usdoj.gov/criminal/cybercrime/cyberethics.htm (US Department of Justice—Computer Crime and Intellectual Property Section)
- http://whatsnewmedia.org/ (What's New Media?)
- http://www.wikipedia.org/ (Wikipedia)

Virtual worlds

- http://www.virtualworldsreview.com/ (Virtual World Reviews)
- http://play.clubpenguin.com (Club Penguin)
- http://ieet.org/index.php/IEET/more/yinjin2005/ (Institute for Ethics and Emerging Technologies)
- http://www.secondlife.com/ (Second Life)
- http://www.cs.waikato.ac.nz/~cbeardon/papers/9201.html (The Ethics of Virtual Reality)

Ethics

- http://www.josephsoninstitute.org/ (Josephson Institute of Ethics)
- http://www.ethicsweb.ca/resources/professional/codes-of-ethics.html (Professional Ehtics)
- http://muse.jhu.edu/journals/kennedy_institute_of_ethics_journal/toc/ken17.1.html (Kennedy Institute of Ethics Journal)
- http://topics.nytimes.com/top/reference/timestopics/subjects/e/ethics/index.html?query=MYSPACE.COM&field=org&match=exact (New York Times Ethics Section)

Media and ethics

- http://freemyspace.com/?P=1 (Free MySpace)
- http://www.naznet.com/ethics/ (Christian Internet Code of Ethics)
- http://wiki.media-culture.org.au/index.php/Computer_Games_-_Ethics:_Gameplay (Computer Games- Ethics: Gameplay)
- http://www.cybercrime.gov/rules/rules.htm (Crimes in Cyberspace)
- http://www.usdoj.gov/criminal/cybercrime/cyberethics.htm (Department of Justice)
- http://connect.educause.edu/blog/StuartYeates/privacyethicsandthei/8497?time=1,185,115,319 (Educause)
- http://usinfo.state.gov/journals/itgic/0401/ijge/gj09.htm (Global Issues—Media and Ethics)
- http://ieet.org/ (Institute for Ethics and Emerging Technologies)

- http://www.globalethics.org/ (Institute for Global Ethics)
- http://www.lessig.org/blog/archives/003,570.shtml (Lawrence Lessig Blog)
- http://librarianinblack.typepad.com/librarianinblack/2005/12/ethics_rules_an.html (Librarianinblack)
- http://www.newmedia.org/articles/37/1/Teens-Set-New-Rules-of-Engagement-in-the-Age-of-Social-Media/Page1.html (New Media Institute)
- http://www.ispub.com/ostia/index.php?xmlFilePath=journals/ijlhe/front.xml (The Internet Journal of Law, Healthcare and Ethics)
- http://www.jmme.org/ (The Journal of Mass Media Ethics)

References

[1] McLuhan M, Fiore Q. The medium is the massage an inventory of effects. New York: Bantam Books, Inc; 1967.
[2] Appadurai A. Disjuncture and difference in the global cultural economy. Public Culture 1990;2(2):1–24.
[3] Jenkins H. Interactive Audiences? In: Harries D, editor. The new media book. London: British Film Institute; 2002. p. 157–70.
[4] Delahunt M. New media. Available at: http://www.artlex.com/ArtLex/n/newmedia.html. Accessed October 23, 2007.
[5] Levinson P. Digital mcluhan a guide to the information millennium. New York: Routledge; 1999.
[6] Among the Audience. The Economist. 2006.
[7] Hilmes M. Cable, satellite and digital technologies. In: Harries D, editor. The new media book. London: British Film Institute; 2002. p. 3–16.
[8] Jenkins H. Convergence Culture. New York: New York University Press; 2006.
[9] Tapscott D, Williams A. Wikinomics: how mass collaboration changes everything. New York: Portfolio; 2006.
[10] Manovich L. Old media as new media: cinema. In: Harries D, editor. The new media book. London: British Film Institute; 2002. p. 209–18.
[11] Uricchio W. Old media as new media: television. In: Harries D, editor. The new media book. London: British Film Institute; 2002.
[12] Joint Statement on the Impact of Entertainment Violence on Children Congressional Public Health Summit
[13] Potter RB. The logic of moral argument. In: Deats P, editor. Toward a discipline of social ethics. Boston: Boston University Press; 1972. p. 93–114.
[14] Christians C, Fackler M, Rotzoll KB, et al. Media ethics: cases and moral reasoning. New York: Addison-Wesley Educational Publishers Inc.; 1998.
[15] Committee AE. AACAP Code of Ethics with Annotations. Available at: http://www.aacap.org/galleries/AboutUs/CodeOfEthics.PDF.
[16] Education AAP-CoP. Media Education. Pediatrics 104; 1999:341–3.
[17] Education AAP-CoP. Media Violence. Pediatrics 2001;108(5):1222–6.

**ELSEVIER
SAUNDERS**

Child Adolesc Psychiatric Clin N Am
17 (2008) 93–111

CHILD AND
ADOLESCENT
PSYCHIATRIC CLINICS
OF NORTH AMERICA

Ethics and the Prescription Pad

Mary Lynn Dell, MD, MTS, ThM[a],*,
Brigette S. Vaughan, APRN[b],
Christopher J. Kratochvil, MD[c]

[a]*Psychiatry and Behavioral Sciences, Emory University School of Medicine, 492 Ponce de
Leon Manor NE, Atlanta, GA 30307, USA*
[b]*Department of Psychiatry, University of Nebraska Medical Center, 985581 Nebraska
Medical Center, Omaha, NE 68198-5581, USA*
[c]*University of Nebraska Medical Center, 985581 Nebraska Medical Center, Omaha,
NE 68198-5581,USA*

The world of bioethics is viewed all too often by practicing clinicians as one or more of the following: an intellectual pursuit of philosophers in the academy, typically sequestered from the realities of clinical medical practice; a relatively new, even annoying, requirement of residency training programs and continuing medical education requirements; or an "add-on" to the list of items to heed related to medical malpractice, though perhaps with less sting than many other issues in the medicolegal category. Although substantial literature exists in the areas of general bioethics, research ethics, ethics concerning the doctor–patient relationship, end-of-life issues, social justice and economic issues in medicine, and pediatric ethics, relatively little has been written about what ethical matters are involved when an individual clinician's pen meets the prescription pad. What are the ethical issues, explicit or subtle, of importance to clinicians, child and adolescent patients, and their families? What ethical considerations influence and inform the recommendations, prescribing practices, and related behaviors of child and adolescent psychiatrists?

Dr. Dell has received funding from the Templeton Foundation and the Louisville Institute.

Dr. Kratochvil is supported by NIMH Grant 5K23MH06612701A1. He also received grant support from Eli Lilly, McNeil, Shire, Abbott and Cephalon, is a consultant for Eli Lilly, Cephalon, AstraZeneca, Abbott and Pfizer, and a member of the Eli Lilly speaker's bureau.

* Corresponding author. 492 Ponce de Leon Manor NE, Atlanta, GA 30307.

E-mail address: dellml@comcast.net (M.L. Dell).

1056-4993/08/$ - see front matter © 2008 Elsevier Inc. All rights reserved.
doi:10.1016/j.chc.2007.08.003

An informed physician: the essential cornerstone for sound prescribing

What qualities, assets, liabilities, and expectations does a child and adolescent psychiatrist bring into the patient contact that influence the act of prescribing psychotropic medication to children? Many would insist that first and foremost is an attitude of beneficence, incorporating a genuine concern for the health, well-being, and happiness of patients they treat. Attitudinally this may be correct, but beneficence and good will alone are insufficient without a sound, sufficiently broad and deep fund of medical knowledge and concerted, intentional efforts to keep current and up-to-date with child and adolescent psychopathology, new medications, emerging indications for those medications, appropriate monitoring of side effects, and multidisciplinary treatments. Intellectual virtues (ie, current scientific knowledge and practical wisdom) must undergird all desirable virtues of character and principled ethical behaviors, lest patients be treated by well-intentioned physicians with outdated, even harmful information and methods [1,2]. After the structured educational environment of residency and formal medical education, clinicians are left largely on their own to determine the content, sources, quality, and methods of delivery—meeting and conference attendance, journal reading, CDs, DVDs, and so forth—of continuing medical education.

The burden of keeping up-to-date for child psychiatrists is arguably greater than for many other disciplines, as information is turning over at an ever-increasing pace, and involves not only the domain of general psychopharmacology, but also overlaps considerably with the multitude of new developments in neuroscience. Currently, with the rare exceptions of buprenorphine and other isolated examples, no specific requirements exist for continuing education in psychopharmacology with particular relevance and application to the type of medical and prescription practices of individual psychiatrists. The American Board of Psychiatry and Neurology recertification process engenders ongoing attention by younger generations of child psychiatrists to newer information and trends in psychiatric prescription practices through the study required for board recertification. American Academy of Child and Adolescent Psychiatry practice parameters provide updated information about developmental, psychodynamic, biologic, family, social, and other important concerns specific to particular disorders that ultimately inform the use of psychotropic medications in actual practice [3]. However, for the foreseeable future, the conscientiousness and attentiveness of the individual clinician regarding factual knowledge and technical fluency with psychotropic medications (eg, the physician's "virtue ethics") remains the primary impetus for the professionalism the psychiatrist brings into each patient encounter.

Psychodynamics and psychopharmacology

Despite perceptions by the general public—and sadly, even many clinicians—to the contrary, the act of prescribing psychotropic medications is one of tremendous psychodynamic significance to children, adolescents, families, and caregivers. Uncovering and appreciating the attributions given to medication can contribute to a better understanding of underlying psychopathology, the real-life contexts that matter to the patient and that affect and are affected by her neuropsychiatric issues, issues that influence adherence to all recommended treatments, and treatment response. Furthermore, even the briefest of encounters with a prescribing physician carries psychotherapeutic weight. Readers are referred to excellent reviews of this topic for more detailed discussions [4,5].

Familiarity with psychodynamic aspects of psychopharmacology is critical to ethical prescribing practices [6,7]. A knowledge of child and adolescent development is also important, medication that is taken from a parent without question by a 6-year-old may become the nidus for a battle of wills if that same child is expected to leave class daily to go to the nurse's office to take that same tablet at 12 years of age, tapping into age-appropriate issues of autonomy, privacy, self-esteem, and acceptance by (and often sameness as) the child's peers. Medication form, substance, size, dosing frequency, and even color and shape may carry attributions and meanings unrelated to the underlying condition itself that nevertheless are important to the child. Depending on the particular disorder and the family and cultural beliefs about psychiatry, taking medication may be a constant reminder to the child that he/she is "bad," "flawed," or "not good enough" in the eyes of others. The psychodynamics of particular families are also important to note. Does the family believe that the child's condition is biologically based, behavioral, deliberately executed by the identified child patient, or a combination? Are there other family members or friends with mental illness who have taken psychotropic medications, and does the child remind them positively or negatively of those individuals? Can the family afford the time and expense of ongoing appointments and pharmacy bills, and will those stresses be reflected in the relationship with the child? Do this child's problems complicate ongoing issues related to divorce, custody, childcare, and finances? Is the child or are other relatives blamed for these additional burdens, either unknowingly or overtly? Does the family feel pressured by the school to have psychotropic medications prescribed for their son or daughter? Is the family influenced by media marketing of psychiatric medications targeted to the general public, and are their opinions formed about medication matters even before they reach the psychiatrist?

The physician brings additional qualities to the prescriber–patient relationship of psychodynamic significance. Is the physician also the psychotherapist or the family therapist? Does the physician prescribe for other members of the family, or perhaps other friends and acquaintances in the same community? Does the physician practice in the same group as the child's psychotherapist, facilitating a longer-term relationship with the child and family, or is the doctor one of several in a larger, perhaps less personal clinic or mental health center? Even if the physician limits his contact with the child to brief medication checks, is he still able to convey a sense of personal interest and investment in the youngster's well-being during those quick, perhaps infrequent encounters? Does the psychiatrist feel pressured by the family, school, institution, or organization that employs him to prescribe medication? Has the psychiatrist been adequately trained in psychodynamics and working as a member of a multidisciplinary team, or does he or she consider medication prescription to be the primary or only role of a child psychiatrist in the mental health care of children and adolescents?

Once a medication is initiated, a clinician's role should extend beyond simple queries into effectiveness, tolerability, and adherence. A savvy prescriber will strive to learn more about the child, the underlying conditions for which medication is being prescribed in the first place, and revisit basic and supplemental elements of the thorough history to see if initial information was inaccurate, incomplete, or if changes have occurred over time. Medication noncompliance should not be seen only as a problem to be fixed, but as a window into the internal life of the child, the psychodynamics of the family, the child's ever-expanding relationships with individuals and groups outside the home, and an opportunity to strengthen the psychotherapeutic alliances of the child with all mental health care providers [8].

In summary, any child and adolescent psychiatrist who writes prescriptions for psychotropic medications for children and adolescents must understand both the obvious and latent meanings of those agents to the identified patient, the family, and relevant school and community organizations whose opinions and voices figure prominently in the child's world. Physicians also must be aware that these meanings can change over time with alterations in family structure, predictable life transitions, moves, unpredictable tragedies, and the trajectory of the child's development over time. In a sense, if a physician serves the child as the medication provider only, his or her fluency in child and family development and psychodynamics must be even more finely honed than nonprescribing clinicians, for there is much less time to elicit and integrate psychodynamic material in service of the child's care than the physician might otherwise enjoy.

General ethical principles applicable to psychotropic medication prescription

Autonomy

Over the past three decades, as the modern discipline of bioethics has developed and gained influence in medical practice and research, the evolution of the concept of *autonomy* has led the field away from the general umbrella of kindly paternalism and "the doctor knows best" philosophy prevalent, if not dominant, until at least the 1960s. Given that patient treatments and interventions in psychiatry historically have included methods that affect patients' bodily freedom, interactions with others, as well as medications and other biologic treatments with serious and potentially long-lasting side effects and sequelae, individual autonomy in the psychiatrist–patient relationship may be even more important—or at least the denial or dismissal of patient autonomy—than in other medical specialties that prescribe medications.

Autonomy refers to an individual's right to have her own opinion, think for herself, behave as she wishes, and make her own health care decisions based on her value system and personal preferences [9]. Most psychiatrists attempt to honor patient preferences and decision-making as much as possible, perhaps trying to influence decisions and behaviors with education about particular treatments and sharing their experiences treating others with similar afflictions if a particular patient at hand is making a decision the clinician does not believe to be in her best interests. In general, especially in countries and cultures that value individualism and independence quite highly, the autonomy of the patient is considered supreme and capable of trumping the wishes health care providers, family, and friends may have for the patient. Psychiatry differs from other medical specialties in that in cases in which psychiatric illness renders one potentially harmful to self or others or so gravely disabled as not to be able to care for one's most basic needs, a patient can be forced to undergo a psychiatric evaluation and/or hospitalization against her wishes. In emergencies, outpatient or inpatient, a patient's autonomy might be limited even further by the administration of psychotropic medications if behavioral and environmental interventions fail to decompress tense situations and the individual is assessed to be imminently harmful to self or others. Physicians should be aware of state, local, and organizational laws and policies applicable to involuntary hospitalization and medication administration in the institutions and states in which they practice.

Assuming that a psychiatrist is prescribing in a nonemergent setting and situation in which the physician determines a particular individual may benefit from psychotropic medication, honoring patient *autonomy* involves having respect for and, at times, enabling the patient to think and act autonomously—even if such autonomy leads to decisions at odds with what the psychiatrist recommends. Respect for autonomy includes a negative obligation not to control or overly influence a patient's choices, as well as a positive obligation to educate and facilitate the patient's ability to make autonomous, and preferably wise and helpful, decisions in the future [10,11].

Children are not considered to be autonomous individuals, at least regarding health care, because from a developmental perspective they cannot understand fully the conditions that are the target of treatment; the potential risks, benefits, and alternatives to a particular treatment; or the longer term consequences of such decisions—in other words, children cannot give informed consent, and even older, more mature adolescents are precluded from doing so in most instances by state statutes. Hence, in most encounters involving the prescription of psychotropic agents to minor children, parents and legal guardians are the agents of autonomy with whom child and adolescent psychiatrists work [12]. However, the clinician's duty to honor and provide a safe setting for the child or adolescent to mature in their own physical, emotional, and moral autonomy places great significance on the youth's assent to medication treatment and the process of informed consent (see later discussion) as both should be tailored to the child's appropriate developmental level, in addition to the cognitive level and sophistication that optimizes the understanding and recognizes the autonomy of the adult decision-maker appropriately.

Beneficence and nonmaleficence

Beneficence and nonmaleficence are intertwined concepts related to a physician's duty to act in the best interests of the patient. *Nonmaleficence*, the duty or obligation not to inflict harm, is the doctor's cardinal rule—*primum non nocere*, or "do no harm." *Beneficence,* the obligation to seek out and do good for patients, is perhaps the greatest positive moral impetus for ethical behavior of health care professionals. Because a few treatments have such minimal risks so as to be considered purely beneficial, and a greater number of interventions carry such high odds of complications or sequelae so as to be deemed dangerous or harmful, the majority of medical decision-making opportunities, and hence ethical dilemmas, involve balancing the potential gains of treatment with risks interventions [12–14].

When prescribing psychotropics for children, the child psychiatrist seeks to do good or benefit those suffering from the neuropsychiatric, emotional, and social distresses inherent to mood, anxiety, attentional, psychotic, and other psychiatric disorders. However, the potential for benefit from these medications must be balanced against the risks of not only physical side effects, but also the social stigma, cost, inconvenience, and even family disapproval that can accompany even the most seemingly clear-cut, evidence-based treatment recommendation. For instance, the potential benefits of a psychostimulant trial for attention deficit hyperactivity disorder, combined type, in a 6-year-old struggling in school must be weighed against potential harm if that child also carries diagnoses of primary pulmonary hypertension with resultant cardiomegaly, cardiac conduction abnormalities, growth retardation, and diminished appetite. When the risks of a particular medication are determined to outweigh possible benefits, physicians and families may find themselves repeating the same process of weighing treatment risks versus benefits, or the principles of nonmaleficence and beneficence, with second and third-line psychopharmacologic agents or non-pharmacologic interventions.

Justice

Philosophers through the years have understood *justice* to mean fairness, or equitable treatment of persons in the same or comparable circumstances.

Often in bioethics, the term justice is more accurately understood as *distributive justice*, or the fair distribution of health care services as guided by norms, policies, or procedures agreed to by society [9,15].

The issue of distributive justice in health care, especially access to quality mental health care for children, the aged, minorities, rural populations—just to mention a few often marginalized groups—is an ever-present concern in the practice of child and adolescent psychiatry. It affects the type of care, the discipline of provider covered, the frequency of follow-up visits, the level and duration of care, and which specific illnesses will be treated or not. Prescription practices are influenced, sometimes even dictated, by which medications in which drug classes, generic versus trade name, are reimbursable or available in hospital and third-party payer formularies. The rate of medication prescription may actually increase when there is limited access to effective non-psychopharmacologic treatment modalities. These complicated webs of relationships are illustrated by recent reports about the rising number of psychotropic prescriptions for preschoolers in general, with Medicaid children overrepresented in the medicated group compared with children insured by HMOs and private insurance through parents' work [16–20].

Many attitudes and proactive behaviors clinicians undertake on behalf of their individual patients for the sake of "justice" are perhaps characterized more accurately under the umbrella of patient advocacy [9]. Although we may know that actual data do not support the advantages of a brand name of a specific medication over its generic form—or a relatively new psychostimulant preparation over an older, less expensive one—as clinicians we sincerely care *about*, not just for, our patients and want each child and family to have the very best of all elements of treatment. When in our offices and clinics prescribing psychotropics to a particular patient, we must not only appreciate where the family sits in relationship to justice politically in health care and third-party payer systems, but also balance these larger-than-life societal debates with what the child's and family's views are of fairness and care that satisfies their collective needs and desires. We must partner with the family to weigh the blessings and burdens of "adequate," "good enough," "acceptable," "highly desirable," and "best" care available, especially regarding the costs of psychotropic medications. Sometimes, less than textbook care is in the best interests of the child, depending on the particular problem and the child's and family's life contexts.

Other concepts relevant to prescribing psychotropic medications to minors

Informed consent, decision-making capacity, and competence

According to a consensus of several disciplines relevant to bioethics, including medicine, psychology, law, and philosophy, *informed consent* is composed of five elements: (1) competence, (2) disclosure, (3) understanding, (4) voluntariness, and (5) consent [10]. The Committee on Bioethics of the American Academy of Pediatrics, building on Appelbaum and colleagues' [21] work on the theory and practice of informed consent, has outlined the components as follows:

1. "Provision of information: patients should have explanations, in understandable language, of the nature of the ailment and condition; the nature of proposed diagnostic steps and/or treatment(s) and the probability of their success; the existence and nature of risks involved; and the existence, potential benefits, and risks of recommended alternative treatments (including the choice of no treatment).
2. Assessment of the patient's understanding of the above information.
3. Assessment, if only tacit, of the capacity of the patient or surrogate to make the necessary decision(s).
4. Assurance, insofar as is possible, that the patient has the freedom to choose among the medical alternatives without coercion or manipulation" [22].

Informed consent is a good example of an ethical concept and duty that has evolved into a legal entity as well. Regulated by the states, informed consent—especially the disclosure of potential risks, benefits, and options of alternative treatments, as well as no treatment—may be judged against what a "reasonable" physician should disclose, what a "reasonable" patient would want to know, or a combination of both [23].

The assessment of a patient's—or, in pediatric prescription-writing, parent's or guardian's—understanding is multifaceted and cannot be separated from the assessment of the capacity of the responsible adult to make necessary decisions. Problems hindering the understanding of factual information offered by the clinician about the medication may be very straightforward and remedied with varying degrees of ease, as with a translator when the parent and physician speak different languages or speaking slowly, in short and simple sentences, avoiding technical jargon when the parent has limited formal education or exposure to medical settings. On the other hand, our training in general psychiatry serves us well in our obligation to assess the decision-making capacity of the parent, especially when the adult's mental status is odd, bizarre, or fluctuating or the adult suffers from inadequately treated psychiatric illness. *Competence* is the legal term describing an adult who has satisfactory decision-making capacity by virtue of their ability to understand basic facts about the medical condition, recommended treatment, alternatives to the recommendations, and possible risks and benefits or recommended and alternative treatments. Competent individuals are also able to reason through their decisions, make choices, and communicate those choices to health care providers [10,24,25]. When a child psychiatrist is not comfortable with the decision-making capabilities of those adults charged with giving informed consent for psychotropic medication treatment of minor patients, he or she should be familiar with the processes in his or her practice location for identifying surrogate decision makers and what is entailed in obtaining legal informed consent for treatment.

Assent

Although parents are presumed to be the most appropriate medical decision-makers for their children, there are several compelling moral and practical arguments for obtaining the *assent*, or agreement, of the child with the recommended treatment plan [12]. First, the very process of assent involves a manner of conversation with the minor that implicitly conveys respect for their developing autonomy and personhood. Assent is an excellent vehicle for educating the child or adolescent about their illness, treatment, and even prognosis on a level commensurate with their cognitive and emotional development. Taking the time to have a two-way conversation about these matters with the patient can increase their comfort level with the care, strengthen the therapeutic alliance, provide opportunities for them to ask questions of importance to them, and give insights into particular family and contextual dynamics relevant to medication and treatment adherence. As with informed consent, the interpersonal, interactive process between child and physician is just as important as the content itself.

The American Academy of Pediatrics has identified four elements of assent that are also applicable to treatment with psychotropic medications:

1. "Helping the patient achieve a developmentally appropriate awareness of the nature of his or her condition.
2. Telling the patient what he or she can expect with tests and treatment(s).
3. Making a clinical assessment of the patient's understanding of the situation and the factors influencing how he or she is responding (including whether there is inappropriate pressure to accept testing or therapy).
4. Soliciting an expression of the patient's willingness to accept the proposed care" [22].

If the child dissents to proposed treatment, the clinician's response should be gauged according to the type and severity of the illness, and the relative risks and benefits of the treatment. One must take the time to understand the specific reasons why the child does not want the treatment, for they may be unrelated to the medication itself and addressed in appropriate other ways. Also, many initial objections can be worked through with additional time and developmentally appropriate education.

An exception to the usual parental informed consent and minor patient assent practice occurs when the identified patient is an *emancipated minor*. This term applies to minors who are married, in the armed forces, are parents themselves, or are living outside their parents' home and are managing their own finances. Emancipated minors are capable of giving their own informed consent. Because exact policies in this area are determined at the state level, physicians should be familiar with the laws applicable in their practice locations [12].

Written information on psychotropic medications for children, adolescents, and parents

Physicians should be familiar with and consider employing written information about child and adolescent psychiatric disorders and psychotropic medications in their informed consent and assent processes. This is helpful when the information is provided at levels appropriate for educational backgrounds of caregivers and the developmental level of the child, in the language best understood by families, and is furnished by reputable professional medical organizations and scholars [26–28].

Cultural and religious issues

The Group for the Advancement of Psychiatry's (GAP) Committee on Cultural Psychiatry defines *culture* as "a set of meanings, behavioral norms, and values used by members of a particular society as they construct their unique view of the world." The GAP expands on this definition, stating that those meanings, norms, and values encompass "social relationships, language, nonverbal expression of thoughts and emotions, religious beliefs, moral thought, technology, and financial philosophy." Additionally, culture is fluid, not fixed, and may bend and change over time from generation to generation [29].

The related concepts of race and ethnicity are also significant for psychopharmacology. *Race* entails the grouping or categorizing of humans based primarily on physical characteristics. Whereas *ethnicity* may include aspects of race, it is the broader view of "belonging to a group of people with a common origin and with shared social and cultural beliefs and practices. It entails the notion of identity and …an individual's self-image and intrapsychic life" [29].

Psychopharmacology is affected by both the biologic features of race and ethnicity and the psychosocial aspects of culture. Cross/ethnic/racial variations occur in the *pharmacokinetics* (absorption, distribution, metabolism, and excretion of drugs) and the *pharmacodynamics* (how medicines act on target organ receptors to produce their effects). Genetics, especially polymorphisms of important enzymes in drug metabolism processes, and nongenetic biologic factors such as diet, smoking, and complementary and alternative medicines, are important factors to consider in clinical work with patients from all ethnic backgrounds. Psychosocial aspects of culture potentially important to the psychotropic prescription process include understandings of disease and mental illness, illness behaviors, attitudes toward physicians, beliefs about traditional healing processes, and meanings attributed to the medication color, form and route of administration [30–36].

Religion and spirituality are important aspects of the worldviews of individual patients, their families, local communities, and broader culture. Whereas religious and spiritual beliefs and practices can be elements of a particular culture (eg, Roman Catholicism as part of the Irish Catholic character of an ethnic neighborhood in an inner city on the east coast of the United States), basic elements of religion and spirituality can also transcend multiple cultures and ethnicities. For instance, those who are from an Irish Catholic background may have religious and spiritual beliefs in common with Catholic Mexican Americans, Puerto Rican immigrants in New York City, and French Canadians who relocate to the upper midwestern United States. In contrast, an American town of 50,000 inhabitants may be culturally homogenous from secular perspectives, including health attitudes and behaviors regarding psychiatric illness and medication management, but be religiously pluralistic and comprised of conservative and mainline Protestant, Catholic, and Jewish residents. Religious beliefs influence understandings of illness in general, and especially mental illness when it includes concerns such as substance abuse and acting out behaviors that overlap with moral and ethical domains also addressed by religions. Spirituality and religion influence family priorities, rituals, how they view care of the body during health and illness, attitudes toward health care providers, medications, authority, discipline—virtually all aspects of child-rearing. Child psychiatrists are well-advised to be aware of how religious, spiritual, and other cultural factors can influence psychopharmacologic treatment of child psychiatric disorders, and delve deeper into these issues whenever the prescriber–patient relationship or treatment adherence need greater reflection [37–40].

Special populations

Children who are in foster care or state wards or who are incarcerated

Prescribing psychotropic medication to any child warrants special care. The clinician must make an assessment based on all available information, working in conjunction with the child and caregivers to make the most appropriate decision regarding the need for medication. In an ideal situation, the child, parent, and clinician will then readily come to consensus with a particular treatment plan; however, in reality, conflicting opinions may present regarding what the optimal plan of care should entail. The process can become even more challenging when the child is placed outside of the home and adults other than parents are given authority for medical decision-making. Decisions to follow a clinician's recommendations to initiate a psychotropic medication can be quite affect-laden in and of itself, but when consent is provided by a case worker or legal guardian other than a parent (and who may have differing views than the parent), the situation can become extremely contentious.

Children who are wards of the state or are in out-of-home placement frequently suffer from significant behavioral and emotional difficulties that lead to consultation with a child psychiatrist. It is not unusual for these children to have mental health problems, which may have contributed to their families' inability to care for them at home, or perhaps as a sequela of the out-of-home placement itself. Additionally, there is a tremendous overlap between youth involved with the legal system and psychiatric disorders, as illustrated by the significant number of incarcerated youth who meet diagnostic criteria for a mental health disorder. For children and adolescents placed outside of the home, a multitude of caregivers may be providing input into psychiatric care, including case workers, group home/residential facility staff, foster parents, attorneys, and parole officers, each with varying degrees of decision-making responsibility. The parents may or may not continue to have parental rights, often lose the ability to consent to treatment for their child, and all too often may not even be consulted regarding treatment decisions. The clinician must then struggle with who to involve in treatment decisions, how to involve them, and how best to reach a consensus knowing that ultimately the parents' wishes may not be honored. This can be a complex, emotional and time-intensive process that is further complicated when all parties are not in agreement. If the clinician uses this time as an opportunity to listen to concerns, answer questions, and hopefully form a therapeutic alliance, there is a greater likelihood of consensus, a treatment plan that serves the best interests of the child, and treatment success. Ultimately, the child's best interest should guide treatment decisions, leaving the clinician to make recommendations as to what is most clinically appropriate, not necessarily what is most "popular."

Unfortunately, in situations where multiple adults are involved in the decision-making process (parents, foster parents, case workers, probation officers, judges, and so forth), all of whom may be asked to provide input and ultimately some of them to consent to a treatment for the child, the child's involvement in the process and assent to treatment can be overlooked. Because he or she may be labeled as a "difficult" or "bad" kid by some, it may be that even less weight is given to his or her opinion. Including the child at a developmentally appropriate level in these discussions is important, although recognition of limitations due to age, immaturity, and potentially limited insight and cognitive ability is warranted.

Children who are developmentally disabled

Children who are developmentally disabled or mentally retarded often have a variety of individuals making decisions on their behalf as well. In some of these cases, the child is able to communicate his or her thoughts about the medication ("It hurts my stomach" or "It makes me feel bad"), but in others the clinician must rely solely on the reports of caregivers. This may be similar to the treatment of a very young child who cannot articulate the positive or negative effects of a medication. The clinician must be watchful for caregivers who may have ulterior motives and want a child medicated for their own convenience, or because pharmacotherapy may simply be "easier" than behavioral therapy, or as is more often the case, caregivers who have unrealistic expectations about what benefits a treatment may potentially hold for their child. As is always the case, the more vulnerable the child, the greater the importance of a careful risk/benefit assessment before making clinical decisions. If the potential benefits to the child do not outweigh the potential risks, then the treatment should be reconsidered.

Off-label prescribing

Pediatric psychopharmacologic research has grown significantly in the last decade; however, clinicians still have a limited database with which to guide evidence-based practice. Even when specific conditions or drugs have been studied, the limited data available can make clear evidence-based recommendations difficult in determining the most appropriate course of treatment. Clinicians, as a result, find themselves sampling from various published guidelines and combing the adult literature for direction in treating children with mental illness. The treating clinician is often left with a question of what to do when they exhaust "agreed upon" recommendations without satisfactory response, particularly in the case of treatment-refractory disorders or comorbidities. This may lead to dosing above approved guidelines, polypharmacy, and frequently, off-label prescribing.

While it would be ideal to adequately study all psychopharmacologic agents before using them in children, research is lacking for many of the medications on the market today. Until such studies are completed, it will sometimes be necessary for practitioners to employ off-label prescribing. Off-label drug use is defined as the use of a drug to treat a condition or a population of patients even though the drug is not specifically approved for an indication by the US Food and Drug Administration (FDA). Although certainly less than ideal, clinicians are frequently forced to simply integrate what limited data are available from controlled pediatric trials, with less rigorous pediatric trials, adult trials, and their own clinical experience in making treatment decisions. The risk/benefit assessment may be particularly complex in these situations, especially for pediatric disorders where even adult data are either not applicable or nonexistent. In complex cases or in the absence of a clear diagnosis, prescribing may become symptom-driven (eg, managing aggression). In these cases, the clinician must take even greater care to ensure that the medication selected is warranted, that other potentially FDA-approved agents or drugs with more available safety and efficacy data have been considered, and that the risk/benefit ratio is favorable. Educating the parents and/or other caregivers about the rationale and potential risks and benefits of the off-label use is the responsibility of the clinician. This information must be delivered in a factual yet understandable manner, with care given to not instill false hope or excessive fear.

Black box warnings

Throughout the past several years, a number of black box warnings have been placed by the FDA on psychotropic medications used in the treatment of children and adolescents. Most pertinent have been the warnings placed on antidepressants, antipsychotics, and medications approved for the treatment of attention deficit hyperactivity disorder. These warnings highlight key safety information and are meant to serve as alerts to clinicians, but as has been recently demonstrated can also have significant unintended consequences. Perhaps the highest profile of the recent black box warnings, and the most controversial, is the warning on antidepressants.

In 2004, the FDA issued its black box warning for suicidality (suicidal thoughts or behaviors) for antidepressant use in the pediatric population [41]. This warning stemmed from meta-analyses of data from 24 pediatric antidepressant trials, which demonstrated a 4% risk of suicidality in patients on active medication compared with 2% in patients on placebo. Despite demonstration of efficacy of antidepressant use in children and adolescents, the FDA determined that the potential increased risk of suicidality was significant enough to warrant the black box warning. The warning extended to all antidepressant medications, and was specific not only to the treatment of depression, but rather anytime the antidepressants were prescribed. The FDA also mandated that a medication guide including information on these risks be provided to parents/guardians with each prescription filled. Guidelines for patient monitoring were established, including face-to-face visits with the clinician weekly for 4 weeks, every other week for 4 weeks, and then monthly.

This highly publicized warning was subsequently correlated with a significant drop in the rate of prescriptions of antidepressants to children and adolescents [42]. Although it may be that in some cases this reflected a more appropriate use of the medication, it also likely reflected greater concern by parents, clinicians, and patients on the use of these medications. Unfortunately, the warnings of potential risks were not necessarily coupled with discussions of potential benefit, which may well have contributed to the subsequent decline in prescriptions. Although one cannot assess causation in this situation, it is important to note that multiple studies have suggested strong correlations with declined rates of completed suicides with increases in antidepressant use in children and adolescents. In fact, the recent decline in antidepressant prescriptions has been demonstrated to be correlated with a recent increase in completed suicides in this same population [43].

These recent issues surrounding the black box warning in antidepressants highlight many of the key ethical issues addressed above:

- Importance of clinician's knowledge of the data. An informed clinician is better able to appropriately weigh the potential risks and benefits of a treatment, particularly when the data are complex and evolving.
- Education of the patient and caregivers. The informed clinician needs to share their knowledge about the treatment to facilitate informed consent and assent, which should address potential risks and benefits, including the potential risks of not treating. Also, as was discussed in the FDA hearings on antidepressants, parents who are not aware of the risks are not aware of the need to monitor, what to monitor for, and the need to communicate concerns with the clinician.
- Flexibility. It is important to meet the family where they are at, providing time to consider the facts, discuss issues with others, and perhaps try appropriate alternatives before proceeding to the clinician's first choice.
- Monitoring. As pointed out in the FDA guidance, appropriate use of antidepressants in children requires close clinician monitoring as well as monitoring by family members.

Closing caveats for ethical prescription of psychotropics for children and adolescents

- Keep up-to-date about developments in neuroscience and psychopharmacology relevant to diagnosis and treatment of children and adolescents.
- Take a detailed medical history of the child, paying close attention to chronic medical conditions and medications prescribed by other physicians. Update this information regularly.
- Document all vitamins, herbs, and over-the-counter medications taken by the child, including frequency and doses. These substances can alter psychotropic drug metabolism and lead to unanticipated drug interactions and toxicities.
- Inquire about other substance use on a regular basis. Don't forget about caffeine, hydrocarbons, and steroids, even in younger children.
- Take thorough family medical and psychiatric histories, with particular attention to past and current psychopharmacologic treatment of close family members.
- Remember the importance of individual psychotherapy, family therapy, behavioral management, group therapy, social skills groups, and other nonpharmacologic treatments.
- Be clear not only about the child's diagnosis, but the specific symptoms the medication is intended to target. This helps in monitoring treatment response.
- Obtain appropriate medical and laboratory testing, with periodic monitoring, as recommended (eg, liver functions, complete blood count with differential, and serum drug levels for valproic acid; electrocardiogram when employing agents with the potential to prolong QTc).

- Monitor and document vital signs, height, and weight on a regular basis.
- Be mindful of variations in pharmacokinetics and pharmacodynamics due to genetics and ethnic diversity.
- As part of the informed consent process, discuss all FDA black box warnings and all other cautions from regulatory agencies, professional medical organizations, and manufacturers with the parents or guardians. Review the need for regular and frequent monitoring and what the child and adult should look for between appointments, then document what teaching has been done and the recommendations given to the family regarding monitoring of these medications.
- Obtain developmentally appropriate assent of the child or adolescent for psychotropic medication. Attention to assent is a great teaching vehicle and strengthens therapeutic alliance. The amount and sophistication of the information provided should be updated as the child matures.
- Document the informed consent/assent process thoroughly in the child's chart, including a notation about the teaching done and any written information provided.
- Whenever possible, obtain permission to share key information about psychotropic medications with significant adults in the child's life, including both parents, step-parents, grandparents, teachers, and child-care providers.
- Obtain permission to communicate information about diagnosis, medications, and possible side effects and drug interactions to the child's primary care physician.
- If prescribing for children seeing other mental health practitioners for nonpharmacologic therapies, obtain permission to implement an effective system of two-way communication of important information.
- Use appropriate instruments for monitoring treatment responses (eg, parent and teacher rating scales for psychostimulant treatment in attention deficit hyperactivity disorder) and medication side effects (eg, abnormal involuntary movement scale for youth-prescribed antipsychotic medications) [44].
- Keep a concise, easily readable medication log sheet in the chart, noting dates of prescription and names, strengths, and forms of medicines prescribed; how often they are to be taken by the patient; and amount to be dispensed by the pharmacy with the number of refills. Include a column for date and reason medication was discontinued.
- Document all telephone calls, e-mail messages, and other communications with parents, guardians, and primary care physicians regarding psychotropic medications, especially the communications between regularly scheduled appointments.
- Document all details of prescriptions and refills given over the telephone or faxed to pharmacies, including names of individuals handling the prescriptions and contact information for those pharmacies.

- Know the price ranges of psychotropics you commonly prescribe, including generic preparations and how those generics compare in efficacy and effectiveness to brand-name preparations. This is helpful when weighing the cost/benefit ratio for prescribing generics for a particular child.
- Become familiar with the medications carried on the formularies of local hospitals and insurance carriers, including generics, as well as appeal processes if payment is denied for a medication you believe to be necessary for your patient.
- Stay up-to-date with all federal, state, local, and institutional regulations and policies regarding the prescription of psychotropic medications to children and adolescents.
- Give parents and children, especially adolescents, your office number, preferred procedures for communicating about prescriptions, and telephone numbers for emergency coverage outside of regular office hours. Document that this information has been given.

By working together as a team, the patient, family, clinician, and other concerned individuals can better serve the child and hopefully lead to better outcomes in the long run.

References

[1] Pellegrino ED, Thomasma DC. Phronesis: medicine's indispensable virtue. In: Pellegrina ED, Thomasma DC, editors. The virtues in medical practice. New York: Oxford University Press; 1993. p. 84–91.
[2] Peteet JR. Introduction. In: Peteet JR, editor. Doing the right thing: an approach to moral issues in mental health treatment. Washington, DC: American Psychiatric Publishing, Inc.; 2004. p. vii–xiv.
[3] American Academy of Child and Adolescent Psychiatry. Available at: http://www.aacap. org/cs/root/member_information/practice_information/practice_parameters/practice_ parameters. Accessed July 25, 2007.
[4] O'Brien JD, Perlmutter I. The effect of medication on the process of psychotherapy. Child Adolesc Psychiatr Clin N Am 1997;6(1):185–96.
[5] Pruett KD, Martin A. Thinking about prescribing: the psychology of psychopharmacology in pediatric psychopharmacology: principles and practice. In: Martin A, Scahill L, Charney D, et al, editors. Pediatric psychopharmacology principles and practice. Oxford (England): Oxford University Press; 2002. p. 417–25.
[6] Coffey BJ. Ethical issues in child and adolescent psychopharmacology. Child Adolesc Psychiatr Clin N Am 1995;4(4):793–807.
[7] Koocher GP. Ethics in child psychotherapy. Child Adolesc Psychiatr Clin N Am 1995;4(4): 779–91.
[8] Lewis O. Psychological factors affecting pharmacologic compliance. Child Adolesc Psychiatr Clin N Am 1995;4(1):15–22.
[9] Lo B. Overview of ethical guidelines. In: Lo B, editor. Resolving ethical dilemmas: a guide for clinicians. 3rd edition. Philadelphia: Lippincott, Williams, and Wilkins; 2005. p. 10–6.
[10] Beauchamp TL, Childress JF. Respect for autonomy. In: Beauchamp TL, Childres JF, editors. Principles of biomedical ethics. 5th edition. New York: Oxford University Press; 2001. p. 57–112.

[11] Miller BL. Autonomy. In: Post SL, editor. Encyclopedia of bioethics, vol. 1. 3rd edition. New York: Macmillan Reference USA; 2004. p. 246–51.

[12] Beauchamp TL, Childress JF. Beneficence. In: Beauchamp TL, Childres JF, editors. Principles of biomedical ethics. 5th edition. New York: Oxford University Press; 2001. p. 165–224.

[13] Churchill LR. Beneficence. In: Post SL, editor. Encyclopedia of bioethics, vol. 1. 3rd edition. New York: Macmillan Reference USA; 2004. p. 269–73.

[14] Lo B. Promoting the patient's best interests. In: Lo B, editor. Resolving ethical dilemmas: a guide for clinicians. 3rd edition. Philadelphia: Lippincott, Williams, and Wilkins; 2005. p. 28–35.

[15] Beauchamp TL, Childress JF. Justice. In: Beauchamp TL, Childres JF, editors. Principles of biomedical ethics. 5th edition. New York: Oxford University Press; 2001. p. 225–82.

[16] Burke MG. Commentary by a child psychiatrist practicing in a community setting. J Child Adolesc Psychopharmacol 2007;17(3):295–9.

[17] DeBar LL, Lynch F, Powell J, et al. Use of psychotropic agents in preschool children: associated symptoms, diagnoses, and health care services in a health maintenance organization. Arch Pediatr Adolesc Med 2003;157:121–3.

[18] Zito JM, Safer DJ, dosReis S, et al. Trends in the prescribing of psychotropic medications to preschoolers. J Am Med Assoc 2000;283:1025–30.

[19] Zito JM, Safer DJ, dosReis S, et al. Psychotropic practice patterns for youth: a 10-year perspective. Arch Pediatr Adolesc Med 2003;157:17–25.

[20] Zito JM, Safer DJ, Valluri S, et al. Psychotherapeutic medication prevalence in Medicaid-insured preschoolers. J Child Adolesc Psychopharmacol 2007;17(2):195–203.

[21] Appelbaum PS, Lidz CW, Meisel A. Informed consent: legal theory and clinical practice. New York: Oxford University Press; 1987.

[22] Committee on Bioethics of the American Academy of Pediatrics. Informed consent, parental permission, and assent in pediatric practice. Pediatrics 1995;95(2):314–7.

[23] Berger JE. Committee on Medical Liability of the American Academy of Pediatrics. Consent by proxy for nonurgent pediatric care. Pediatrics 2003;112(5):1186–95.

[24] Grisso T, Appelbaum PS. Assessing competence to consent to treatment: a guide for physicians and other health professionals. New York: Oxford University Press; 1998. p. 1–30.

[25] Lo B. Informed consent. In: Lo B, editor. Resolving ethical dilemmas: a guide for clinicians. 3rd edition. Philadelphia: Lippincott, Williams, and Wilkins; 2005. p. 17–27.

[26] American Academy of Child and Adolescent Psychiatry. Facts for families. Available at: http://www.aacap.org/cs/root/facts_for_families/facts_for_families. Accessed July 1, 2007.

[27] Dulcan MK, editor. Helping parents, youth, and teachers understand medications for behavioral and emotional problems: a resource book of medication information handouts. 3rd edition. Washington, DC: American Psychiatric Press, Inc.; 2007.

[28] National Institute of Mental Health. Available at: http://www.nih.nimh.gov/public/medicate.cfm. Accessed July 25, 2007

[29] Committee on Cultural Psychiatry of the Group for the Advancement of Psychiatry. Cultural assessment in clinical psychiatry. Washington, DC: American Psychiatric Press, Inc.; 2002. p. 6–7.

[30] Gaw AC. Cross-cultural psychopharmacology. In: Cross-cultural psychiatry. Washington, DC: American Psychiatric Press, Inc.; 2001. p. 117–40.

[31] Gaw AC. Cultural context of nonadherence to psychotropic medications in psychiatry patients. In: Cross-cultural psychiatry. Washington, DC: American Psychiatric Press, Inc.; 2001. p. 141–64.

[32] Munoz R, Primm A, Ananth J, et al. Disparities. In: Life in color: culture in American psychiatry. Chicago: Hilton Publishing Company; 2007. p. 165–81.

[33] Munoz R, Primm A, Ananth J, et al. Remedies in color. In: Life in color: culture in American psychiatry. Chicago: Hilton Publishing Company; 2007. p. 105–25.

[34] Smith MW. Ethnopsychopharmacology. In: Lim RF, editor. Clinical manual of cultural psychiatry. Washington, DC: American Psychiatric Publishing, Inc.; 2006. p. 207–35.
[35] Tseng W-S. Culture, ethnicity, and drug therapy. In: Handbook of cultural psychiatry. San Diego (CA): Academic Press; 2001. p. 505–11.
[36] Tseng W-S. Ethnicity, culture, and drug therapy. In: Clinician's guide to cultural psychiatry. Boston: Academic Press; 2003. p. 343–52.
[37] Josephson AM. Formulation and treatment: integrating religion and spirituality in clinical practice. Child Adolesc Psychiatr Clin N Am 2004;13(1):71–84.
[38] Josephson AM, Dell ML. Religion and spirituality in child and adolescent psychiatry: a new frontier. Child Adolesc Psychiatr Clin North Am 2004;13(1):1–15.
[39] Mabe PA, Josephson AM. Child and adolescent psychopathology: spiritual and religious perspectives. Child Adolesc Psychiatr Clin N Am 2004;13(1):111–25.
[40] Sexson SB. Religious and spiritual assessment of the child and adolescent. Child Adolesc Psychiatr Clin N Am 2004;13(1):35–47.
[41] Food and Drug Administration. Avaialble at: http://www.fda.gov/cder/drug/antidepressants/SSRIlabelchange.htm. Accessed July 25, 2007.
[42] Nemeroff CB, Kalali A, Keller MB, et al. Impact of publicity concerning pediatric suicidality data on physician practice patterns in the United States. Arch Gen Psychiatry 2007;64: 466–72.
[43] Hamilton BE, Minino AM, Martin JA, et al. Annual summary of vital statistics: 2005. Pediatrics 2007;119:345–60.
[44] Rapoport J, Connors C, Reatig N. Rating scales and assessment instruments for use in pediatric psychopharmacology research. Psychopharmacol Bull 1985;21:713–1111.

**ELSEVIER
SAUNDERS**

Child Adolesc Psychiatric Clin N Am
17 (2008) 113–125

CHILD AND
ADOLESCENT
PSYCHIATRIC CLINICS
OF NORTH AMERICA

Conflicts of Interest Between Physicians and the Pharmaceutical Industry and Special Interest Groups

Diane H. Schetky, MD

*University of Vermont College of Medicine at Maine Medical Center,
Portland, Rockport, ME 04856, USA*

Ethical foundations

The physician–patient relationship is a fiduciary one, in which the patient's interests are kept foremost and should never be exploited for self-gain on the part of the physician. Fiduciary relationships instill trust and are the hallmark of professional organizations. They serve to protect the professional relationship and the image of the profession. Conflicts of interest arise when "judgment concerning a primary interest tends to be unduly influenced by a secondary interest" [1].

The pharmaceutical industry (PI), like many for profit businesses, is beholden to stock holders, and its primary interest is making money. In contrast to the practice of medicine, there is no fiduciary duty to the patients that it serves. At the interface between these two different worlds is the physician, who determines what medications to prescribe to which patients and in what dosage. For years, the intermediary was the "detailman," also known as the "drug rep" or, more recently, as a pharmaceutical representative (PR). The PI's sphere of influence has expanded beyond one-on-one contact with physicians to direct advertising to patients, underwriting continuing medical education (CME) programs, sponsoring educational speakers, lavish drug displays at conventions, free gifts, and research and consulting relationships. Until recently, there was little concern about these interactions and few ethical guidelines to govern them.

Dr. Schetky has not had any ties to the pharmaceutical industry other than small investments, which she does not control or monitor. She is retired from clinical practice and most recently from the Maine State Forensic Service.

E-mail address: arcticpoppy@verizon.net

Drug company dependencies

I recall my excitement, as a medical student in the 1960s, upon receiving a black bag with my name inscribed upon it from a pharmaceutical company. It was complete with my very own stethoscope, otoscope, tuning fork, and a percussion hammer; the black bag remained at my side throughout my clinical rotations. I do not recall the name of the pharmaceutical company donor, and this undoubtedly was my first attempt at dissociating pharmaceutical company gifts from companies and their products. I naively believed that this might somehow confer immunity from undue influence should I choose to accept their gifts. In private practice, like many of my colleagues, I met with PRs and gladly accepted their free samples for my indigent patients, along with coffee mugs and pens. I also accepted, and sometimes relied upon, their biased handouts regarding the latest research studies involving their drugs. I recall how a charming, East Indian PR, aware of my fondness for Indian food, would ply me with Indian goodies made by his mother.

Only gradually did I begin to realize that many patients could not afford these new drugs, once their free samples ran out, and that Medicaid would not approve them. Despite their touted improvements over the old standby drugs, the superior efficacy of these new products would become questionable. I attended a few local drug-sponsored dinners at some of our nicer restaurants and hospital talks with speakers sponsored by drug companies. I noted that the product of the company sponsoring the speaker always fared better than the competition. I noted lavish drug company displays at professional meetings and attendees leaving with free gifts in bags adorned with the logo of a pharmaceutical company. Logos also decorated the free canvas bags given out at registration, and, unwittingly, 15,000 psychiatrists at American Psychiatric Association (APA) meetings would be transformed into walking billboards for the PI. Some bold patients began to wonder about all of the pharmaceutical company logos decorating waiting rooms and their physicians' office and notepaper and began to question whether their physician was working for them or for the pharmaceutical companies.

I began to purge myself of drug company goodies, distance myself from their advertising, and try to get more facts about pharmaceutical companies. It soon became apparent that the problem lies not just with seduction by pharmaceutical representatives, but with the growing dependency of physicians, medical organizations, and academic medical centers (AMCs) upon these companies for the funding of educational materials, programs, CME activities, research, and conferences.

Pharmaceutical company revenues and expenditures

Pharmaceutical companies continue to be the most profitable stocks. In 2006, the pharmaceutical market grew 8.3% (an increase from 5.4% the previous year due to Medicare prescription benefits), for sales totaling $275 billion [2]. In 2001, the profit margin of the top nine United States drug companies was 16% of their revenues or about three times that of other Fortune 500 industries [3]. These profits stem from new products and extended patents as well as from increasing the number of prescriptions written and the cost of prescriptions and by getting physicians to shift to using newer, more expensive drugs. The PI is the largest lobby in Washington, DC, and it contributes heavily to congressional campaigns. It has effectively used its influence to extend drug patents, create enormous tax breaks for the PI, and influence legislation to benefit the PI. Examples of this abound, including getting Congress to authorize Medicaid to pay for off-label medication use, Medicare drug benefits, and eliminating the ability of Medicare to bargain for lower-priced drugs. The PI spends $12 billion per year on marketing to physicians, or about $11,000 to $13,000 per physician on promotions each year [4]. This includes $3.5 million of free lunches each year [5]. The average return on each dollar spent on detailing physicians is $10.29 [6].

Despite the claims of the PI about the high cost of developing new drugs, it spends twice as much on marketing [3,6]. The PI began to rely on publicly funded research in 1980 with the passage of the Bayh-Dole Act, which paved the way for the patenting of National Institute of Mental Health–funded research and exclusive licensing to pharmaceutical companies in exchange for royalties. At least one third of licensed drugs are now acquired from sources outside of the PI. In 1984, Congress passed the Hatch-Waxman Act, which extended monopoly rights for brand name drugs, and in the 1990s, it passed laws that extended the patent life of brand-named medications. In 1992, Congress passed the 1992 Drug User Fee Act, which, in return for a substantial fee, hastened the process of drug approval. In 1997, the Food and Drug Administration (FDA) dropped most restrictions on direct-to-consumer advertising of prescription drugs [3].

Between 1996 and 2001, the pharmaceutical sales force in the United States doubled to 90,000 [3]. Marketing research firms began purchasing prescription data from pharmacies and selling them to the PI, thereby enabling PRs to track the prescribing practices of physicians. This invasion of patient and physician privacy seemed to slip by under the radar screen. Access to prescription records enabled PRs to get feedback on their marketing techniques and focus on high prescribers. Not surprisingly, studies found that visits to physicians by PRs netted more prescribing of their products. As competition between companies increased, so did incentive pay to PRs, such as bonuses of $30,000 to $50,000. As noted by Elliot [6], detailmen became replaced by Pharma Barbies and Pharma Kens, whose good looks and culinary skills often exceeded their medical knowledge. PRs began pursuing physicians more aggressively by wooing them and their office staffs with gifts and free meals and parties to gain access and influence. PRs soon learned that, "Bribes that aren't considered bribes "..." are the essence of pharmaceutical gifting" and that the more gifts a doctor takes the more likely the doctor is to believe that they have no effect on him" [6].

PRs know that developing a relationship with a doctor is key to effective selling. Some may push the limits of ethically acceptable behavior to promote their product aggressively [6]. This may include distorting research data, minimizing side effects, or promoting questionable drugs or the off-label use of products, in addition to offering lavish gifts, trips, or expensive tickets to sporting events. Warner-Lambert (now Pfizer) aggressively marketed Neurontin for bipolar disorder and migraine, neither of which was an approved use of the drug, at recommended dosages higher than those that had been studied. It also initiated a shadowing program in which physicians were paid $350 per day for allowing PRs to sit in as they examined patients [8]. In another case involving the promotion of off-label use, Lilly, in its "Viva Zyprexa" campaign, was marketing the drug to primary care physicians for use in dementia, despite a lack of evidence for any efficacy for this condition. Within 3 months of initiating this campaign in 2001, PRs had motivated physicians to write 49,000 new prescriptions for Zyprexa, and total sales doubled [9,10]. PRs who meet their quotas are rewarded handsomely, with salaries up to $90,000 per year plus bonuses [8]. These incentives may contribute to biased presentations; however, one PR lamented that they often are the last to be informed about potential problems of the medications that they are promoting [6].

Clinicians

Many physicians continue to view small gifts from pharmaceutical companies as innocuous. They see themselves as being more impervious to their influence than are their colleagues. Numerous studies have countered the assumption that small gifts do not influence physician behavior [9]. PRs use gifts to exploit the finding that even the smallest gift leads to the impulse to reciprocate. Gifts to physicians typically result in physicians writing more prescriptions and even a sense of entitlement. Elliott [6] described "the delicate balance of pretense and self deception," in which the PRs try to influence physicians and pretend that they are giving impartial information while the physicians pretend that they are not being influenced and that they are not customers.

PRs are particularly likely to target psychiatrists because psychotropic drug accounts are among their most profitable ones and constitute a significant percentage of their sales. Studies have shown that industry promotions have more influence on physicians than do collegial consultations or the scientific literature [4,11]. Information presented by PRs may be inaccurate, yet most physicians fail to recognize this [12].

Direct advertising indirectly affects physicians because it leads to demands by patients for the drugs they see advertised on television that promise to improve their lives. These ads are fraught with messages that appeal to popularity, authority, emotion, and celebrity influence [12]. Many consumers fail to appreciate that the newest purple pill being touted for acid reflux is essentially the same as the one whose patent just expired and went generic, except for a few tweaked molecules and a name change. The phenomenon of "me too drugs" (ie, variations on the old ones) has become common as pharmaceutical companies try to hold onto their share of the market [7]. Of concern, many physicians, afraid to say no for fear of alienating their patients, concede to their patients' requests for specific medications. The United States and New Zealand are the only countries that permit direct-to-customer advertising [7]. Of interest, medical group practices that limit physician interactions with drug reps have lower prescription costs for their patients [13].

Academic medical centers

The PI has become a powerful presence in medical education, ranging from drug lunches, CME events, and social events to financial support for residents attending meetings and research. PRs are all too eager to shape the habits and minds of trainees and know that free pizza assures good attendance at presentations. Trainees may underestimate their influence and lack the skills necessary to critique the data provided. The Web site Nofreelunch.org has taken an active role in trying to raise residents' awareness of pharmaceutical company influence.

Increasingly, faculty members have become dependent upon money from pharmaceutical companies to augment their salaries or underwrite their research. A disturbing trend is the prevalence of AMCs—reported as two thirds in one study—that have equity interests in companies that underwrite their research [14]. Such dual agency can easily lead to conflicts of interests or bias among faculty in considering therapeutic options, such as favoring psychopharmacology over other interventions and choice of drugs. Bias may be a problem if faculty members with financial ties to industry serve on hospital formulary committees. Stanford University Medical School released figures for 2005 showing that of the more than 700 faculty members, 299 had potential conflicts of interest related to their research. Among the 10 members of the school's Conflicts of Interest Committee, 7 revealed financial relationships with medical companies. The author notes that this situation is not unique and that Stanford's rules regarding conflicts of interest are more stringent than are those of other medical schools [15]. Additional sources of conflict may include equity or stock in pharmaceutical companies.

Bias related to conflicts of interest can affect research designs and results and lead to the decision not to publish unfavorable results. Researchers with ties to industry are more likely to publish results favorable to the products of companies with whom they have ties than are researchers with no such ties [16]. Numerous scandals in recent years have heightened unethical

practices by pharmaceutical company researchers, and some have impli-
cated academic psychiatrists, as well. Typically, these cases have involved
suppressing unfavorable results, such as weight gain from atypical antipy-
schotics or the suicide risk associated with giving selective serotonin
reuptake inhibitors to young patients. Outrage over the withheld antidepressant data has led to call for change and more transparency of drug research
data in order to work toward protecting the integrity of clinical research
[17]. Pharmaceutical companies also may refuse to turn over data to the researchers who participated in the research [18]. Yet another problem is the
increasing number of ghostwritten papers being published that have been
authored by PI personnel, rather than the respected academicians whose
names appear on them.

The *New England Journal of Medicine*, in 1984, became the first major
medical journal to require authors to disclose any significant financial ties
that they might have to companies whose products were discussed in their
submissions. An even stricter policy was initiated in 1990 for editorial
writers, which required that they have no ties to companies whose products
they discussed. Angell [19] noted that disclosure alone does not absolve one
of bias and that it has become difficult to find editorialists without financial
ties to the PI. She goes on to note that AMCs are "growing increasingly
beholden to industry" and depend on drug companies for making up budget
shortfalls.

Continuing medical education and annual meetings

Medical specialty organizations have become heavily dependent upon
pharmaceutical companies financing their annual meetings, and they seem
to have no exit strategies. For instance, exhibits, most of which were by
pharmaceutical companies, accounted for 45% of revenues at a recent
meeting of the American Academy of Family Physicians Annual Scientific
Society [20]. At the 2002 annual meeting of the APA, there were 23 pharmaceutical companies occupying only 12% of assigned booths but using 79%
of the booth area. There were 46 industry-supported symposia for which the
APA received about $50,000 each, for a total of $3.15 million [21]. Without
such support, registration fees would be prohibitively expensive, leading to
low attendance. The APA notes that although approximately half of its
convention revenue comes from the PI, 80% of it goes toward covering
the cost of the meetings, thus APA keeps only 20 cents of every dollar
that it gets from the PI. Drug company revenues constitute 29% of APA
income. About half comes from advertisements and the other half comes
from symposia, grants, fellowships, and awards.

Pharmaceutical displays take up proportionately more space (often the
size of a football field) in exhibit halls than do book vendors and tend to
be more elaborate and eye catching. Lurie and colleagues [22,23] conducted
a study of 24 drug exhibit booths at the 2002 APA convention in an attempt

to determine whether they had followed Pharmacy Research and Manufacturers of America (PhRMA) guidelines and APA exhibit rules. PhRMA states that interactions between pharmaceutical companies and health care providers inform healthcare professionals about products, their risks and benefits, provide scientific and educational information and support medical research and education. This voluntary marketing code, which went into effect in April 2002 before the APA convention, states that gifts intended for the personal benefit of physicians should not be offered. Nonetheless, 27% of exhibitors gave out gifts, including invitations to meals and entertainment, without an educational component. More than half of the exhibitors violated the APA or FDA rules regarding permissible displays. Four companies were promoting the off-label use of drugs counter to FDA regulations [21].

Drug advertisements adorn shuttle buses, public spaces, and local maps at annual meetings, causing the public and patients to raise eyebrows and wonder if the medical profession has sold out to the PI. Picketers, many of them disenchanted patients, get into the fray and denounce psychiatrists as drug killers. Industry-sponsored CME activities draw many attendees with the added incentive of fulsome free breakfasts and receptions that accompany these symposiums. Presently, the pharmaceutical industry pays more than half of the cost of CME for physicians [23]. Pharmaceutical companies sponsor attendees from foreign countries and pay for their travel, rooms, meals, and registration at conventions. At the 2006 APA annual meeting in Toronto, international registrants—only a fifth of whom were members—outnumbered members of the APA from the United States [24]. Those registrants who accept financial help from pharmaceutical companies state that they would not be able to attend these meetings without it. They also believe that this funding does not affect their prescribing habits, a view that is not shared by other attendees. Of interest, many of these sponsored registrants come from countries in which new drugs are initially introduced.

A related problem at professional meetings is the matter of physicians on pharmaceutical speakers' bureaus. Typically, they are well-known academic researchers who are perceived as influential. Their fees may be in the range of several thousand dollars per talk, and it is not unusual for physicians to be on the speaker rosters of multiple pharmaceutical companies. In 2004, there were nearly 240,000 talks sponsored by pharmaceutical companies, which represented a fourfold increase over the previous 6 years [25]. Ethical integrity is compromised when speakers read Power Point Presentations prepared by pharmaceutical companies with data about which they have no first-hand knowledge or when they vary the content of their presentations to be favorable to the company sponsoring that particular talk. Although speakers are not obligated to mention the sponsor's product, they are paid handsome sums and may feel a sense of obligation to the sponsor and a need to be accountable to the company's PR who is sitting in on the talk. They also may wish to remain on the company's speakers' roster to be able to pay for their children's college tuition. Incidents have been cited of physicians on Merck's speakers' bureau being threatened by a senior vice president to stop discussing the risks of Vioxx [26,27].

Physicians consulting with industry

The number of physicians consulting with the investment industry has increased by 75% in the last 8 years. Almost 1 in every 10 physicians is now engaged with the investment industry in some capacity, such as serving on advisory boards, as consultants, and educators or even being engaged to make presentations to potential investors [28]. Unlike collaborations between industry and academia that are intended to benefit patient care, these newer collaborations are intended to increase profits and benefit investors. The physician is reimbursed generously and may even receive stock options. Ethical problems may arise if physicians who are engaged in research leak confidential information to investment firms, thereby violating insider-trading laws. Conflicts of interest arise if a physician invests in funds for which he advises or receives compensation related to the profitability of a fund. Rarely are these relationships disclosed in medical publications or to the press, yet they should be made public [29]. In Minnesota, one of the few states to have laws requiring pharmaceutical firms to disclose payments made to physicians, more than 20% of the state's licensed physicians received money from pharmaceutical companies [29].

There has been growing concern that many advisors to the FDA are on the payroll of pharmaceutical companies. In 2005, the FDA voted to allow Vioxx back on the market, despite concerns about cardiovascular toxicity. Of 10 members of the panel with financial ties to the industry, 9 voted to bring the drug back. In contrast, panel members without industry ties voted 12 to 8 against its return [30]. The FDA recently announced that expert advisors to the government who consult for pharmaceutical companies or makers of medical devices would be barred from voting on whether to approve that company's product if they receive more than $50,000 per year from the company [31].

Guidelines

In 1998, the American Academy of Child and Adolescent Psychiatry (AACAP) approved Guidelines for Commercial Contributions to the AACAP [31]. This document deals with commercial support of Academy-related activities, name lending for profit, use of advertising in AACAP publications, use of corporate and nonprofit logos, and exhibits at AACAP activities. The policy gives the Academy considerable control over content, format, and selection of speakers in commercially supported educational activities; demands that programs be for scientific and educational purposes only; and bans the promotion of products. It prohibits the serving of any food or beverages at commercially supported activities that are not also served at regular Academy Programs. It places restrictions on promotional and novelty giveaways at exhibitor booths and stresses that they must be related to professional activities. The Guidelines note the risk for developing dependence on corporate funds and insist that AACAP maintain sufficient financial independence to enable the Academy to decline commercial funding. This forward-looking document has resulted in AACAP showing considerably more restraint in its dealings with the PI than has occurred in other professional organizations [31].

As noted by Anders [17], there is need for more transparency in pharmaceutical research so that data are accessible to all. Trainees should learn how to critique research studies, and all physicians should be encouraged to find objective sources for obtaining drug information. A few good sources are The Medical Letter (www.medicalletter.com), Prescriber Letter (www.prescriberletter.com), and Therapeutics Initiative (www.ti.ubc.ca).

The American Medical Association put forth guidelines concerning Gifts to Physicians from Industry, which was updated in 2005 [32]. The guidelines stress that gifts primarily should benefit the patient and not be of substantial value. Gifts of minimal value are considered permissible if related to the physicians' work (eg, pens and note pads). Gifts with strings attached should not be accepted. Regarding CME, appropriate disclosure of financial support and any financial conflicts of interest should be made. Subsidies that are intended to underwrite costs of CME are permissible in as much as these meetings can contribute to patient care; however, the subsidy should go to the conference sponsor. Subsidies should not be accepted directly or indirectly to pay for the costs of travel, lodging, and personal expenses of those attending meetings. These guidelines note that honoraria and reimbursements of expenses of faculty are acceptable. Support to enable medical students and residents to attend meetings is permissible if funds are made to the academic institution to be dispersed to the trainees.

The Prescription Project was started recently by Community Catalyst, a health care consumer advocacy group in Boston, and the Institute of Medicine as a Profession, a research group at Columbia University. The Project, funded with a $6 million grant from the Pew Charitable Trust, seeks to end conflicts of interests that may arise from the marketing of products to physicians by pharmaceutical companies. The project promotes evidenced-based medicine and tries to counter the bias of drug marketing. It calls for AMCs to tighten their policies governing ties with industry and to restrict gifts from PRs and their contact with trainees. Thus far, several major AMCs, such as Yale, University of Pennsylvania, Stanford, and Tufts New England Medical Center, have initiated restrictions [33].

Brennan and colleagues [34] called for more stringent regulations in AMCs, in addition to bans on gift giving and the acceptance of free samples of the newest drugs from PRs. They suggested that a system of vouchers could be implemented for low-income patients. Physicians with ties to the PI should be excluded from hospital formulary committees. Manufacturers should not be permitted to support CME activities directly or indirectly; however, if they wish to support these programs they should do so through a central repository, which would disperse funds to Accreditation Council for Graduate Medical Education (ACCME)-approved programs. They noted that this was likely to result in a dramatic decrease in contributions to CME programs. They recommend that faculty at AMCs not serve on speakers' bureaus for the PI, because in doing so they become "an extension of manufacturers' marketing apparatus" [35]. Faculty also should be prohibited from publishing any articles or editorials that have been ghostwritten by PI employees. The investigators recognized the need for consulting and research contracts with industry, but like others, they stressed the need for more open communication and transparency.

In 2002, the ACGME mandated the development of curricula and policies to address these issues. In a separate document by the Task Force on Financial Conflicts in Research, it addresses issues regarding conflicts of interest in research [36]. Regarding relationships with industry, the ACGME Principles to Guide the Relationships between Graduate Medical Education and Industry recommends (1) an ethics curricula dealing with the issues of gift-giving to physicians; (2) full and appropriate disclosure of sponsorship and financial interests in all program- and institution-sponsored events and full disclosure of research interests; and (3) that programs and sponsoring institutions determine what contact, if any, is suitable between residents and industry. They stress the need for an objective, evidenced-based learning environment in which to promote clinical skills and judgment. Further, residents need to be aware of how promotional activities affect judgment in prescribing decisions and research activities. They demand that residents consider the cost-benefit analysis as a component of prescribing and that attention to costs be part of advocacy for patient rights within the health care system. The Principles stress that teaching institutions need to find appropriate funding sources to sustain their programs.

The American Student Medical Association recommends abolishing industry gifts, meals, lectures, and industry-sponsored CME. Students are urged to sign a Pharmfree pledge [37].

The PhRMA Code on Interactions with Health Care Physicians, although well intended, is voluntary, and studies suggest that it is violated often. As long as detailing physicians is profitable there will be incentives to disregard the code. Dresser [38] recommends the push for academic detailing, also known as "counterdetailing." These programs supply independent, evidence-based information to physicians. Geppert calls for all professional organizations to provide ethics instruction to members regarding relationships with pharmaceutical companies [39].

Some of the above guidelines have not had a great deal of impact, whereas others have made significant inroads. The American Medical Association guidelines on gifting have come under attack because they were supported by money from the PI. As noted by Geppert [39], much of the focus in the past was on gift giving, but there is now increasing emphasis on identifying and rectifying other problematic relationships between professional organizations and the PI.

Government regulations

Lobbyists for the PI hold enormous sway over government and were responsible for passage of the Medicare prescription benefits, which was a windfall for the PI. As noted by Angell [3], the FDA, which approves new drugs, receives half of its support from drug companies in return for quick reviews. We need a better system of checks and balances and a system that does not condone dual agency. Recent legislation is beginning to address conflicts of interest at this level.

Summary

Given the fact that the PI is now paying for 60% of the cost of CME [23], many critics note an association between CME sponsorship and spiraling prescription prices. They assert that it is not fair for consumers to be paying indirectly for much of the cost of medical education and research in this country and that the PI profits in the process. Marketing to physicians is a major factor in increasing medication costs. A free pizza is not free, and more individuals are concerned that increasing numbers of patients are unable to afford medications even as more is spent on physician marketing. Some marketing practices are viewed as encroaching on boundaries and violating ethical standards.

Medical trainees, physicians, and the public need to be alerted to the pervasive conflicts of interest that exist in the relationships between physicians and the PI. Physicians need to be more reflective about their interactions with the PI and see the bigger picture beyond the point of their free drug company pens. The medical profession must become more self-regulating and clear about the codes of ethical behavior relative to the PI and PRs and how they impact on patient care. Professors and researchers need to become role models for trainees and be more vigilant about conflicts of interest. Unless medicine's drug company dependency is curtailed, there is the risk that physicians will rely on less than objective information about medications, and patient care will suffer.

Angell [3] recommends numerous reforms in the PI, including having it focus on innovative drugs rather than on "me too" drugs, and she urges that they "open their books." She adds that legislators are "so beholden to the pharmaceutical industry that it will be exceedingly difficult to break its lock on them." She admonishes academia to take back full responsibility for medical education and urges professional societies to be self-supporting.

AMCs and the medical profession must end their drug company dependencies and find less tainted sources of funding. This, of course, is easier said than done. Greater attention must be given to ethics in medical education, and physicians need to come to terms with their sense of entitlement and adjust to leaner professional meetings. Practitioners need to turn to more objective sources of information about the medications that they prescribe. When in doubt about what constitutes appropriate conduct with the PI, physicians should confer with the Ethics Committees of their professional organizations.

Acknowledgment

Thanks to Patty Kahn, medical librarian at Penobscot Bay Medical Center, for assistance with the references.

References

[1] Thompson DF. Understanding financial conflicts of interest. N Engl J Med 1993;329(8): 573–6.
[2] IMS Health Financial, business and trade releases. Available at: http://www.IMS_Japan. cojp/industry_trends_press_releases_2007. Accessed September 4, 2007.
[3] Angell M. The truth about drug companies. New York: Random House; 2005.
[4] Wazana A. Physicians and the pharmaceutical industry. Is a gift ever just a gift? JAMA 2000; 283:373–80.
[5] Saul S. Doctors and drug makers: a move to end cozy ties. New York: New York Times 2007. p. C1.
[6] Elliott C. The drug pushers. The Atlantic Monthly. April 2006; 82–93.
[7] Public Citizen Congress Watch. 2002 Drug industry profits: hefty pharmaceutical company margins dwarf other industries. Available at: http://www.citizen.org/congress/reform/drug_ industry/coproratearticles.cfm?ID=9923.
[8] Peterson M. Suit says company promoted drug in exam rooms. New York Times. May 15, 2001;1.
[9] Orlowski JP, Wateska L. The effects of pharmaceutical firm enticements on physician prescribing patterns. There's no such thing as a free lunch. Chest 1992;02(1):270–3.
[10] Berenson A. Drug files show maker promoted unapproved use. New York Times. December 18, 2006; A1.
[11] Brodkey A. The role of the pharmaceutical industry in teaching psychopharmacology: a growing problem. Acad Psychiatry 2005;29:222–9.
[12] Wilkes MS, Doblin BH, Shapiro MF. Pharmaceutical advertisements in leading medical journals: experts' assessments. Ann Intern Med 1992;116(11):912–9.
[13] Galt K, Rich E, Kralewski J. Group practice strategies to manage pharmaceutical cost in an HMO network. Am J Manag Care 2001;7:1081–90.
[14] Bekelman E, Yan L, Gross P. Scope and impact of financial conflicts of interest in biomedical research. JAMA 2003;289:454–65.

[15] Jacobs P. How profits, research mix at Stanford. Available at: http://www.matr.net/article_19768html1-18k.

[16] Bodenheimer T. Uneasy alliance: clinical investigators and the pharmaceutical industry. N Engl J Med 2000;342:1539–44.

[17] Anders T. Enhancing transparency of research: antidepressant medications for children and adolescents. Statement from Thomas Anders, M.D. President of the American Academy of Child and Adolescent Psychiatry. Washington, DC, February 6, 2007. Available at: http://www.aacap.org, media, press releases. Accessed September 5, 2007.

[18] Meier B. Contracts keep drug research out of reach. New York Times. November 29, 2004. 2004; 29

[19] Angell M. Is academic medicine for sale? N Engl J Med 2000;342:1516–8.

[20] Standbridge JB. Of doctor conventions and drug companies. Fam Med 2006;38:518–21.

[21] Lurie P, Tran T, Manuel S, et al. Violations of exhibiting and FDA rules at an American Psychiatric Association Annual Meeting. J Public Health Policy 2005;26:389–99.

[22] Kassirer JP. Doctors and drug companies. Boston Globe. July 6, 2005; 15.

[23] Relman A. Defending professional independence. ACGME's proposed new guidelines for support of CME. JAMA 2003;14:03.

[24] APA Annual Report 2006 Arlington, VA: American Pspychiatric Association.

[25] Hensley D, Martinez B. Speaker programs come under the microscope again. To sell their drugs, companies increasingly rely on doctors. Wall Street Journal 2005; section A: 1.

[26] Kassirer JP. When physician-industry interactions go awry. J Pediatr 2006;149:S43–6.

[27] Topol E, Blumenthal D. Physicians and the investment industry. JAMA 2005;293:2654–7.

[28] Harris G, Robert J. Doctor's ties to drug makers are put on close view. New York Times. March 21, 2007; A1.

[29] Harris G. Ten voters on panel backing pain pills had industry ties. New York Times 2005; 24:A1.

[30] Harris G. FDA rule limits role of advisers tied to industry. New York Times. March 22, 2007; A1.

[31] American Academy of Child and Adolescent Psychiatry. Guidelines for commercial contributions to the AACAP. Available at: http://www.aacap.org.

[32] American Medical Association. Ethical opinions and guidelines. 2005. Updated clarification on Opinion E-8.061: Gifts to physicians from industry.

[33] Cooney E. Project seeks to limit ties between doctors, drug companies. White Coat Notes: news from the Boston medical community [Boston Globe]. Available at: http://boston.com/yourlife/health/blog/2007/02/prescription-pr.html. Accessed September 5, 2007.

[34] Brennan TA, Rothman DJ, Blank L, et al. Health industry practices that create conflicts of interest: a proposal for academic medical centers. JAMA 2006;295(4):429–30.

[35] Accreditation Council for Continuing Medical Education. Standards for commercial support: standards to ensure independence of CME activities. Available at: http://www.accme.org/index.cfm. Accesssed September 5, 2007.

[36] American Student Medical Association. Principles regarding pharmaceuticals and medical devices 2005. Available at: http://www.amsa.org/ppp/pharm.cfm. Accessed September 4, 2007.

[37] Pharmaceutical Research and Manufacturers of America, "Code on Interactions with Health Professionals." Available at: http://www.phrma.org/code-on=-interractions-withhealthcare-professionals/. Accessed September 4, 2007.

[38] Dresser R. Pharmaceutical company gifts: from voluntary standards to legal demands. Hastings Cent Rep 2006;8–9.

[39] Geppert C. Medical education and the pharmaceutical industry: a review of ethical guidelines and their implications for psychiatric training. Acad Psychiatry 2007;31:32–9.

ELSEVIER
SAUNDERS

Child Adolesc Psychiatric Clin N Am
17 (2008) 127–148

CHILD AND
ADOLESCENT
PSYCHIATRIC CLINICS
OF NORTH AMERICA

Ethical Issues in Psychiatric Research on Children and Adolescents

Jinger G. Hoop, MD, MFA[a],*, Angela C. Smyth, MD[b],
Laura Weiss Roberts, MD, MA[a,c]

[a]*Department of Psychiatry and Behavioral Medicine, Medical College of Wisconsin,
8701 Watertown Plank Road, Milwaukee, WI 53226, USA*
[b]*Department of Child and Adolescent Psychiatry, University of Chicago,
5841 S. Maryland Avenue, MC2077, Chicago, IL 60637, USA*
[c]*Health Policy Institute, Medical College of Wisconsin, 8701 Watertown Plank Road,
Milwaukee, WI 53226, USA*

Psychiatric illness in children and adolescents places an enormous burden on individuals, families, and society [1,2]. The lack of scientific data regarding the treatment of child psychiatric illnesses is a significant barrier to adequate care for young people who have mental disorders [3–5]. In the absence of scientific evidence, clinicians must deprive children of treatment or subject them to the risks of untested therapies, often by extrapolating from what is known to be effective in adults. Indeed, a significant proportion of medications used in child psychiatry are prescribed "off-label" [6].

Childhood and adolescence involve major changes in growth and development of the structure and functioning of the brain, and our knowledge about how this developmental process affects clinical signs and symptoms of psychopathology, drug metabolism, and treatment efficacy is still limited [5,7]. Treatments that are considered safe and effective in adults may be neither in children. The incidence of lamotrigine-induced Stevens-Johnson syndrome [8] and suicidality associated with antidepressants [9,10] are examples of differential risk profiles in the two populations. Furthermore, drugs with efficacy in adults do not necessarily benefit children. Controlled studies of tricyclic antidepressants in depressed children, for example, have not shown efficacy over placebo [7,11].

Dr. Hoop gratefully acknowledges support from NARSAD: The Mental Health Research Association, and Dr. Roberts gratefully acknowledges support from the National Institutes of Health.

* Corresponding author.
E-mail address: jhoop@mcw.edu (J.G. Hoop).

Recognition of these issues has led to an increased emphasis on the inclusion of children and adolescents in clinical treatment trials [3,5]. Simultaneously, studies to investigate the biology of psychiatric illnesses are using increasingly complex methodologies, such as genome scans [12] and functional neuroimaging [13]. During this time of growing interest in psychiatric research involving children, and in new theoretic and methodological paradigms, it will not be unusual for clinical child and adolescent psychiatrists to have some involvement in research, be it as principal investigators, collaborators, or referring clinicians. In these roles, psychiatrists have a professional obligation to develop an awareness of the ethical issues that are involved in research on children.

The aim of this article is to provide child and adolescent psychiatrists with practical information about ethically relevant aspects of research trials. We describe the regulations and safeguards that have been developed to protect research participants. We explain how clinicians can critically evaluate experimental protocols so that they can advise families about research participation in a manner that is attuned to the family's needs. Throughout, we are mindful of the psychiatrist's role in advocating for a better evidence base for practice and in working with researchers to design and implement ethical protocols that benefit patients and society while respecting the rights of patient participants.

Background: research ethics and regulation

The ethics of medical research has been formulated over the past half century, in a series of documents that were prompted by research-related scandals and that each address ethical issues in human subjects research in a slightly different fashion. The infamous Nazi experiments on concentration camp inmates led to the creation of the Nuremberg Code, a 10-point document that calls for the voluntary consent of research participants and the need to balance the risks of research with the potential benefits to the subjects [14,15]. The World Medical Association's Declaration of Helsinki [16], first issued in 1964, elaborated and expanded upon the concepts in the Nuremberg Code and described the potential vulnerability of certain research subjects to coercion.

Historically, the enrollment of children in research has raised serious ethical concerns. In the 1950s and 1960s, for example, investigators deliberately infected a group of mentally retarded children with hepatitis at the Willowbrook State Hospital in Staten Island, New York [17]. The children's parents provided consent; however, the voluntarism of their consent has been questioned because admission to the overcrowded hospital depended on agreement to participate in the study. Other examples of ethically problematic research involving children include the US government–sponsored radiation experiments of 1944 to 1974, in which children and adults were intentionally exposed to ionizing radiation through a variety of means. After the experiments came to public attention in the early 1990s, an Advisory Committee appointed by President Bill Clinton recommended greater safeguards for human research participants and called for clarification of the acceptable parameters of research involving children [18].

Perhaps the single most important guideline for the ethical conduct of research is *The Belmont Report*, published by the US National Commission for the Protection of Human Subjects of Biomedical and Behavioral Research in 1979 [19]. *The Belmont Report* identified three principles as the moral and philosophical foundation for ethically sound medical research: respect for persons, beneficence, and justice. These ethical principles will be touchstones throughout this article. Respect for persons encompasses a deep regard for the worth and dignity of all human beings and a particular emphasis on respect for human autonomy (ie, the right to personal self-governance). To be autonomous, an individual must be able to make independent decisions voluntarily, free from the coercion of others [20]. Respect for persons is demonstrated most clearly in the research setting in the process of informed consent for research participation. The second concept, beneficence, is the ethical ideal of doing good. In research, this translates to the obligation to maximize benefits and minimize potential harms to individual research participants and to society. The third principle, justice, refers to the notion that equals generally should be treated equally and that the benefits and burdens of social activities should be distributed fairly across members of society. Justice is demonstrated in the design of research protocols, especially in the selection of research subjects [19].

To understand what makes medical research ethical, it is necessary to define how clinical research differs from clinical care. From an ethical perspective, clinical care is devoted exclusively to enhancing the well-being of individuals, whereas clinical research focuses more broadly on improving the human condition. This distinction is articulated in the US Department of Health and Human Services and the US Food and Drug Administration regulations regarding human subjects' protection [21,22]. Although laws and regulations are not necessarily created to uphold ethical principles, these federal regulations can be considered to represent a community standard with broad-based support [23]. The guidelines define "human subjects research" as a "systematic investigation ... designed to develop or contribute to generalizable knowledge" that pertains to living individuals "about whom an investigator ... obtains (1) data through intervention or interaction ... or (2) identifiable private information" [21]. This definition determines whether an activity is governed by federal protections for research participants and whether it requires approval by an appropriate institutional review board (IRB) [21].

In the United States, IRBs exist in any facility or system in which research using government funds is conducted and in many private sector organizations. Each IRB consists of a group of individuals, including scientists, physicians, community members, and clergy, who represent a variety of perspectives, both scientific and lay. Such boards meet regularly to review the scientific, legal, and ethical merits of clinical research protocols. National Institutes of Health guidelines call for an IRB to review and approve protocols before any human participants are enrolled. IRBs also are charged with periodically reviewing ongoing studies, and they have the power to suspend or halt protocols if concerns arise [21].

Two key elements of the legal definition of human subjects research are embodied by the phrases "systematic investigation" and "generalizable knowledge." Ordinary psychiatric clinical practice, even though it may involve the off-label use of medications, is not necessarily an intentional, systematic investigation designed to contribute to generalizable knowledge and, therefore, is not necessarily considered a form of medical research. Systematic investigations that are designed to gather data for purposes other than yielding generalizable knowledge also are not necessarily research. An example of such an activity is conducting a survey of patient satisfaction with the services at a particular mental health clinic when the intention is not to contribute to generalizable knowledge but to gather data to be used internally for quality assurance purposes [24].

The boundary between research and clinical innovation often is less than sharp, however, particularly in medical specialties with a limited scientific evidence base for treatments. A psychiatrist who publishes a case report about the unusual clinical presentation and treatment of a single patient may not be engaging in medical research; however, if the psychiatrist plans to offer patients an innovative treatment and subsequently to publish a case series, the activity seems to meet the "systematic investigation" and the "intent to contribute to generalizable knowledge" criteria for research. Clinicians, in such circumstances, have an ethical duty to consult with the appropriate IRB for peer review and oversight [21]. Consultation with an IRB also is appropriate in cases in which it is not clear whether an activity should be considered clinical innovation or research.

In addition to defining human subjects research, federal regulations mandate certain protections for vulnerable research participants, including children [25]. The concept of vulnerability in the research setting traditionally was associated with reduced capacity to consent to medical research participation freely and knowingly [14,19], although the definition has expanded to include many other factors that increase the possibility of exploitation [20,26]. The federal regulations provide special protections for children that control the allowable levels of risk that participants may experience and the process of informed consent [21,25]. These topics are discussed in detail below.

Finally, "children" is defined by the federal guidelines for research protections as persons who are younger than the local jurisdiction's legal age to consent to the treatments and procedures involved in research. The legal age of majority varies across jurisdictions, and it is reduced in some localities for treatment associated with reproductive health, substance abuse, and mental health [25].

Ethically important aspects of research

All ethical studies have certain characteristics that demonstrate their investigators' commitment to the principles of respect for persons, beneficence, and justice [19,27–29]. According to Emanuel and colleagues [27], to be ethical, a clinical research study must have seven characteristics: social and scientific value, scientific validity, fair subject selection, a favorable risk/benefit ratio, independent review, informed consent, and respect for potential and enrolled participants. Roberts' [28] conceptual analysis of the ethical acceptability of psychiatric research protocols focuses specifically on a slightly different set of dimensions, including scientific merit and design; expertise, commitment, and integrity; risks and benefits; confidentiality; participant selection and recruitment; informed consent and decisional capacity; incentives; institution and peer/professional review; and data presentation (Box 1). Because of its special applicability to mental health research, the Roberts format is used in this article to highlight the ethical issues pertinent to child psychiatry research studies.

Scientific merit and general design

To be ethical, a study must yield valuable knowledge, and to do so, it must be scientifically sound [19,27,28,30]. Even a minimal risk study involving adults should have scientific merit to justify the time and effort expended by the participants—an expression of the ethical ideals of respect for persons as well as justice in the use of scarce resources. The scientific value of a study is related to the importance of the research question that is posed and the methodology used to answer it. The design should use accepted scientific methods and test hypotheses adequately to yield meaningful data [28].

In research involving children, the scientific value of the study must be especially great for studies that involve more than minimal risk and for studies that offer no possibility of direct benefit for the participant. Protocols in which both of those pertain must, according to the federal guidelines, be "likely to yield generalizable knowledge about the subjects' disorder or condition which is of *vital importance* for the understanding or amelioration of the subject's disorder or condition (emphasis added)" [25]. The scientific evidence base in child psychiatry is still so modest that an enormous number of vitally important research questions are as yet unanswered, and a multitude of protocols on these topics could meet the ethical standard of high scientific value [7]. For example, studies involving molecular and epidemiological genetic techniques have the potential to yield vital information about the genetic and environmental causes of child psychiatric illnesses, such as autism, attention deficit disorder, and learning disabilities [12]. Functional and structural neuroimaging studies may help to reveal the biologic basis of neuropsychiatric diseases as well as inform

Box 1. Evaluating the ethical acceptability of child and adolescent psychiatric research protocols

Scientific issues
Is the study scientifically valuable?
Will the hypotheses be tested adequately?
Can the design yield meaningful data?
Does the protocol use accepted scientific methods?

Research team and institutional issues
Does the investigative team have enough expertise and
    institutional and other support to complete the experiment
    successfully?
Are the researchers aware of research ethics issues and potential
    problems related to the protocol?
Are they in good standing within the scientific and professional
    communities?
What conflicting roles and conflicts of interest exist in relation to
    this protocol? How will they be dealt with?
Are the documentation features of the protocol adequate to
    monitor procedures and the professional accountability of the
    research team?

Design issues related to risk and benefit
Does the design minimize experimental risks to participants? Do
    alternative designs pose less risk?
Does the protocol pose excessive risk to individual participants,
    the community, or larger society?
If participants are likely to have emerging symptoms as a result
    of protocol involvement, have appropriate mechanisms for
    following symptom progression been developed? Are there
    clear criteria for disenrollment, and have alternative
    mechanisms for treatment been provided?
What benefits exist for participants? Is the likelihood of benefit
    described accurately?
Is it expected that any benefits derived from the protocol will be
    applicable to the specific population being studied?

Confidentiality
Is participant information safeguarded carefully during the
    collection, storage, and analysis stages of the study?
Are the participant and his or her guardians aware of potential
    disclosure obligations of the researchers?
Are research records kept separate from clinical records? If not, is
    there a sound justification for this practice?

Are there important "overlapping relationships" between investigative staff and participants? How will these be dealt with in terms of confidentiality protections?

Participant selection and recruitment issues

Does the process of selection, exclusion, and recruitment ensure that children and adolescents are included in a manner consistent with federal guidelines and only if essential to the study's scientific hypotheses?

Are understudied populations inappropriately excluded from participation (ie, are selection and recruitment practices potentially biased)?

Is the recruitment process itself noncoercive?

Informed consent, assent, and permission

Is the consent form concise, readable, accurate, and understandable?

Does the informed consent disclosure process include all relevant information, such as:

the study's purpose and the nature of the illness or the phenomenon being studied

who is responsible for the scientific and ethical conduct of the study

why the individual may be eligible for participation

the proposed intervention and its associated risks and benefits and their relative likelihood

alternatives to participation

key study design features (eg, placebo use, randomization, medication-free intervals, frequency of visits, confidentiality, plans for use of data)

What procedures are in place to ensure that participants provide assent or consent to participation, if capable of doing so?

Is there reasonable assurance that children and parents will not experience coercive pressure to participate in the project or continue in the project?

Incentive issues

Are incentives for participation sufficient and timed so that they compensate research participants without being coercive?

If health care is an incentive, how will the patient's health care needs be met if disenrollment becomes necessary?

Institutional and peer/professional review issues

Is the institutional context sufficient to allow the research to be conducted successfully?

Has the protocol undergone appropriate scientific and ethical
review?
Should the protocol undergo any additional review steps (eg, by
community leaders)?
Does the protocol have features (eg, high risk) that merit ongoing
external monitoring?

Data presentation issues
Will the presentation of the data describe the ethical safeguards
used in the protocol?
Will the presentation of the data meet current ethical standards
(eg, authorship, accurate disclosure of conflicting roles and
conflicts of interest)?
Will participants' identities be protected adequately in data
presentation?

Adapted from Roberts L. Ethical dimensions of psychiatric research: a constructive, criterion-based approach to protocol preparation. The research protocol
ethics assessment tool (RePEAT). Biol Psychiatry 1999;46:1117–19; with
permission.

our understanding of normal development [13]. Well-designed treatment trials and services research are urgently needed to inform evidence-based clinical practice.

Over time, as information gaps begin to close, standards for scientific
merit will naturally shift and evolve. For this reason, the scientific value
of longitudinal protocols should be reevaluated periodically. Studies that
are designed to seek to answer the vital scientific questions of today may
be wholly irrelevant (and therefore, unethical) tomorrow [7].

Expertise, commitment, and integrity

Related to the issue of the scientific value of a protocol is the ability of the
research team to carry out the protocol in a scientifically competent manner,
with appropriate attention to ethical matters [18,19,28,30]. The team of investigators must have sufficient expertise and support for the study and
should be members in good standing of the scientific and professional community [28]. For protocols that use new scientific methodologies, it may not
be possible for any investigator to claim deep expertise in the methodology,
but all should demonstrate a commitment to pursing excellence in the execution of their work. A well-designed and important study will produce un-
usable data if it is implemented in a sloppy fashion. So too will a poorly
designed study, even if well executed. Both instances are counter to the ethical ideals of justice and respect for persons, because they waste resources
and negate the contribution of human participants.

The investigative team should be knowledgeable about the ethical conduct of research [18,31,32], and any overlapping roles or obligations that might pose conflicts of interest should be acknowledged (eg, academic researchers with financial ties to industry or researchers who provide clinical services to their research subjects). In some cases, conflicts of interest may be avoided or minimized by the creation of specific safeguards, such as separating the roles of clinician and researcher. If conflicts cannot be avoided, they should be disclosed to potential participants and their guardians [32,33].

Risks and benefits

The relationship of research risks and benefits is a crucial ethical issue for all medical research protocols [18,19,21,27,28,31,34]. Every study involving human volunteers should be designed in a way that minimizes the experimental risks to each individual participant and maximizes benefits [18,27,28,31,34]. Doing so upholds the ethical principles of nonmaleficence (do no harm) and beneficence. Distributive justice also should be taken into account when considering design issues that are related to risks and benefits, and investigators should attempt to minimize risks and maximize benefits that may accrue to specific communities and populations as a result of the research [19].

The issue of risks and benefits is key to the ethical conduct of research involving children. Federal guidelines on medical research involving children are based on the level of risk and whether there is the possibility of a direct benefit to participants (Table 1) [25]. The federal regulations state that medical research protocols whose procedures carry no more than minimal risk are acceptable in children so long as appropriate consent procedures are followed. Minimal risk is defined as "the probability and magnitude of harm or discomfort anticipated in the research are not greater in and of themselves than those ordinarily encountered in daily life or during the performance of routine physical or psychologic examinations or tests" [25].

The interpretation of this definition varies among researchers and among IRBs. Procedures such as interviews regarding noncontroversial topics and venipuncture are widely considered minimal risk, although the latter might be extremely distressing to some children [29]. Some, but not all, IRBs also would define studies involving low-level radiation exposure through positron emission tomography scanning, the use of anxiolytic medication during imaging procedures (eg, MRI), and lumbar puncture without sedation as having "minimal risk" [35].

Under two circumstances, protocols that involve procedures with more than minimal risk may be acceptable in children. The first pertains to studies that have the potential to benefit participants directly. Such studies include those involving treatment, intervention, or monitoring procedures that are likely to contribute to participants' well-being [25]. These studies may be

Table 1
United States federal guidelines for allowable risks in research on children

Amount of risk in protocol	Research with potential benefit for participants	Research without potential benefit for participants
Minimal risk	Acceptable if adequate provisions are made for soliciting the assent of the children and the permission of parents/guardians	Acceptable if adequate provisions are made for soliciting the assent of the children and the permission of parents/guardians
Minor increase over minimal risk	Acceptable if • The risk is justified by the anticipated benefit to the participants • The relation of the anticipated benefit to the risk is at least as favorable to the participants as that presented by available alternative approaches • Adequate provisions are made for soliciting the assent of the children and the permission of parents/guardians	Acceptable if • The intervention or procedure presents experiences to subjects that are reasonably commensurate with those inherent in their actual or expected medical, dental, psychologic, social, or educational situations • The intervention or procedure is likely to yield generalizable knowledge about the subject's disorder or condition which is of vital importance for the understanding or amelioration of the subjects' disorder or condition • Adequate provisions are made for soliciting the assent of the children and the permission of parents/guardians
More than minor increase over minimal risk	Acceptable if • The risk is justified by the anticipated benefit to the participants • The relation of the anticipated benefit to the risk is at least as favorable to the participants as that presented by available alternative approaches • Adequate provisions are made for soliciting the assent of the children and the permission of parents/guardians	Requires review and approval by the Secretary of the US Department of Health and Human Services

From U.S. Department of Health and Human Services: Code of Federal Regulations: title 45 public welfare, Department of Health and Human Services, part 46 protection of human subjects, Subpart D, additional protections for children involved as subjects in research, 2005. Available at: http://www.hhs.gov/ohrp/humansubjects/guidance/45cfr46.htm#subpartd. Accessed April 27, 2007.

acceptable if there is a favorable risk/benefit ratio for the participants and if that ratio is at least as favorable as available alternatives [25].

The second circumstance pertains to studies of more than minimal risk that do not have the possibility of direct benefit to the children who participate. Only studies that involve a "minor increase over minimal risk" are possible (without express authorization of the Secretary of the Department of Health and Human Services), and the protocols must meet the following criteria: the level of risk and the experiences of children enrolled in the study must be comparable to those of children who have the same disorder or condition who are not enrolled in the study, and study participation must be likely to create generalizable knowledge about the child's disorder or condition that is vital to understanding or treating the disorder or condition [25].

These guidelines have been interpreted to mean that healthy children may participate only in minimal-risk research, because research involving a greater level of risk must offer some potential benefit or must be aligned with the experiences of other children with the same "disorder or condition" as those enrolled in a trial; however, some experts have defined "condition" loosely, to include having a family history of a disorder. This definition allows, for example, presently healthy children to participate in certain family-based genetic studies with more than minimal risk [35].

Confidentiality

The protection of personal information about patients and research participants is an expression of the ethical ideal of respect for persons [27]. Confidentially is a privilege in our society, linked with the right to privacy. Confidentiality differs from anonymity, with the latter being more absolute (ie, no one anywhere is able to link the personal information with the appropriate individuals).

Confidentiality is vital to mental health research on children because study procedures and resulting data could lead to stigma and discrimination. Therefore, information about participants should be safeguarded carefully throughout study protocols (eg, by storing data without personal identifiers, such as name or date of birth, and by keeping data in password-protected computer files and locked filing cabinets). Participants and parents should be informed about whether any information gathered in the study will be disclosed and under what circumstances [28]. If study procedures may uncover evidence of child abuse or neglect, investigators should inform parents about the reporting procedures that study personnel will follow.

In the United States, the "Privacy Rule," a federal regulation under the Health Insurance Portability and Accountability Act of 1996, provides specific legal guidelines for the use of health-related data in the research setting [36]. Health-related data concerning deceased individuals as well as living persons are covered by the Privacy Rule.

Protocols that gather highly stigmatizing or discriminatory information may require additional safeguards for the confidentiality of data. One such protection is a Certificate of Confidentiality issued by the National Institutes of Health [37]. These certificates allow study personnel to refuse to disclose identifying information on research participants if it should be requested in the course of civil or criminal proceedings at the federal, state, or local level.

Participant selection and recruitment

To be ethical, research studies should demonstrate fairness in their selection of subjects [19,27,28]. Fairness in subject selection is an expression of the ethical principle of justice, which holds that equals generally should be treated equally and that the benefits and burdens of social activities should be distributed fairly across members of society [19]. In the past, some medical research was conducted among institutionalized groups, such as prisoners or mental hospital patients, not because those populations were uniquely relevant to the scientific aims of the study, but because they were convenient to study because of their diminished ability to refuse participation [27,38]. This is not acceptable. Inclusion criteria for a research study should be appropriate to meeting the aims of the study while protecting groups that are vulnerable to exploitation [18,19].

Fairness also should characterize the exclusion criteria for studies. Populations that could stand to benefit from study findings should be included if appropriate to the study aims and not particularly vulnerable to exploitation. Persons should not be excluded solely because of age, gender, or ethnic/cultural background, for example, unless there is a sound scientific reason for doing so. In the past, many treatments were studied systematically primarily in white men, and the ability to generalize the findings of those studies to children, women, and members of other ethnic groups may be limited [39]. A major emphasis in United State's funding of medical research is to reduce disparities in health care by including more groups in medical research when scientifically appropriate and when doing so does not create undue burdens for those populations [40,41]. In the case of child psychiatry research, protocols that involve children must do so only because the inclusion of children is essential to the study's scientific aims, not simply because the study would be more expedient or efficient to conduct in this population. Consideration also must be given to the need for favorable risk/benefit profile in research in children [35].

Informed consent, assent, and permission

Since the formulation of the Nuremburg Code, informed consent has been seen as a cornerstone of the ethical conduct of medical research [18,19,28,31]. By obtaining participants' informed consent, researchers demonstrate their respect for the autonomy of potential subjects, encouraging them to freely and knowingly make an important choice about their bodies and their lives. Rather than the mere signing of a document, informed consent ideally is a dynamic process of information sharing between participant or guardian and researcher. Children (defined as those under the legal age of majority) are not recognized as being capable of giving legally binding consent to research participation. As a consequence, the Department of Health and Human Services guidelines stipulate that a parent or guardian may provide permission through a process that is equivalent in its scope and thoroughness to the informed consent process [23]. In this context, the children may provide assent to the choice made by the guardian. Assent is defined as providing affirmative agreement to participate and not merely failing to object [25]. The federal regulations allow IRBs to determine which children are capable of assenting to research participation, "taking into account the ages, maturity, and psychological state of the child" [25]. Although there is a lack of consensus regarding the "assent process" [42], expectations related to assent typically relate to the age of the child (eg, the "rule of 7s" suggests that cognitively normal children are capable of simple assent or refusal of research participation at about age 7 years, and at age 14, they become capable of a more sophisticated level of cognition required for participation in the informed consent process).

Informed consent in adults has been conceptualized as having three elements: information sharing, decision-making capacity, and voluntariness [43]. Information sharing occurs when researchers provide potential participants with all relevant information about the research protocol. Such information must include the purpose, the procedures involved, any foreseeable risks, and potential benefits. Participants or guardians must be educated about the usual standard of care and which study procedures are experimental. Alternatives to research participation also must be described [18,28,44].

The second component of the informed consent process is the decision-making capacity of the person facing the choice. The phrase "decision-making capacity" differs from the legal term "competency," which is a formal determination made through a legal process. Decisional capacity—as it is generally defined—consists of four abilities: to communicate a preference, to comprehend the information necessary for the decision, to appreciate the significance of the choice being made in the context of one's life, and to reason (ie, to weigh information, compare options, and consider consequences) [45,46].

The third component of informed consent is voluntarism, the ability to make a free, uncoerced decision. Four domains of influence affect an individual's ability to make a voluntary decision, including developmental factors; illness-related factors; psychologic, cultural, and religious factors; and external features and pressures [20].

For children who have mental illness, there are many threats to independent, authentic, and free decision making. This is particularly true for young children, who are not able to form decisions based on experiences and mature cognitive capacities, which older adolescents and adults have. The process of gaining assent for pediatric research should take into account the complexities introduced by the dynamics of the guardian–child relationship and the developmental stage of the child [25,47,48]. Investigators should look for opportunities to enhance the voluntariness of a young person's decision by taking care not to rush the decision or use coercive incentives and by presenting information about the study in a manner congruent to the child's cognitive development [25,49,50]. Similarly, offering opportunities for open and informative discussions without guardians present may be essential for the process of obtaining uncoerced assent for a teenager [20].

Incentives for participation

Ideally, offering compensation for research participation is an expression of respect for persons that is given in a fair and equitable manner, thereby fulfilling the ethical ideal of justice. Financial incentives for research participation should compensate the study volunteers but should not be so large as to be coercive (ie, the potential research subject should not feel that the money is "an offer I cannot refuse," even though the study or its procedures may be personally objectionable) [28,51,52]. The potential for coercion makes the use of any financial incentive for research on children and adolescents controversial, however, so much so that it has been banned in the European Union [53].

Many child psychiatry research protocols offer health care or clinical monitoring to participants, and this may be a strong incentive to participation, especially in communities in which there is limited access to child psychiatry treatment providers and for diseases for which there are no standard treatments. This is not to say that such protocols are unethical, but careful attention should be paid to minimizing the risks and maximizing the benefits of the study and to making plans for the care of participants who must be disenrolled during the study [28].

Institutional and peer/professional review

Trials involving human participants should be reviewed by independent experts who are empowered to approve, reject, or revise the protocols [21]. The approval of an IRB that is not subject to the conflicts and pressures that may influence any given investigator provides an extra layer of protection for human study volunteers and is an act of social accountability [27]. Protocols involving highly vulnerable or stigmatized populations may benefit from additional review by community members [28]. Federal regulations require certain protocols, typically multisite intervention trials, to have on-going oversight by specially constructed committees called data safety and monitoring boards (DSMB) in addition to IRB review [4,28,54]. Typically, a DSMB is a group of experts without ties to the research team that is charged with ongoing monitoring of the integrity of study data and the safety of participants.

Data presentation

A final ethical component of research involves the publication of the data gathered in the course of the work. For society to gain knowledge from a study, its findings must be made known [27,28]. All study data should be made public in some fashion, even so-called "negative findings" that do not support the investigators' hypotheses or demonstrate an investiga-tional drug's efficacy and safety. Clinical trial registries have been estab-lished to ensure that data are presented or published and that negative results are not "buried" [55]. When data are presented, the ethical safe-guards used in the study should be described so that they are subject to peer review and public scrutiny [28]. Presentation should include an accurate disclosure of any significant overlapping roles and conflicts of interest among the participants [56]. If conflicts of interest have been managed in a manner beyond mere disclosure, this should be acknowledged. Finally, data should be publicized in such a way that individual confidentiality is protected appropriately.

Special ethical issues in child and adolescent psychiatry research

Randomized, controlled treatment trials

The risks and benefits that pertain to specific design features in pediatric and psychiatric research have been the subject of much discussion and con-troversy and perhaps none more so than the randomized, controlled treat-ment trial. Randomized, controlled trials (RCTs) generally are considered the gold standard for demonstrating treatment efficacy and safety [57,58], but these trials pose specific concerns, especially when placebo is used in the control arm [59–64]. First, does the randomization process harm patients, who might otherwise receive treatment that is tailored to their indi-vidual needs? Second, is there sufficient evidence of the safety and efficacy of the treatment under study to justify its use in children randomized to the treatment arm [65]? Third, are the risks and benefits of the treatment arm and the control arm well balanced (ie, does "equipoise" exist regarding the study's research question) [66]? Fourth, if subjects are blinded to their assign-ment to various arms of the trial, can truly informed consent be achieved [59]? Although the dearth of empiric evidence for the treatment of child psy-chiatric disorders makes RCTs of high scientific value, these ethical concerns have limited their use and public acceptability [67], particularly for psycho-pharmacologic studies and for studies involving young children [5].

In a 2007 commentary, Carandang and colleagues [54] propose that a solution to this impasse could be found by identifying "high-risk" child psychiatry RCT treatment protocols and providing them with an additional layer of oversight in the form of data safety and monitoring boards. They characterize as high-risk those studies with the following characteristics: high-risk features of the illness (eg, suicidality); high-risk features of the intervention (ie, behavioral inhibition or regression); high-risk features of the research environment (eg, inexperienced investigators); novel cohorts (eg, first use of a therapy in children or adolescents); or novel interventions (ie, untested pharmacologic agents).

To provide an empiric measurement of the acceptability of the risks and benefits in specific child psychiatry RCTs, a few investigators have conducted so-called "social validity" surveys. The first such study published [68] involved a questionnaire survey of 40 parents of children who had mental retardation or borderline IQ and had taken part in two double-blind, placebo-controlled, crossover pharmaceutical trials, one involving methylphenidate and the other fenfluramine. The survey demonstrated that 4 weeks after the trial ended, 88% of the parents were satisfied with the specific conclusions of the study regarding pharmacotherapy for their children, and an equal proportion said that they would join the study again if presented with the same opportunity. Many of the few social validity studies in the child psychiatry literature have assessed protocols involving treatment for attention-deficit/hyperactivity disorder and generally found high levels of parental satisfaction with the study procedures (reviewed in Refs. [69,70]).

Older children and the ability to consent

It is reasonable to assume that intellectually normal adolescents have the decisional capacity necessary to make certain choices about research participation [48,50,71], although the federal regulations pertaining to research do not address the concept of "mature minors" who have the capacity to consent, despite being younger than the legal age [25,72]. There is a lack of consensus among researchers and IRBs about whether it is ethically appropriate to obtain informed consent (as opposed to assent to parental wishes) from these individuals in the research setting [47,73]. Some protocols with adolescent research participants may require both the adolescent and the parent to provide informed consent [74].

It also is unclear how often parents and adolescents make congruent choices about research participation. In a University of New Mexico study of 36 adolescents who had asthma and their parents [74,75], the adolescents were less willing to have parents make decisions regarding research than the parents assumed [74]. The parents were more likely to cede decision-making authority to sons than to daughters. Parent and adolescent opinions about participation were concordant only about 60% of the time [75].

The "therapeutic misconception"

Despite careful adherence to the process of informed consent, research participants of any age may overestimate the personal therapeutic benefits of the study, a phenomenon termed "therapeutic misconception" [45]. The therapeutic misconception has been demonstrated among psychiatric and nonpsychiatric research participants and is expressed as an unwarranted belief about how individualized the treatment is and how likely the subject is to receive a therapeutic benefit. The desperation and hope experienced by parents of suffering children may make them particularly susceptible to this misconception regarding their children's research participation. Limited data seem to support this idea. A 1995 report by researchers in Australia [76] described a questionnaire survey of 62 parents whose infants and toddlers had recently completed a randomized, double-blind clinical trial for an investigational oral asthma drug. The informed consent process for the study was by all accounts unusually thorough, involving a telephone interview by a registered nurse, followed by written information sent to the parents' homes and two 20- to 40-minute in-person information-sharing sessions, one performed by a pediatrician and the other by a nurse. The parents were interviewed 1 to 3 months after the completion of the trial about their understanding of the research process. Only about 13% understood that a purpose of the trial was to determine drug safety as well as efficacy, and nearly half believed that there were no risks to the study [76].

Several strategies have been proposed in the literature to minimize the impact of the therapeutic misconception [77–80]. The informed consent process should clearly educate parents and children about how the scientific aims of research differ from the goals of clinical care, although this may not be sufficient. As objective, trusted authorities, treating child psychiatrists may have an extremely important role to play in helping parents and children come to a rational understanding of the risks, benefits, and therapeutic potential of research trials. In the University of New Mexico study of 36 adolescents who had asthma and their parents described above, both groups expressed high regard for the advice of physicians regarding research participation [74]. Similar findings were demonstrated in a survey of 863 expectant parents in Uppsala County, Sweden [81], in which more than 80% of those polled believed that an attending physician should be "fully involved" in evaluating the level of risk that children should be exposed to in clinical research. This level of trust places a great responsibility on physician researchers; hence the critical importance of integrity, professionalism, and preparation for the ethical aspects of human subjects research.

Conflicts of interest arising from incentives for referrals

As professionals who are worthy of public trust, clinicians have a fiduciary responsibility to use their skills on behalf of their patients. Therefore, it is increasingly seen as a conflict of interest for clinicians to accept financial incentives for referring their patients to research trials [33,82,83]. Although it is arguably ethical to accept reimbursement for the actual administrative cost of the referral [82], such costs are presumably low, whereas incentives as high as $5000 have been reported in the literature [33]. Such incentives pose a conflict between the financial self-interest of the clinician and his or her fiduciary responsibility toward patients [33,82,83]. The conflict may distort the clinician's judgment without his or her awareness.

Summary

Scientific neglect of childhood disorders, especially mental and emotional illness, can be seen as an ethical failure—the lack of beneficence toward this important population, which represents humanity's future. Therefore, the current heightened research interest in pediatric disorders is ethically justified; however, just as caring for children who have mental illness is ethically challenging in ways that may not be seen when working with adults, conducting research on childhood psychiatric conditions and treatment through research also poses unique ethical difficulties. Child and adolescent psychiatrists need to be mindful of these challenges because they play an increasing role in referring children for clinical trials and advising families of the implications of participation in research.

To accomplish this, psychiatrists first need to be acutely aware of how disempowered families may be: minors have minimal power to determine their treatment, and parents may be desperate to help their children in the face of limited resources and few options. Second, to protect and advocate for their patients, psychiatrists must be aware of the ethical dimensions of research involving human participants, which stem from the core principles of respect for persons, beneficence, and justice. Third, to be able to advise families adequately, clinicians should familiarize themselves with research trials currently underway and become knowledgeable about new and emerging methodologies. This may involve contacting researchers for more information, helping families review consent forms, consulting with investigators about the appropriateness of individual patients as study participants, and even collaborating in the design of research protocols.

In addition, psychiatrists need to acquire the knowledge and skills to effectively communicate to families the significance of participating in a research trial. This discussion typically emphasizes that participation is voluntary, that withdrawal from the study is an option, that the decision to participate in research will not exclude them from getting alternative clinical care, and that research-related care does not necessarily provide the individualized treatment found in routine care. Finally, it is important that all physicians obtain education in ethics and professionalism and develop self-awareness regarding their motivations for referring patients to clinical trials. Integrity is needed to ensure that recommendations are in the best interests of the patient, and courage may be required to step in to protect the patient when circumstances require it. In all of these ways, clinicians can work toward an improved evidence base for psychiatric practice while remaining fully committed to the well-being of children in their care.

Acknowledgments

The authors thank Brian Fisch, Josh Reiher, and Ann Tennier for their assistance in the preparation of this manuscript.

References

[1] Angold A, Messer SC, Stangl D, et al. Perceived parental burden and service use for child and adolescent psychiatric disorders. Am J Public Health 1998;88(1):75–80.

[2] Blanchard LT, Gurka MJ, Blackman JA. Emotional, developmental, and behavioral health of American children and their families: a report from the 2003 national survey of children's health. Pediatrics 2006;117(6):e1202–12.

[3] Laughren TP. Regulatory issues in pediatric psychopharmacology. J Am Acad Child Adolesc Psychiatry 1996;35(10):1276–82.

[4] NIH policy and guidelines on the inclusion of children as participants in research involving human subjects. Available at: http://grants.nih.gov/grants/guide/notice-files/not98–024.html. Accessed March 6, 1998.

[5] Greenhill L, Jensen P, Abikoff H, et al. Developing strategies for psychopharmacological studies in preschool children. J Am Acad Child Adolesc Psychiatry 2003;42(4):406–14.

[6] Hepper F, Fellow-Smith E. Off-label prescribing in a community child and adolescent mental health service: implications for information giving and informed consent. Clinician in Management 2005;13(1):29–34.

[7] Vitiello B, Jensen P, Hoagwood K. Integrating science and ethics in child and adolescent psychiatry research. Biol Psychiatry 1999;46:1044–9.

[8] Dooley J, Camfield P, Gordon K, et al. Lamotrigine-induced rash in children. Neurology 1996;46(1):240–2.

[9] Simon G. The antidepressant quandary—considering suicide risk when treating adolescent depression. N Engl J Med 2006;355(26):2722–3.

[10] Bridge JA, Iyengar S, Salary CB, et al. Clinical response and risk for reported suicidal ideation and suicide attempts in pediatric antidepressant treatment: a meta-analysis of randomized controlled trials. JAMA 2007;297(15):1683–96.

[11] Ryan ND, Varma D. Child and adolescent mood disorders–experience with serotonin-based therapies. Biol Psychiatry 1998;44(5):336–40.

[12] Plomin R. Finding genes in child psychology and psychiatry: when are we going to be there? J Child Psychol Psychiatry 2005;46(10):1030–8.

[13] Abou-Saleh MT. Neuroimaging in psychiatry: an update. J Psychosom Res 2006;61(3): 289–93.

[14] National Institutes of Health. Regulations and ethical guidelines. The Nuremberg Code. Available at: http://ohsr.od.nih.gov/guidelines/nuremberg.html. Accessed May 1, 2007.

[15] Annas GJ, Grodin MA. The Nazi doctors and the Nuremberg Code. New York: Oxford University Press; 1992.

[16] The World Medical Association. Declaration of Helsinki, 1964. Available at: http://www.
     wma.net/e/policy/b3.htm. Accessed April 27, 2007.
[17] Krugman S. The Willowbrook hepatitis studies revisited: ethical aspects. Rev Infect Dis
     1986;8(1):157–62.
[18] The President's Advisory Committee on Human Radiation Experiments. The human radi-
     ation experiments. New York: Oxford University Press; 1996.
[19] National Commission for the Protection of Human Subjects of Biomedical and Behavioral
     Research: The Belmont Report: ethical principles and guidelines for the protection of human
     subjects of research, 1979. Available at: http://www.hhs.gov/ohrp/humansubjects/guidance/
     belmont.htm. Accessed June 12, 2006.
[20] Roberts LW. Informed consent and the capacity for voluntarism. Am J Psychiatry 2002;
     159(5):705–12.
[21] U.S. Department of Health and Human Services: Code of Federal Regulations: Title 45
     public welfare, Department of Health and Human Services part 46 protection of human
     subjects, 2005. Available at: http://www.hhs.gov/ohrp/humansubjects/guidance/45cfr46.htm.
     Accessed April 27, 2007.
[22] U.S. Department of Health and Human Services: Code of Federal Regulations: title 21 Food
     and Drug Administration, Department of Health and Human Services. Part 50 protection of
     human subjects and Part 56 institutional review boards, 2001. Available at: http://www.
     access.gpo.gov/nara/cfr/waisidx_01/21cfrv1_01.html. Accessed April 27, 2007.
[23] Levine RJ. Respect for children as research subjects. In: Lewis M, editor. Child and adoles-
     cent psychiatry. Baltimore, MD: Williams and Wilkins; 1991. p. 1229–38.
[24] Roberts LW, Hoop JG, Anderson TT, et al. Professionalism and ethics: a self-assessment
     guide for medical professionals. Washington, DC: American Psychiatric Press, Inc.; in press.
[25] U.S. Department of Health and Human Services: Code of Federal Regulations: title 45 pub-
     lic welfare, Department of Health and Human Services, part 46 protection of human sub-
     jects, Subpart D, additional protections for children involved as subjects in research, 2005.
     Available at: http://www.hhs.gov/ohrp/humansubjects/guidance/45cfr46.htm#subpartd.
     Accessed April 27, 2007.
[26] Levine C, Faden R, Grady C, et al. The limitations of "vulnerability" as a protection for
     human research participants. Am J Bioeth 2004;4(3):44–9.
[27] Emanuel E, Wendler D, Grady C. What makes clinical research ethical? JAMA 2000;
     283(20):2701–11.
[28] Roberts L. Ethical dimensions of psychiatric research: a constructive, criterion-based ap-
     proach to protocol preparation. The research protocol ethics assessment tool (RePEAT).
     Biol Psychiatry 1999;46:1106–19.
[29] Munir K, Earls F. Ethical principles governing research in child and adolescent psychiatry.
     J Am Acad Child Adolesc Psychiatry 1992;31:408–14.
[30] President's Commission for the Protection of Human Subjects in Biomedical and Behav-
     ioral Research. Protecting human subjects. Washington, DC: Government Printing Office;
     1981.
[31] Brody BA. The ethics of biomedical research: an international perspective. London: Oxford
     University Press; 1998.
[32] Levine RJ. Clinical trials and physicians as double agents. Yale J Biol Med 1992;65(2):
     65–74.
[33] Morin K, Rakatansky H, Riddick FA Jr, et al. Managing conflicts of interest in the conduct
     of clinical trials. JAMA 2002;287(1):78–84.
[34] Appelbaum PS. Rethinking the conduct of psychiatric research. Arch Gen Psychiatry 1997;
     54(2):117–20.
[35] Chen D, Miller F, Rosenstein D. Ethical aspects of research into the etiology of autism.
     Research Reviews 2003;9:48–53.
[36] United States Department of Health and Human Services. Code of Federal Regulations, title
     45 public welfare, Department of Health and Human Services, part 160 and Subparts A and

E of part 164, privacy rule 2000. Available at: http://www.hhs.gov/ocr/regtext.html. Accessed April 27, 2007.

[37] National Institutes of Health. Certificates of confidentiality: background information, 2003. Available at: http://grants1.nih.gov/grants/policy/coc/background.htm. Accessed April 27, 2007.

[38] Beecher HK. Ethics and clinical research. N Engl J Med 1966;274:1354–60.

[39] Dresser R. Wanted: single, white male for medical research. Hastings Cent Rep 1992;22: 24–9.

[40] Institute of Medicine. Guidance for national healthcare disparities report. Washington, DC: National Academy Press; 2002.

[41] United States Department of Health and Human Services. Healthy people 2010: understanding and improving health. 2nd edition. Washington, DC: Government Printing Office; 2000.

[42] Miller VA, Nelson RM. A developmental approach to child assent for nontherapeutic research. J Pediatr 2006;149:S25–30.

[43] Faden RR, Beauchamp TL, King N. A history and theory of informed consent. New York: Oxford University Press; 1986.

[44] Roberts LW, Geppert C, McCarty T, et al. Evaluating medical students' skills in obtaining informed consent for HIV testing. J Gen Intern Med 2003;18:112–9.

[45] Appelbaum P, Roth L, Lidz C. The therapeutic misconception: informed consent in psychiatric research. Int J Law Psychiatry 1982;5(3–4):319–29.

[46] Appelbaum PS, Grisso T. The MacArthur competence study I, II, III. Law Hum Behav 1995;19:105–74.

[47] Oesterheld J, Fogas B, Rutten S. Ethical standards for research on children. J Am Acad Child Adolesc Psychiatry 1998;37(7):684–5.

[48] Gaylin W. The competence of children: no longer all or none. Hastings Cent Rep 1982;12(2): 33–8.

[49] Arnold LE, Stoff DM, Cook E Jr, et al. Ethical issues in biological psychiatric research with children and adolescents. J Am Acad Child Adolesc Psychiatry 1995;34:929–39.

[50] Rosato J. The ethics of clinical trials: a child's view. J Law Med Ethics 2000;28:362–78.

[51] Dresser R. Mentally disabled research subjects. The enduring policy issues. JAMA 1996;276: 67–72.

[52] Levine RJ. Ethics and regulation of clinical research. Baltimore (MD): Urban & Schwartzenberg; 1981.

[53] Scherer DG, Brody JL, Annett RD, et al. Financial compensation to adolescents for participation in biomedical research: adolescent and parent perspectives in seven studies. J Pediatr 2005;146(4):552–8.

[54] Carandang C, Santor D, Gardner D, et al. Data safety monitoring boards and other study methodologies that address subject safety in "high-risk" therapeutic trials in youths. J Am Acad Child Adolesc Psychiatry 2007;46(4):489–90.

[55] Horton R. Trial registers: protecting patients, advancing trust. Lancet 2006;367(9523): 1633–5.

[56] International Committee of Medical Journal Editors. Uniform requirements for manuscripts submitted to biomedical journals: writing and editing for biomedical publication. 2005. Available at: http://www.icmje.org/icmje.pdf. Accessed May 1, 2007.

[57] Lader EW, Cannon CP, Ohman EM, et al. The clinician as investigator: participating in clinical trials in the practice setting: appendix 1: fundamentals of study design. Circulation 2004; 109:e302–4.

[58] Leber P. The placebo control in clinical trials (a view from the FDA). Psychopharmacol Bull 1986;22:30–2.

[59] Schaefer A. The ethics of the randomized clinical trial. N Engl J Med 1982;307:719–25.

[60] Rothman KJ, Michels KB. The continuing unethical use of placebo controls. N Engl J Med 1994;331:394–8.

[61] O'Leary KD, Borkovec TD. Conceptual, methodological, and ethical problems of placebo groups in psychotherapy research. Am Psychol 1978;33:821–30.

[62] Levine RJ, Schafer A. The use of placebos in randomized clinical trials. IRB 1985;7(2):1–6.

[63] Bok S. The ethics of giving placebos. Sci Am 1974;231(5):17–23.

[64] Klerman GL. Scientific and ethical considerations in the use of placebo controls in clinical trials in psychopharmacology. Psychopharmacol Bull 1986;22:25–9.

[65] Derivan A, Lventhal B, March J, et al. The ethical use of placebo in clinical trials involving children. J Child Adolesc Psycholpharmacol 2004;14(2):169–74.

[66] Freedman B. Equipoise and the ethics of clinical research. N Engl J Med 1987;317(3):141–5.

[67] Caldwell P, Butow P, Craig J. Parents' attitudes to children's participation in randomized controlled trials. J Pediatr 2003;142(5):554–9.

[68] Aman M, Wolford P. Consumer satisfaction with involvement in drug research: a social validity study. J Am Acad Child Adolesc Psychiatry 1995;34(7):940–5.

[69] Bukstein OG. Satisfaction with treatment for attention-deficit-hyperactivity disorder. Am J Manag Care 2004;10(4 Suppl):S107–16.

[70] Tierney E, Aman M, Stout D, et al. Parent satisfaction in a multi-site acute trial of risperidone in children with autism: a social validity study. Psychopharmacology (Berl) 2007;191: 149–57.

[71] Melton GB. Parents and children: legal reform to facilitate children's participation. Am Psychol 1999;54:935–44.

[72] Belitz J. Caring for children. In: Roberts LW, Dyer AR, editors. Concise guide to ethics in mental health care. Washington, DC: American Psychiatric Publishing; 2004. p. 119–35.

[73] Dorn LD, Susman EJ, Fletcher JC. Informed consent in children and adolescents: age, maturation and psychological state. J Adolesc Health 1995;16(3):185–90.

[74] Brody JL, Scherer DG, Annett RD, et al. Family and physician influence on asthma research participation decisions for adolescents: the effects of adolescent gender and research risk. Pediatrics 2006;118:356–62.

[75] Brody JL, Annett RD, Scherer DG, et al. Comparisons of adolescent and parent willingness to participate in minimal and above-minimal risk pediatric asthma research protocols. J Adolesc Health 2005;37(3):229–35.

[76] Harth S, Thong Y. Parental perceptions and attitudes about informed consent in clinical research involving children. Soc Sci Med 1995;40(11):1573–7.

[77] Appelbaum PS, Grisso T. Assessing patients' capacities to consent to treatment. N Engl J Med 1988;319:1635–8.

[78] Lidz CW, Appelbaum PS, Grisso T, et al. Therapeutic misconception and the appreciation of risks in clinical trials. Soc Sci Med 2004;58:1689–97.

[79] Roberts LW, Warner TD, Anderson CT, et al. Schizophrenia research participants' responses to protocol safeguards: recruitment, consent, and debriefing. Schizophr Res 2004; 67:283–91.

[80] Roberts LW, Hammond KA, Warner TD, et al. Influence of ethical safeguards on research participation: comparison of perspectives of people with schizophrenia and psychiatrists. Am J Psychiatry 2004;161:2309–11.

[81] Rodriguez A, Tuvemo T, Hansson M. Parents' perspectives on research involving children. Ups J Med Sci 2006;111(1):73–86.

[82] Fleischman A, Klein J. Clinical research in the private office setting—ethical issues. Trans Am Clin Climatol Assoc 2002;113:126–36.

[83] Roa JN, Cassia LJ. Ethics of undisclosed payments to doctors recruiting patients in clinical trials. BMJ 2002;325:36–7.

ELSEVIER
SAUNDERS

Child Adolesc Psychiatric Clin N Am
17 (2008) 149–163

CHILD AND
ADOLESCENT
PSYCHIATRIC CLINICS
OF NORTH AMERICA

Publishing Ethics in Child and Adolescent Psychiatry: Essentials for Authors and Readers

Garry Walter, MD, PhD[a,b,*],
Joseph M. Rey, MD, PhD[a], Nerissa Soh, PhD[b],
Sidney Bloch, MD, PhD[c]

[a]University of Sydney, Victoria Street, Potts Point, Sydney,
New South Wales, 2006, Australia
[b]Child and Adolescent Mental Health Services, Coral Tree Family Service,
Northern Sydney Central Coast Health, P.O. Box 142, North Ryde,
New South Wales 1670, 2006, Australia
[c]Department of Psychiatry and Center for Health and Society, University of Melbourne,
St. Vincent's Hospital, 46 Nicholson Street, Fitzroy, Melbourne,
Victoria 3065, Australia

As is Dr. Faith's custom, he peruses the latest issue of his favorite child and adolescent psychiatry journal and selects the papers he will read. He is pleased to note the review of adolescent depression, because he is scheduled to talk to a community group on this topic. Two articles on attention-deficit/hyperactivity disorder (ADHD) appeal because patients who have this disorder make up a large part of his practice. When he reads these contributions, Dr. Faith is not concerned with a few authors' statements of having received pharmaceutical industry support or that one of the articles resembled a paper by the same group that he recalled reading in another journal. The review has an unusually long authorship list, but Dr. Faith is more interested in whether he knows any of the authors rather than being perturbed about whether all those named actually contributed to the paper's preparation.

Most colleagues, like Dr. Faith, probably concentrate on the content of the journals they read, giving short shrift to "publishing ethics." Notwithstanding

This work was supported by the McGeorge Bequest, University of Sydney, Sydney, Australia.

*Corresponding author. Child and Adolescent Mental Health Services, Coral Tree Family Service, Northern Sydney Central Coast Health, P.O. Box 142, North Ryde, New South Wales 1670, 2006, Australia.

E-mail address: gwalter@mail.usyd.edu.au (G. Walter).

the growing interest in psychiatric ethics [1–3], the ethical dimension of publishing in psychiatry remains neglected [4]. This applies equally to the subspecialties, such as child and adolescent psychiatry [5]. It is timely to address pertinent ethical issues that arise in publishing in this field.

Ethical issues in child and adolescent psychiatric publishing

A concerted effort to identify and deal with ethical issues in scientific publishing began 30 years ago with the establishment of the International Committee of Medical Journal Editors (ICMJE) [6]. The Committee on Publication Ethics (COPE) [7], World Association of Medical Editors [8], and Council of Science Editors [9] followed in its wake, all committed to the same purpose. Congresses on scientific publishing, which concern ethical themes, have taken place every 4 years since 1989, the most recent in Chicago in 2005 [10]. Articles and books have emerged on the subject [11,12]. Although a few medical journals have produced position statements on publishing ethics [13,14], child and adolescent psychiatric publications have rarely been among them.

Ethical problems in scientific publishing include conflict of interest, bias, reporting fraudulent or inhumane research, redundant publication, plagiarism, a range of concerns about authorship, and insensitive language. Drawing on our previous work [4], we examine these issues in child and adolescent psychiatry.

Conflict of interest

Conflicts of interest are of crucial importance. The ICMJE [6] states that they exist "when an author (or the author's institution), reviewer or editor has financial or personal relationships that inappropriately influence (bias) his or her actions (such relationships are also known as dual commitments, competing interests or competing loyalties)."

The subject has garnered much recent attention. Lester Crawford, a former US Food and Drug Administration commissioner, was found guilty in 2007 of false reports concerning shares he held in pharmaceutical companies; he was sentenced to 3 years of supervised probation and fined $90,000 [15]. Although rarely reaching such a criminal level, conflicts of interest are common in health-related fields, and child and adolescent psychiatric publishing is not immune. Research funded by the pharmaceutical industry reported in psychiatric journals has increased steadily, possibly by 50% in recent years [16]. Moreover, positive outcomes are reported much more commonly in trials so funded (78%), compared with those without industry sponsorship (48%) or those financed by a competitor (28%) [16]. The obvious issue arises as to the extent to which industry-funded research influences findings and to what degree, if at all, one can trust such work. Recent controversies about selective reporting of the effectiveness of antidepressant medication in young people and the medication's association with suicidal behavior [17,18] highlight this matter.

Conflicts of interest are not restricted to drug trials. For example, *The Lancet* published a study that suggested a link between autism and the measles-mumps-rubella (MMR) vaccine [19]. The report sent shock waves around the globe and frightened parents and medical practitioners. As a consequence, MMR vaccination rates in England declined by 10% in the following 5 years, whereas cases of measles almost quadrupled [20]. A journalist later established that the principal author, Andrew Wakefield, had not disclosed that the Legal Aid Board had commissioned him to determine, for a sizable fee, if evidence sufficed to support a legal action by parents of children allegedly harmed by the vaccine. *The Lancet* retracted the article, in part, and the General Medical Council opted to examine the author's fitness to practice. Subsequent research conclusively refuted any link between the vaccine and autism [21].

As the ICMJE statement indicates, conflicts of interest may affect reviewers and editors. Two senior editors of the *Canadian Medical Association Journal* were dismissed, ostensibly because they had published material contrary to the Association's perceived interests [22]. Many physicians were appalled, voicing their concerns about the breaching of editorial independence [23,24].

By and large, medical practitioners may prefer to believe that drug company funding or gifts, for example, do not influence their judgment or behavior, which is not true [25]. It also warrants stressing that extraneous factors that contribute to a potential conflict of interest may be subtle, including, for example, academic rivalry and intellectual passion.

Conflicts of interest are not inherently improper and may be unavoidable. Similarly, disclosure of competing interests is not an admission of wrongdoing [20]. It is the editor, on behalf of authors and readers, who is obliged to determine whether these conflicts are sufficiently serious to deny publication of a report. Typical instances are shown in Box 1. Many journals require an explicit disclosure of these matters, a requirement once regarded by some as the "new McCarthyism" [26], but now accepted as *de rigueur*.

Bias

Bias in publishing is linked inextricably to conflicts of interest. Editors may be inclined to publish their preferred topics. They also may be reluctant to publish negative results [27], thus distorting the "evidence base" for certain treatments. Submissions from the developing world may be viewed prejudicially as lacking scientific thoroughness [28]. Reviewers also are vulnerable; for example, they may act unfairly because an author's conceptual approach does not coincide with their own or through professional envy. Bias may manifest in subtle ways, such as when reviewers unconsciously

Box 1. Summary of disclosure obligations for authors, reviewers, and editorial staff

Authors should

State explicitly whether potential conflicts do or do not exist

Describe the role of the study sponsor, if any, in study design; in the collection, analysis, and interpretation of data; in the writing of the report; and in the decision to submit the report for publication

Report ownership of stock or other financial instruments of companies whose products are mentioned in the article or who manufacture competing products ("product" can be a drug, questionnaire, device, therapy, and so forth)

Report paid consultancy or employment with a company or a competitor whose products are mentioned in the article

Report honorarium or other compensation for writing the article, for participating in the development of the article, or for conducting research related to material contained in the article

Report speaker fees or educational grants[a]

Report travel assistance to attend meetings[a]

Reviewers should

Be asked to state explicitly whether conflicts do or do not exist

Disclose to editors any conflict of interest that could bias their opinions of the manuscript

Not use knowledge of the reviewed work before its publication to further their own interests

Editors and relevant editorial staff should:

Avoid selecting peer reviewers with obvious potential conflicts of interest (eg, those who work in the same department or institution as any of the authors). Authors often provide editors with the names of persons they believe should not be asked to review a manuscript because of potential conflicts of interest; authors should give the reasons for the editor to judge their validity.

Have no personal, professional, or financial involvement in any of the issues they might judge

Not use the information gained through working with manuscripts for private gain

---

[a] Usually in the previous 2 years.

Modified from International Committee of Medical Journal Editors. Uniform requirements for manuscripts submitted to biomedical journals: writing and editing for biomedical publication 2006. Available at: http://www.icmje.org; with permission.

procrastinate in returning assessments or modify their own research on the basis of a report reviewed.

Publication of fraudulent research

Fraud, characterized by an intention to deceive, is the "antithesis" of ethically sound scientific behavior. Colleagues must be able to trust reports of methods used and results found [29].

Sir Cyril Burt, one of the most influential educational psychologists of his time, who proposed that intelligence is largely inherited, has been cast by contemporary leading scientists as a notorious perpetrator of fraud [30]; however, it is the case of Stephen Breuning which provides a landmark, in that it probably was the first with grave implications for patients which led to criminal prosecution [31,32]. Breuning (eg, Ref. [33]) claimed that, in mentally retarded children, tranquilizers were less effective and produced more side effects than stimulants and decreased their response to behavioral treatment. The purported finding shaped management policies toward the use of psychotropic medication in these patients [31,34]. Incredibly, no research was performed. Breuning's sentence included several hundred hours of community service and a ban from professional practice, among other penalties. The fallout affected unsuspecting coauthors, one remarking of the perpetrator [35], "Our interactions have tarnished my reputation, and caused me pain." Perhaps the only "positive" to ensue was a radical decline in citations to the offending articles once they were exposed, showing that researchers can purge the literature of falsified work [4,31].

Publishing inhumane research

If you could ease the suffering of a teenager who had intractable schizophrenia or cure another who had a degenerative brain disorder by applying results of research that had been performed by sadistic scientists using barbaric procedures on young people, would you proceed? Sharing Beecher's [36] sentiments about the cruel Nazi experiments, "this loss [of experimental data]...would be less important than the far reaching moral loss to medicine if the data were to be published," we echo the Declaration of Helsinki on biomedical research, which states that "reports of experimentation not in accordance with the principles in this Declaration should not be accepted for publication" [37]. It is worth noting that the scientific quality of inhumane studies often is poor, rendering them unethical from a second standpoint [38,39].

Redundant publication

The essence of this practice, variously termed fragmented, multiple, divided, and "salami" publication and reporting in "least publishable units" [40], is generating more articles from a body of "data" than is objectively warranted [4]. The practice is undesirable in that it squanders journal space, may distort meta-analyses, and inflates curriculum vitae deceptively.

Occasionally, republishing a "classic" paper, a journal article as a chapter, or an article in a journal whose readers may not have had access to the original is permissible. Acknowledgment of the source material is required, and in these situations, "redundant publication" is a misnomer [41].

Redundant publication in psychiatry that has attracted editorial comment includes two papers, with much overlapping data, on postpartum mental illness [42–45] and two cases relating to antidepressant trials [46–53] where identical (or near-identical) papers were published by a research group, without the editors' knowledge [4]. Occasionally, as occurred with the *Journal of the American Academy of Child and Adolescent Psychiatry* [54], editors have been able to intercept potentially redundant publications before printing and have commented on the matter in their journal.

If authors harbor doubts about the degree of overlap between two or more of their papers, they ought to provide the editor with a copy of the published article, alongside their submission, to permit an objective judgment.

Like other forms of publishing misconduct, redundant publication may undermine more than one ethical principle [4]. For instance, it wastes space and is an abuse of reviewers', editors', readers', and indexers' time—a violation of "distributive justice"—and may spoil the reputation of the journal, host institution, or unsuspecting coauthors.

Plagiarism

Plagiarism refers to "the use of others' published and unpublished ideas or words (or other intellectual property) without attribution or permission, and presenting them as new and original rather than derived from an existing source" [8].

Several cases of plagiarism have been detected in psychiatric journals. For example, an academic resigned following the revelation that he had plagiarized large sections of four review articles [32,55]. When lecturing, he was apt to quote extensively from published material by colleagues, but omitted attribution when he converted these lectures into publications [4,55]. In another case, a paper reporting on a treatment for tics and ADHD [56] was slavishly copied [57]; when challenged, the perpetrator said that he "had been impressed by the [earlier] study and based his study upon it" [58]. In a further example, a paper on "equine-facilitated psychotherapy" for children [59] was largely copied from someone's Master's thesis [60]. In a fourth case, part of an article on insulin binding in anorexia nervosa [61] was plagiarized by a reviewer [62]; on exposure, he returned to his native country—his supervisor forfeiting an academic appointment—and the person whose work had been misused abandoned a career in research in a state of bitterness [4,63,64].

More controversial is self-plagiarism, whereby authors use portions of their previous publications on the same topic in another publication, instead of quoting them formally. This may be done unwittingly and, further, there are limited ways to make an essentially similar statement about a topic. Although this violates copyright assigned to the publisher, its characterization as a form of scientific misconduct remains unsettled.

Assuming authorship

Authorship is regarded by researchers as a reward for their "blood, sweat, and tears," a mark of academic worth, and essential for academic progression. Therefore, its nature has been much debated and its potential abuse noted [4].

The ICMJE [6] posits that authorship should be based on all of the following criteria: substantial contributions to the study's conception and design, or acquisition of data, or their analysis and interpretation; drafting the article or revising it critically; and approval of the final draft. Some journals stipulate information about the contribution made by each author.

Although controversy continues about who qualifies for authorship, unequivocally withholding it is straightforward [4]. "Guest" (or "honorary" or "gift"), "planted," or "ghost" authorship is considered unethical. A guest author is one who is knowingly listed as an author, for example to influence reviewers (if they are not blind to the authors), as a professional favor, or to seek some kind of benefit (eg, reciprocal guest authorship). Planted authorship refers to that conferred without the person's knowledge. In ghost authorship, a person, not uncommonly working on behalf of a company, has made a substantial contribution to a paper but is not credited as an author.

The order of authors listed needs brief comment. First-named authorship carries the most prestige. Readers also may believe that a paper's first author has assumed greater responsibility than the others listed. This premise was quashed a few years ago when an article had to be retracted [65,66] because of unsound methodology, and the host university blamed all of the authors [4]. Nevertheless, certain journals request a "guarantor" who will take responsibility for the integrity of research, from inception to publication [6].

Entitlement to, and ordering of, authorship is best determined at the outset of a project, or early in the process, although decisions may change later. Public airing of grievances are not in a profession's best interests. Fortunately, to our knowledge, no such grievances have found their way into child and adolescent psychiatry journals.

Sensitive use of language

It is vital to use language sensitively and responsibly [4]. Increasingly, journals (eg, Ref. [67]) alert authors to unacceptable pejorative terms, like "psychotics," and suggest more suitable ones ("patients with psychosis"). Some expressions in child and adolescent psychiatry have unfairly apportioned blame and remained in use for extended periods. Notorious illustrations are "schizophrenogenic mother," coined by Frieda Fromm-Reichmann

[68] and "refrigerator parent," promoted by Bruno Bettelheim on the basis of Leo Kanner's formulation of autism [4,69]. Such language may cause harm unintentionally. For example, the use of the expression "adolescent turmoil" may well have contributed to those in need of treatment not receiving it, because they were deemed to be going through a normal developmental phase [4].

A journal's editorial and correspondence columns often are fora for intense debate. This is a healthy aspect of academic exchange, but debate should focus on the subject and strenuously avoid *ad hominem* criticism; offensive language invariably distresses its target, and any later retractions and apologies (eg, Ref. [70]) are embarrassing.

How can we understand unethical publishing?

Identifying contributory factors to unethical publishing and typical categories of perpetrators is the first step to curbing it. Two offender groups have emerged [4,32,71]. Bright, ambitious people embarking on a scientific career, working in prestigious institutions governed by a "publish or perish" ethos and unable to access supervision or mentorship readily, may publish at a frenetic pace. They are much affected by expectations to generate "positive" data; the declining status of replication studies (which might uncover fraud); and the association of publication productivity with academic self-esteem, tenure, promotion, and securing grants. A second category consists of isolated professionals, mostly clinicians, who are recruited by pharmaceutical companies to serve as associate investigators in drug trials; they are prone to fabricating data.

It is salutary to point out that anyone who participates in one or another aspect of publishing is at risk of acting unethically. A recent study found that retractions in the biomedical literature were more than twice as likely to result from genuine mistakes than from intentional scientific misconduct [72]. As Goodstein [29] put it, "....minor deceptions arise in virtually all scientific papers, as they do in other aspects of human life." Such behavior, he argues, may not be laudable, but is not the equivalent of scientific misconduct. Nevertheless, "lesser" infringements are common and can seriously undermine the integrity of science. This is reflected in the results of a survey of more than 3000 American researchers [73]. Whereas only 0.3% of the respondents admitted to falsifying data, 5% reported publishing the same results in various publications, 6% did not present data that contradicted their previous research, 10% had assigned authorship inappropriately, 12% overlooked colleagues' use of flawed data, and 15% had dropped observations from analyses based on a "feeling" that they were inaccurate.

These sorts of findings clearly highlight the need to examine and modify the research environment overall, including reducing institutional and competitive pressure [73].

Table 1
Ethical issues in child psychiatric research

Ethical principle	General research with children	Child psychiatry research
Respect for person	Children's developmentally limited ability to consent/assent	Informed consent doubly limited: cognitive immaturity and impaired cognitive processing
	Developmental aspects of decision making; suggestibility	Developmental and emotional impact on decision making
	Parents' rights and natural protective role	Parents' protective role colored by emotional stress of disturbed child
	Coercive inducement; child's view of $ amount	Coercion from harassed parent and reimbursement
Beneficence	Conflict between need for placebo control and the right to best proven treatment	Need for placebo to determine effective treatment when no or poor evidence base
Justice, equity	Need for research with children to help "research orphans"	Need for child psychopharmacologic research to guide ongoing psychopharmacotherapy for children
	Children's vulnerability	Double vulnerability: children and mental impairment
	Fair reimbursement for research burden of parents	

Modified from Spetie L, Arnold LE. Ethical issues in child psychopharmacology research and practice: emphasis on preschoolers. Psychopharmacology 2007;191:16; with permission.

Special issues concerning publishing of research involving minors

It is beyond the scope of this article to examine in detail ethical issues concerning research involving minors, which is dealt with elsewhere in this issue (see the article by Hoop and colleagues) and summarized in Table 1. Insofar as such research will be disseminated through scholarly journals, how that research is described is crucial. For example, in child and adolescent psychiatry research, participants usually lack the legal capacity to give consent, and parents or guardians do so as proxies (although the young person's assent often is desirable). Published reports should summarize this aspect of a study. Similarly, the use of placebo controls in general psychiatric research frequently raises ethical concerns because participants on placebo may be deprived of effective treatment, yet such a design may be justified in child psychiatry research because treatments of well-established efficacy and safety are lacking (eg, Ref. [74]). In the child and adolescent psychiatry literature, summarizing the (lack of) evidence base which justifies the use of placebo is necessary. In all reports, it is desirable to cite ethical matters which have attended a particular research project.

Box 2. Strategies to promote ethical publishing in child psychiatry

Developing guidelines on publishing ethics

Teaching publishing ethics and scientific probity to mental health professionals and students in the field

Individual child psychiatry journals paying greater attention to the subject of publishing ethics

Child psychiatry journals forming consortia to tackle ethical problems

Learned institutions discouraging redundant and other wasteful publication

Harnessing information technology to promote ethical standards of publishing

Detecting and reporting publishing misconduct

Imposing penalties for transgressors

Conducting research on the subject

Adapted from Walter G, Bloch S. Publishing ethics in psychiatry. Aust N Z J Psychiatry 2001;35:28–35; with permission.

Recommendations to promote ethical publishing

Given the scope of ethical problems that may dog publishing in child and adolescent psychiatry and the various factors underpinning them, it is likely that several strategies will be required to promote ethical publishing (Box 2).

Guidelines on publishing ethics in medicine are rare; specific ones for child and adolescent psychiatry do not exist. Development of the latter is sorely needed. Professional organizations in this domain have a role here and should go beyond what usually happens—alluding briefly to publishing ethics under the rubric of research ethics (or not mentioning publishing ethics at all). In 2006, COPE contributed substantially in this regard by producing an excellent series of flow charts, detailing, for example, recommended responses to suspected undisclosed conflict of interest, fabricated data, redundant publication, plagiarism, and requests to add or remove an author [75]. These charts could be applied readily, with appropriate modification, to the discipline of child and adolescent psychiatry.

Teaching publishing ethics might prevent improper conduct in future generations of investigators, but this is rarely done [76]. To our knowledge, the only routine course in the child and adolescent mental health field is offered as part of the child and adolescent psychiatry training program in Sydney, Australia. Its curriculum covers all of the topics addressed above, with liberal use of case illustrations (Garry Walter, MD, PhD, unpublished data).

Child and adolescent psychiatric journals have a major role to promote ethical standards. For example, the profile of publishing ethics could be raised by encouraging editorials and articles on the subject, "Instructions for Authors" could encompass ethical guidelines, and, when papers are submitted, editors could remind authors and reviewers of their ethical responsibilities. Facilitating reports of negative findings could help to offset the long-standing prejudice against them. This, in turn, would allow readers to appraise the evidence base more accurately [27]. Editors need to be mindful of the ethical ramifications of each journal section. For example, in those journals that publish case reports, preventing potential harm by ensuring that authors obtain the parent's or guardian's permission and the child's assent and by preserving patient anonymity through omitting identifying information, is recommended.

Given the inadequate reporting of antidepressant trials in children and adolescents [77], editors should heed the advice of editors' organizations (eg, Refs. [78,79]) and require prior registration of all therapeutic trials published in their journals, so countering selective release of outcome data.

Editors, together with senior members of their editorial boards, can play a vital role in counseling authors who have acted unethically, perhaps unwittingly, thus helping them to appreciate the relevant issues and preventing recurrence.

Child and adolescent psychiatric journals, the *Journal of the American Academy of Child and Adolescent Psychiatry*, *The Journal of Child Psychology and Psychiatry*, and the *European Journal of Child and Adolescent Psychiatry*, among others, could consider forming a consortium to address ethical aspects of publishing. Their editors and editorial boards also would benefit by membership of various organizations dealing with publishing ethics and participation in available electronic discussion groups (eg, Ref. [80]).

University departments of child and adolescent psychiatry and other academic institutions should inform their staff about unethical publication practices. The "publish or perish" pressure would be reduced if candidates for tenure or promotion were considered on the basis of their best work, rather than on the number of their publications. In the absence of universally agreed methods to measure the quality of published articles, clarifying what constitutes high quality would be useful [81].

Information technology should be harnessed to promote better publishing. Apart from e-mail discussion fora mentioned above, software to detect plagiarism and open Internet-based peer review are two measures that may improve ethical standards.

Child and adolescent psychiatry academics and all those who work in the field are duty-bound to report cases of publishing misconduct. Crucially, whistleblowers need protection from possible adverse consequences. A trainee in child and adolescent psychiatry who discovers that an article by her seniors stems from fraudulent research would face a stormy period if she disclosed this to the editor. A foolproof remedy is not at hand to deal with this situation.

Regrettably, serious publishing misconduct calls for sanction to prevent further harm and to deter the offender from recidivism and others from following suit. Depending on the nature of the offense, the penalty may include reprimand, deregistration, job loss, ineligibility for research grants, a ban from publishing in the particular child and adolescent psychiatry journal, and perhaps other journals too, and circulating a 'blacklist' of discredited persons among editors [4]. Legal liability for such measures warrants careful consideration.

Finally, negligible research has been done on unethical publishing in child and adolescent psychiatry. Systematic study of factors contributing to it and the usefulness of measures to curb it would be likely to exert a salutary effect on authors and all members of the "publishing community."

Summary

Authors and readers need to be aware of appropriate ethical standards of publishing in child and adolescent psychiatry and appreciate the essence of such aspects as conflict of interest, bias, reporting fraudulent or inhumane research, redundant publication, plagiarism, assuming authorship, insensitive use of language, and the special circumstances of publishing research about young people They also should contribute, in whatever ways that they can, to the enhancement of ethical publishing.

References

[1] Ballantyne R. Mental health ethics: the new reality. Journal of Ethics in Mental Health Care 2006;1:1.
[2] Green SA, Bloch S. An anthology of psychiatric ethics. New York: Oxford University Press; 2006.
[3] Robertson M, Walter G. Overview of psychiatric ethics I: profession ethics and psychiatry. Australas Psychiatry 2007;15:201–6.
[4] Walter G, Bloch S. Publishing ethics in psychiatry. Aust N Z J Psychiatry 2001;35:28–35.
[5] Morgan GA, Harmon RJ, Gliner JA. Ethical issues related to publishing and reviewing. J Am Acad Child Adolesc Psychiatry 2001;40:1476–8.
[6] International Committee of Medical Journal Editors. Uniform requirements for manuscripts submitted to biomedical journals: writing and editing for biomedical publication. Available at: http://www.icmje.org. Accessed April 2, 2007.
[7] Committee on Publication Ethics. Available at: http://www.publicationethics.org.uk. Accessed April 2, 2007.
[8] World Association of Medical Editors. Available at: http://www.wame.org. Accessed April 2, 2007.
[9] Council of Science Editors. Available at: http://www.councilscienceeditors.org. Accessed April 2, 2007.
[10] Fister K. At the frontier of biomedical publication. Br Med J 2005;331:838–40.

[11] Jones AH, McLellan F. Ethical issues in biomedical publication. Baltimore (MD): The Johns Hopkins University Press; 2000.

[12] Smith R. The trouble with medical journals. J R Soc Med 2006;99:115–9.

[13] Roberts JG. Publishing in our journals: ethics and honesty. Anaesth Intensive Care 1991;19: 163–4.

[14] Barker KL. Editorial: implementing ethical guidelines for publication of research in Endocrine Society journals. Endocrinology 1994;134:3–4.

[15] Yen H. FDA ex-chief spared jail time. Available at: http://washingtontimes.com/metro/20070228-122725-9081r.htm. Accessed April 22, 2007.

[16] Kelly RE, Cohen LJ, Semple RJ, et al. Relationship between drug company funding and outcomes of clinical psychiatric research. Psychol Med 2006;36:1647–56.

[17] Jureidini JN, Doecke CJ, Mansfield PR, et al. Efficacy and safety of antidepressants for children and adolescents. Br Med J 2006;328:879–83.

[18] Rey JM, Dudley M. Depressed youth, antidepressants and suicide: no reason to panic but an opportunity to improve clinical practice. Med J Aust 2005;182:378–9.

[19] Wakefield A, Murch SH, Anthony A, et al. Ileal-lymphoid-nodular hyperplasia, non-specific colitis, and pervasive development disorder in children. Lancet 1998;351:637–41.

[20] Chew M. What conflict of interest? Med J Aust 2004;181:4–5.

[21] Demicheli V, Jefferson T, Rivetti A, et al. Vaccines for measles, mumps and rubella in children. Cochrane Database Syst Rev 2005;4:CD004407.

[22] Kassirer JP. Assault on editorial independence: improprieties of the Canadian Medical Association. J Med Ethics 2007;33:63–6.

[23] Shuchman M, Redelmeier DA. Politics and independence–the collapse of the Canadian Medical Association Journal. N Engl J Med 2006;354(13):1337–9.

[24] Wilson MH. The CMA's legitimation crisis. Br Med J 2006;332:854.

[25] Moynihan R. Who pays for the pizza? Redefining the relationships between doctors and drug companies. 1: entanglement. Br Med J 2003;326:1189–92.

[26] Rothman KJ. Conflict of interest: the McCarthyism in science. JAMA 1993;269:2782–4.

[27] Gilbody SM, Song F. Publication bias and the integrity of psychiatry research. Psychol Med 2000;30:253–8.

[28] Saxena S, Sharan P, Saraceno B. Research for change: the role of scientific journals publishing mental health research. World Psychiatry 2004;3:66–72.

[29] Goodstein D. Scientific misconduct. Academe 2002;88:28–31.

[30] Gillie O. Crucial data was faked by eminent psychologist. London: Sunday Times; 1976.

[31] Garfield E, Willjams-Dorof A. The impact of fraudulent research on the scientific literature: the Stephen E. Breuning case. J Am Med Assoc 1990;263:1424–6.

[32] Lock S, Wells F. Fraud and misconduct in medical research. 2nd edition. London: BMJ Publishing; 1996.

[33] Breuning SE, Davis VJ, Matson JL, et al. Effects of thioridazine and withdrawal dyskinesias on workshop performance of mentally retarded young adults. Am J Psychiatry 1982;139: 1447–54.

[34] Aman MG, Teehan CJ, White AJ, et al. Haloperidol treatment with chronically medicated residents: dose effect on clinical behavior and reinforcement contingencies. Am J Ment Retard 1989;93:52–60.

[35] Poling A. The consequences of fraud. In: Miller DJ, Hersen M, editors. Research fraud in the behavioral and biomedical sciences. New York: Wiley; 1992. p. 140–57.

[36] Beecher HK. Ethics and clinical research. N Engl J Med 1966;274:1354–60.

[37] World Medical Association. Declaration of Helsinki. J Am Med Assoc 1997;277:925–6.

[38] Hunter E. The snake on the caduceus: dimensions of medical and psychiatric responsibility in the Third Reich. Aust N Z J Psychiatry 1993;27:149–56.

[39] Bogod D. The Nazi hypothermia experiments: forbidden data? Anaesthesia 2004;59:1155–6.

[40] Susser M, Yankauer A. Prior, duplicate, repetitive, fragmented, and redundant publication and editorial decisions. Am J Public Health 1993;83:792–3.

[41] Walter G. Salami: kosher and unkosher [letter]. Aust N Z J Psychiatry 1999;33:766–7.

[42] Abou-Saleh MT, Ghubash R. The prevalence of early postpartum psychiatric morbidity in Dubai: a transcultural perspective. Acta Psychiatr Scand 1997;95:428–32.

[43] Ghubash R, Abou-Saleh MT. Postpartum psychiatric illness in Arab culture: prevalence and psychosocial correlates. Br J Psychiatry 1997;171:65–8.

[44] Kerr A. Original publications. Br J Psychiatry 1998;172:193.

[45] Wilkinson G. Duplicate publication. Br J Psychiatry 1998;172:278.

[46] Claghorn JL, Kiev A, Rickels K, et al. Paroxetine vs. placebo: a double-blind comparison in depressed patients. J Clin Psychiatry 1992;53:434–8.

[47] Dunbar GC, Claghorn JL, Kiev A, et al. A comparison of paroxetine and placebo in depressed outpatients. Acta Psychiatr Scand 1993;87:302–5.

[48] Gelenberg AJ, Ottosson JO. Duplicate publication. J Clin Psychiatry 1995;56:81.

[49] Gelenberg AJ, Ottosson JO. Editorial statement. Acta Psychiatr Scand 1995;91:145.

[50] Schone W, Ludwig M. A double-blind study of paroxetine compared with fluoxetine in geriatric patients with major depression. J Clin Psychopharmacol 1993;13:34S–9S.

[51] Schone W, Ludwig M. Paroxetine in der Depressionalsbehandlung geriatrischer Patienten— eine doppelblinde Vergleichsstudie mit Fluoxetin [German]. Fortschr Neurol Psychiatr 1994;62:16–8.

[52] Geretsegger C, Bohmer F, Ludwig M. Paroxetine in the elderly depressed patient: rando- mised comparison with fluoxetine of efficacy, cognitive and behavioural effects. Int Clin Psychopharmacol 1994;9:25–9.

[53] Shader RI, Greenblatt DJ. Twice may be too many: redundant publications. J Clin Psycho- pharmacol 1996;16:1–2.

[54] Dulcan MK. Editor's note: duplicate or divided publication? J Am Acad Child Adolesc Psychiatry 2004;43:245.

[55] Culliton BJ. Harvard psychiatrist resigns. Science 1988;242:1239–40.

[56] Scahill L, Chappell PB, Kim YS, et al. A placebo-controlled study of guanfacine in the treatment of children with tic disorders and attention deficit hyperactivity disorder. Am J Psychiatry 2001;158:1067–74.

[57] Niederhofer H, Staffen W, Mair A. A placebo-controlled study of lofexidine in the treatment of children with tic disorders and attention deficit hyperactivity disorder. J Psychopharmacol 2003;17:113–9.

[58] Bailey JE. An exceptional case of plagiarism!. J Psychopharmacol 2004;18:291–2.

[59] Rothe EQ, Vega BJ, Torres RM, et al. From kids and horses: equine-facilitated psycho- therapy for children. International Journal of Clinical and Health Psychology 2005;5: 373–83.

[60] Taylor SM. Equine facilitated psychotherapy: an emerging field. Available at: http://www. equnefacilitatedpsychotherapy.org. Accessed April 18, 2007.

[61] Wachslicht-Rodbard H, Gross HA, Rodbard D, et al. Increased insulin binding to erythro- cytes in anorexia nervosa. N Engl J Med 1980;300:882–7.

[62] Soman VR, Felig P. Insulin binding to monocytes and insulin sensitivity in anorexia nervosa. Am J Med 1980;68:66–71.

[63] Broad W, Wade N. Betrayers of the truth. New York: Simon and Schuster; 1982.

[64] Kohn A. False prophets. Oxford (UK): Blackwell; 1986.

[65] Stahl SM, Thiemann S, Faull KF, et al. Neurochemistry of dopamine in Huntington's dementia and normal ageing. Arch Gen Psychiatry 1986;43:161–4.

[66] Stahl SM, Thiemann S, Faull KF, et al. Retraction. Arch Gen Psychiatry 1989;46:758.

[67] Australian and New Zealand Journal of Psychiatry. Instructions for authors. Available at: http://www.tandf.co.uk/journals/authors/ianpauth.pdf. Accessed April 15, 2007.

[68] Fromm-Reichmann F. Notes on the development of treatment of schizophrenics by psycho- analytic psychotherapy. Psychiatry 1948;11:263–73.

[69] Wing L. The history of ideas of autism: legends, myths and realities. Autism 1997;1: 13–24.

[70] Gabbard GO, Williams P. A retraction and apology. A boycott by passport. Int J Psychoanal 2006;87:263.

[71] Farthing MJG. Ethics of publication. In: Hall GM, editor. How to write a paper. London: BMJ Publishing; 1998. p. 122–31.

[72] Nath SB, Marcus SC, Druss BG. Retractions in the research literature: misconduct or mistakes? Med J Aust 2006;185:152–4.

[73] Martinson BC, Andersohn MS, de Vries R. Scientists behaving badly. Nature 2005;435: 737–8.

[74] Spetie L, Arnold LE. Ethical issues in child psychopharmacology research and practice: emphasis on preschoolers. Psychopharmacology (Berl) 2007;191:15–26.

[75] Committee on Publication Ethics. Flow charts. Available at: http://www.publicationethics.org.uk/flow-charts. Accessed April 2, 2007.

[76] Eastwood S. Ethical scientific reporting and publication: training the trainees. In: Jones AH, McLellan F, editors. Ethical issues in biomedical publication. Baltimore (MD): The Johns Hopkins University Press; 2000. p. 250–75.

[77] Whittington J, Kendall T, Fonagy P, et al. Selective serotonin reuptake inhibitors in childhood depression: systematic review of published versus unpublished data. Lancet 2004;363: 1341–5.

[78] World Association of Medical Editors. WAME policy statements: the registration of clinical trials. Available at: http://www.wame.org/resources/policies#trialreg. Accessed April 23, 2007.

[79] Council of Science Editors. CSE endorsement of principles: ICMJE's statement on clinical trial registration. Available at: http://www.councilscienceeditors.org/editorial_policies/endorsementofprinciples.cfm. Accessed April 23, 2007.

[80] World Association of Medical Editors. WAME listserve discussions. Available at: http://www.wame.org/resources/wame-listserve-discussion. Accessed April 2, 2007.

[81] Walter G, Bloch S, Hunt G, et al. Counting on citations: a flawed way to measure quality. Med J Aust 2003;178:280–1.

ELSEVIER
SAUNDERS

Child Adolesc Psychiatric Clin N Am
17 (2008) 165–185

CHILD AND
ADOLESCENT
PSYCHIATRIC CLINICS
OF NORTH AMERICA

Ethical Issues in Local, National, and International Disaster Psychiatry

Paramjit T. Joshi, MD[a],*,
Marc E. Dalton, MD, MPH[a],
Deborah A. O'Donnell, PhD[b]

[a]Department of Psychiatry and Behavioral Sciences, Children's National Medical Center,
111 Michigan Avenue, NW, Washington DC, 20010, USA
[b]Department of Psychology, St. Mary's College of Maryland, 18952 East Fisher Street,
St. Mary's City, MD 20686, USA

Any war, act of terror, or a natural disaster as a sudden, unpredictable, and dramatic event that one is forced to endure has a tremendous negative impact at various levels, including the community, family, and individual. Usually, children are affected most by these experiences and are being exposed to trauma and violence in ever-increasing numbers, resulting in a global epidemic [1]. Exposure to trauma-related events often leads to marked disruptions in the contextual and social fabric within which one lives. Becoming a witness or victim to such acts also stirs an array of powerful human emotions. Regardless of the specific character of any particular war or act of terror, such circumstances, by definition, involve destruction, pain, and death. Although these physical losses can be reconstructed or replaced, with the accompanying pain and sorrow gradually diminishing, the psychological scars the trauma and the horrifying images and memories do not heal as easily. Survival is perhaps most challenging and complex for children whose age and psychological immaturity render them more vulnerable to the effects of overwhelming and inescapable stressors initiated by disastrous events; however, the often-intertwined contributions of psychosocial, economic, political, cultural, religious, and community variables have come to be appreciated as confounding factors having an enormous psychological impact.

* Corresponding author. Department of Psychiatry and Behavioral Sciences, Children's National Medical Center, 111 Michigan Avenue, NW, Washington DC, 20010.
E-mail address: pjoshi@cnmc.org (P.T. Joshi).

1056-4993/08/$ - see front matter © 2008 Elsevier Inc. All rights reserved.
doi:10.1016/j.chc.2007.07.010
childpsych.theclinics.com

Until recent times, little attention has been paid to the psychological well-being of the victims of war, terrorism, and natural disasters. The resulting paucity of psychological interventions often gives rise to feelings of hopelessness and helplessness, increased incidences of alcohol and drug use, delinquency, and conduct problems. These factors have a negative impact on society at large. In an environment characterized by such suffering, deprivation, and violence, the developmental aspects of childhood are severely affected. Sometimes one meets survivors of war or torture who have been victims of terror and relive their trauma, frequently transmitting trauma to the next generation. War veterans, who endure and shoulder the burden of posttraumatic stress for years to come, frequently are being "retraumatized" by recurring terrifying events, such as terrorist attacks [2].

In the last decade there is a more or less circumscribed body of research that brings together the various aspects of trauma work. The recent wars in the Balkans, Afghanistan, and the Middle East and natural events such as a Tsunami and hurricanes are good examples of the array of traumatic global events that result in the victims being displaced from their homes and communities and forced to live in refugee camps or in exile. The situation in other parts of the world, such as South Africa and southeast Asia, also illustrates the strife, war, and trauma that many young lives come to know too well. Because children are not "miniature adults," exposure to persistent violence and danger sets into motion a cascade of effects on normal development, putting them at higher risk for the development of mental illness [3]. In addition to the expected posttraumatic stress reactions, traumatic stress can have an even more insidious impact on children and adolescents, affecting many domains of normal child development (eg, prosocial behavior and citizenship at school, in the home, and in the community). Children who are exposed to war and terrorism simultaneously face the tasks of growing up and confronting numerous losses and traumas. Often, they are pulled in many directions, which distorts or interrupts the developmental process. Teenagers, unlike young children, have developed the ability to think abstractly. Along with this capacity comes an increased focus on religion, morality, and ethics, which can affect their understanding of and response to war and terrorism [3]. Ideas and knowledge have changed and expanded dramatically over the past 50 years. Accordingly, so has our ability to make children's lives better. The ultimate goal is to diminish and ease the psychological impact of such disastrous events.

Rights of children

Few human tragedies stir sympathy and public concern more deeply than seeing children suffer secondary to war or terrorist attacks. The trend to make children targets of atrocities is one of the biggest human tragedies that stirs outrage, while simultaneously mobilizing spontaneous humanitarian impulses of wanting to help, perpetuated by the images in the media of children in anguish and pain [4]. To foster and promote the well-being of individuals worldwide, the General Assembly of the United Nations adopted and proclaimed "The Universal Declaration of Human Rights" on December 10, 1948. This Declaration included 30 Articles. Article 1 states, "All human beings are born free and equal in dignity and human rights. They are endowed with reason and conscience and should act towards one another in a spirit of brotherhood." Article 26 specifically speaks to the rights of children and states: i) "Everyone has the right to education. Education shall be free, at least in the elementary and fundamental stages. Elementary education should be compulsory. Technical and professional education shall be made generally available and higher education shall be equally accessible to all on the basis of merit." ii) "Education shall be directed to the full development of the human personality and to strengthening of respect for human rights and fundamental freedoms. It shall promote understanding, tolerance and friendship among all nations, racial or religious groups, and shall further the activities of the United Nations for the maintenance of peace." iii) "Parents have a prior right to choose the kind of education that shall be given to their children" [5].

Further, the International Covenant on Civil and Political Rights was adopted by the United Nations Session on December 16, 1966 and made operative a decade later on March 23, 1976. Article 6 states "All human beings have the natural right to live, which should be protected by laws, and which they are not to be deprived of." Article 23 states "A family is a natural and basic social unit enjoying the right of being protected by society and a state." Article 23 also states, "Every child, regardless of race, color, gender, language, religion, national or social origin, possession or parentage is entitled to such protective measures provided by his family, society and state, as required by his condition of a minor." Despite the declaration and proclamation of such rights, they continue to be violated constantly in many parts of the world [5].

Ethical dilemmas

Health professionals face numerous challenges when involved in trauma work of any kind; however, mental health professionals, in general, and psychiatrists, in particular, face ethical dilemmas every day. They are in the unique position of fulfilling the roles of a doctor as well as being agents of social control. A psychiatrist, through the authority vested in him/her, has the power to deprive individuals of their liberty and to treat them against their will, for the good of the patient and the public [6]; however, when involved in disaster work, whether it is local, national, or international, other factors play a role, especially those that are social and political in nature. The ability of a psychiatrist to conduct a psychiatric examination and to make a clinical diagnosis, even with current advances in biologic psychiatry, is still heavily influenced by cultural and social norms. This was expressed well by Mechanic [7]:

> "Because psychiatry deals with deviance in feeling states and behavior, its conceptions run parallel to societal conceptions of social behavior, personal worth, and morality. Conceptions of behavior can be viewed from competing vantage points, and thus they are amenable to varying professional stances. In the absence of clear evidence of an etiology or treatment, personal disturbance can be alternatively viewed as biological in nature, as a result of developmental failures, as a moral crisis, or as a consequence of socioeconomic, social or structural constraints. Remedies may be seen in terms of biological restoration, moral realignment, social conditioning or societal change. Although all these elements may be present in the same situation, the one that the psychiatrist emphasizes has both moral and practical implications. There is no completely neutral stance. Diagnostic and therapeutic judgments have political and social implications."

Therefore, it seems unavoidable for anyone involved in trauma work (especially international) to pretend that one works in an ethical and political vacuum. The remainder of this article addresses some of the ethical issues that one should be thinking of when indulging in such trauma work, whether it is local, national, or international.

Confidentiality issues

Issues of confidentiality pose their own unique ethical issues. Although much credence is given to the patient–clinician relationship and confidentiality in the West, this is not a well-understood or respected notion in many other parts of the world. Health Insurance Portability and Accountability Act of 1996 (HIPPA) violations in the West can result in regulatory sanctions against the particular clinician or institution. Conversely, when one is providing such services in a refugee camp, shelter, or war zone, one is faced with interviewing or counseling individuals without such privacy provisions. Trying to balance such issues is a continuing dilemma. The overriding decision-making process rests on "what helps the most" or "what causes less harm." Although providing services under such circumstances is not ideal, at the same time, to listen to a young child or teenager describe his or her harrowing experiences of a traumatic scenario provides validation of that experience, even if it is in the presence of others. In some cultures, parents believe that it is their right to know everything that their child may be sharing with a mental health professional and have no qualms in sharing that with extended family members or friends and teachers. Therefore, it is important to understand the local culture, values, child-rearing practices, and religious influences that might have an impact on how we work with and be helpful to traumatized youngsters.

Issues of autonomy and informed consent

It has been stressed that the well-being of the individual patient is paramount and comes before any other consideration. This makes sense, given the centrality of trust to the doctor–patient relationship. Trust is essential; without it, patients would not wish to abdicate that degree of autonomy that may be necessary for physicians to take any kind of therapeutic action (ie, to put their lives, or at least their well-being, in another person's hands). When it comes to children and adolescents in many parts of the world, this autonomy is not culturally granted to the young, and every decision is based on what the care-taking adult wants. How does one respect the child's right to his/her autonomy while respecting the cultural norms of the society? This is particularly true when dealing with a delicate situation of physical/sexual abuse, substance use, or the revelation of any criminal activity. In many cultures, "the parents often demand to know" and have little regard for the privacy of their child. Further, there may be no statutory rulings that one can "hide behind" as a professional. These moral and ethical issues come up again when children are separated from their parents or caregivers.

Autonomy and informed consent are two ethical imperatives that become complicated and open to interpretation when working in disaster psychiatry. Autonomy is a concept found in moral, political, and bioethical philosophy. Within these contexts it refers to the capacity of a rational individual to make an informed, uncoerced decision. This capacity for informed decision making changes during times of disaster, because it often is impossible to be fully apprised and aware of conditions [8,9]. In medicine, respect for the autonomy of patients is considered obligatory for doctors and other health care professionals. When working in disaster settings, especially in international settings, it is important to recognize the family embeddedness of people and the strict hierarchical structure within many families. From an applied perspective, each family should be regarded as its own cultural unit [10]. An individual's experience of self-determination is also influenced by their culture [11].

Similar ethical issues arise with informed consent. Individuals from cultures with strong oral traditions may be especially confused by all of the written documents [10]. In the context of many developing countries, written informed consent and signing official documents prepared by foreign institutions is a foreign concept and can be unsettling and confusing [12]. Asking participants to sign any document, including an informed consent letter, when they cannot read or fully comprehend its contents can be threatening to participants who only sign or use thumbprints for official documents [13].

The relationship between community consent and individual consent also is essential to consider. Village elders are powerful decision makers and protective units in many societies. Individual village dwellers place tremendous trust and respect in these elders, and it is common for the elders to be held responsible for making decisions that impact village dwellers. In a village, it is important to get permission from the leaders of the community [14]. One way to ensure that the individual is truly capable of making an informed decision is to bring in another party. The community elders provide another level of assurance to villagers in times of disaster and uncertainty [15].

Hospitalization decisions

The decision to hospitalize a patient who has mental illness, whether voluntarily or involuntarily, is a difficult task. Over the years, the argument over preserving the rights of a patient versus the good of others has been a difficult one to undertake. Often, the duty to protect and warn versus the rights of a patient are at odds with one another. Additionally, these discussions usually occur in mainstream society in the context of a tragic event, such as a disaster, child abuse/abduction case, or a workplace/school shooting; however, discussions during these times are highly emotional and only tend to illustrate the lack of knowledge when it comes to mental health treatment and delivery, which can lead to further stigmatization.

The principles of beneficence and utilitarianism are two of the ethical principles that intersect in times of a disaster. Regardless of age, examination of a psychiatric patient during a disaster still requires the examining mental health professional to explore whether the patient is posing harm to him/herself or others and whether the patient has the capacity to make treatment decisions for him/herself. In cases involving children up to 18 years of age, if a parent is available and the examining psychiatrist believes that hospitalization is warranted, the parents and the physician ideally can come to that decision together. The more complex situation arises when there is no parent readily identifiable and psychiatric treatment or hospitalization is warranted. According to the *Ethics Primer of the American Psychiatric Association* [16], the Constitution of the United States provides the legal basis for involuntary hospitalization. Involuntary hospitalization is based on two legal concepts: police power and *parens patriae* power. As stated in the primer:

> "..for the benefit of society, governments are responsible for protecting each citizen from other persons' injurious actions. This is called the police power, and the issue here is dangerousness of the individual and protection of citizens from the individual in question. Second, governments have the power and duty to protect individuals who can not do so themselves. This is the principle of *parens patriae*, when governments are the parent of last resort for each citizen."

The ethics primer is clear in its explanation that the *parens patriae* is a benevolent power so that the government can assume "the care of a disabled person as loyally as a parent would care for a child." One can assume that this would be of paramount importance in times of disaster, given the inherent chaos. This has been illustrated in recent times when disasters, such as tsunamis, earthquakes, and hurricanes, have produced situations where the structure of the family is disrupted because of separation or death of the caregivers of children. In these settings, it may be difficult to identify parents or there may be others who have taken responsibility for children when parents are not available. It is during these times that a physician's medical opinion might allow him/her to step in as a parent to care for a child.

Given the above discussions about hospitalizations, there are additional ethical concerns that arise during a disaster. If hospitalization or treatment is needed, numerous questions need to be explored with regard to delivery of care. The ethical principles of beneficence, informed consent, and confidentiality must be recognized. During times of crisis, numerous volunteer health professionals come to the aid of victims of disaster. Most of those who present to provide care are licensed professionals; however, there is room for fraud and incompetence among those who are treating the vulnerable at this time. Specifically, the question of training and credentialing must be considered. After the 2005 hurricane season, Sen. Barack Obama, D-Ill., introduced the Hurricane Katrina Emergency Health Workforce Act in the Senate [17]. The bill did not become law; however, it addressed some interesting and important ethical questions with regard to providing a competent volunteer health care workforce that protects and is competently able to provide the needed health care in times of disasters. It explored topics such as distribution of a volunteer workforce and licensure of that workforce. The ethical concepts of beneficence and utilitarianism are evoked with respect to delivering quality health/mental health care for children in times of disaster for the good of the society; however, issues regarding informed consent remain. Psychiatric care of children is a highly specialized skill. Having trained physicians and therapists who are skilled at working with children, as opposed to adults, is essential. Additionally, in accordance with *parens patriae*, ensuring that persons who are working with children have had adequate background checks becomes paramount to provide for the safety of the child. Specifically, to provide proper informed consent, there needs to be individuals who are trained in psychiatric medicine to give accurate and appropriate information to parents to ensure that they understand the treatment offered. In the absence of parents, those who assume the care of a child should have the knowledge base to make such decisions or at a minimum have that information readily accessible.

Hospitalization during times of disaster also demands that issues of confidentiality be maintained and that a system for communication between treating facilities be supported. There are many who show up to work with patients during times of disaster, but they all should be educated before their interaction with patients during this difficult time to respect the autonomy of the patient and provide care within the bounds of ethics. As is evident when involved in international trauma work, however, many of the issues raised by Senator Obama are not even considerations, many times leaving victims in the hands of unqualified, unlicensed, and, at times, potentially harmful people. When Western professionals work in areas of the world where there is little regard for the above, how does one ethically and morally deal with such circumstances? To whom does one report any problems? The local government? The military? International watch groups? A recent example that was raised by the Marines working in Iraq had to do with observing young children being exploited by the Iraqi army to work as child labor or even being exploited in other ways. The ethical question is how to address these breaches that would be immoral and illegal in the West.

The other vexing problem arises when mass evacuation occurs in the same country, as in the United States after natural disasters (eg, hurricanes). All states require medical professionals to be licensed in their state. How does a physician write prescriptions when not licensed in the state to which he/she has been deployed to assist the victims? There are no federal laws that govern this. Telemedicine faces the same challenges. The Canadian health system and the Armed Forces of the United States have been able to overcome these issues by having protocols addressing these situations.

Ethical considerations when working internationally or with political refugees

Various paradigms have been used to understand the ethical issues that are involved in disaster work with international and refugee populations. Sociocultural perspectives on disaster impact emphasize the extent to which disaster victims' sense of identity suffers as a result of the loss of familiar surroundings, jobs, and social networks. This is especially true for political refugees. The violence-induced identity shifts that many refugees experience can be exacerbated by severed social bonds. This can translate into anger and distrust, but usually ultimately gives way to the creation of new connections and the rebuilding of social bonds [18]. Systemic perspectives focus on the ways that organizations and societies exhibit stress responses in the face of disaster in terms of immediate and delayed reactions [19].

Other clinicians have constructed a transcultural framework as the basis for analysis of the ethics of disaster work through the use of a common language for ethical analysis. This framework consists of eight steps of structured ethical evaluation, including listing ethical arguments for the proposed action, defining the most important ethical principle in the situation, defining potential harm or hurt, and considering how much time is available to accumulate information about these ethical questions. This ethical decision-making process should be used for autonomy, nonmaleficence, beneficence, and justice [10].

The inclusion of local clinicians and researchers in international disaster work is central to intervention success. Collaboration with these local peoples, however, gives rise to unique ethical considerations when working with political refugee populations. In refugee communities, a clinician can inadvertently be perceived as being associated with a feared or despised group. Clinicians also must be sensitive to the potential risk that they put people at by asking questions [20]. The befriending of locals may make one's departure more stressful for the community [8]. Unintended consequences of such interactions may not become apparent until long after the clinician has left, making the dictate to "do no harm" difficult to control [20].

Conceptualizations of illness and trauma

Cultural frameworks for understanding disease

From a phenomenological perspective, the way that people conceptualize and express the nature of their distress and illness has implications for their experience of self and other. Exploring this conceptual discourse can serve as a means of entry into the models that diverse peoples use to make sense of emotional and psychological problems. This exploration better allows for culturally sensitive intervention, especially in times of disaster. Explanatory models of illness organize symptoms and beliefs about causation, associated psychological processes, precipitating situations, and treatment alternatives [21,22]. These models also influence attitudes toward mental health services. In addition, views of the self as independent or interdependent are culturally embedded and can impact health messages, health values, and help-seeking behaviors [23]. Because the trauma response often involves alteration in self in the context of an impaired society, collectivism and individualism become important worldviews to distinguish.

To be effective in promoting health behaviors, intervention strategies must take into account social, cultural, and economic reasons for current practices, including local understandings of risk and the corresponding actions that are seen as helpful in countering risks [24]. For example, many studies have found that people will diagnose an illness based more on the circumstances under which they fell ill than on the actual symptoms of the illness [25]. Ideas about what is valued, what behaviors should be engaged in and avoided, and the rules of social interaction are encoded in culture [26]. Ethical practice dictates that disaster psychiatrists should work to the best of their abilities to educate themselves on cultural understandings of illness and apply this knowledge in their clinical work.

An especially important ethical consideration in international and political refugee trauma work involves the inclusion of religion in mental health discourse [27]. Although this type of spirituality-based approach often is seen as inappropriate in Western medicine, religious sources of strength are central to many worldviews. This can engender confusion and misunderstanding in clinicians who are unfamiliar with local customs and practices [10]. Such local values may involve status differentials based on gender, age, and education that are displeasing to the clinician. Local understandings of illness also make it important for disaster psychiatrists to remember that the diagnosis of posttraumatic stress disorder (PTSD) implicitly follows a Western ontology and value system that may be inappropriate in categorizing the suffering of international residents or political refugees [28,29]. In this regard, the challenges and dilemmas that one faces have to do with how the same symptoms of PTSD may be identified to have divergent meanings in different societies. In some cultures, for example, nightmares may convey messages from ancestors. Survivor guilt may be seen as an essential preliminary to ritual reparations for the dead. Making the diagnosis of PTSD may pathologize coping strategies that are essential to survival [6]. Hypervigilance, especially in a war or terrorist situation, can help an individual to distinguish an incoming from an outgoing bomb, for example, and may mean the difference between life and death. Numbing and denial also may allow a person to endure and muster the psychological strength necessary to deal with the immediate aftermath of a horrific event, as well as make possible courageous acts of nonviolent resistance. While avoiding the complexities of political and social causation, one might argue that the creation of a construct, such as PTSD, and of psychological therapies, such as debriefing, answer the needs of mental health workers to make an immediate response to suffering and helps to maintain detached objectivity that is the professional ideal [6].

Clinical issues

Clinical issues relate to the intervention process itself, diagnostic and assessment issues, and triage in the immediate aftermath of a disaster. Clinical work is made complex by the sometimes conflicting goals of immediate intervention and long-term healing. Tradeoffs often exist between the interests of present and future people [30]. Most trauma symptom inventories are based on Western populations. The construct validity of many Western-based survey tools is questionable when used in non-Western contexts [8]. There is a need for the development, validation, and implementation of culturally adapted symptom inventories and other diagnostic scales and measures. Several of these scales were developed recently by organizations such as the International Psycho-social and Socio-Ecological Research Institute-Uganda, International Rehabilitation Council for Torture Victims-Malawi, and the World Health Organization [31]. When working to clinically diagnose and classify psychopathology, it is best to screen for a spectrum of disorders with continuous scales of measurement, especially because Western diagnostic categories may not apply [29].

Clinicians also should be aware of the many indigenous practices and beliefs in international settings. Indigenous clinicians may have differing understandings of a client's condition, diagnosis, and appropriate treatment approaches. In this respect, clinicians may experience role confusion and ambiguity [27].

It is important to consider the resilience-building aspects that are inherent in most indigenous belief and healing frameworks [29]. Indigenous approaches are characterized often by spontaneously generated therapeutic community interventions. Some indigenous belief systems place importance on deceased ancestors, pollution, animism, and human ill wishers. Indigenous ritual is central to healing. Dreams and visions often are experienced as illuminating and cleansing [32].

Clinicians involved in disaster work have wondered whether combining Western and indigenous approaches to treatment could dilute both, serving to diminish efficacy and potentially confuse the client. In attempting to reconcile different healing frameworks, interventionists may compromise treatment standards [8,32]. In efforts to bridge communication gaps, children sometimes have been used as interpreters. This practice should be avoided whenever possible, because it is not clinically efficacious to put a vulnerable child between a clinician and his or her non-English–speaking parents, especially in situations of organized violence [33].

Multiple unique ethical considerations arise when working with political refugees or evacuees, as opposed to victims of natural disaster. Family members may have different wants regarding repatriation [33]. Disaster clinicians may be called to treat perpetrators who also are victims, creating moral issues for the clinician. These victims-turned-perpetrators represent the reproduction of oppression in the oppressed themselves. These separate characteristics of being a victim and a perpetrator can confuse clinicians and make them feel uncomfortable [27].

Disaster psychiatry should be sensitive to the cultural bases of trauma that involve the role of social support in trauma recovery, the importance of understanding the systems of meaning within which victims' experiences are embedded, and appreciation of ethnicity [32]. This framework emphasizes the personal impact of interpersonal violence, making the distinction between sociopolitical questions and clinical ones murky. Notions of intergenerational trauma and "unspeakability" also must be considered [27].

In disaster work, it often is helpful for the clinician to relabel victims as survivors. An individual's very identity, complete with the multiple layers of internal and external forces, needs to be targeted in this kind of work. Trauma healing involves cultural constructions of traumatic memory and healing on individual and collective levels [27].

Clinical competence and cultural competence

Another important, but frequently overlooked, aspect of the ethics of disaster psychiatry involves the mental health status of clinicians. Because the horrors of disaster can result in vicarious traumatization among health professionals and journalists who are working in war zones [34], it is important for these professionals to monitor their own internal state closely, develop resilient coping strategies, and be strong enough to recognize and admit when the stresses of disaster work have become too much.

Conducting research

Where does research fit into trauma and disaster work? The prime objective in trauma work should not be gathering research data, regardless of how important that might be; however, most academic centers have a tripartite mission of providing clinical care, teaching, and doing research. Although research has an important role in the identification of new and innovative approaches to any kind of work, for it to be the primary motive and objective in this kind of situation is not appealing to the recipients of these interventions. Research methodology can always be built into any evaluation and intervention strategies or programs that are put into place, with the prime objective of being of assistance to the affected population, rather than selfish motives of obtaining research data and furthering one's own academic cause. This certainly raises ethical and moral dilemmas for any academician who is involved in such work [4].

At the same time, it is our responsibility to disseminate knowledge through research and scientific publications. This becomes a tricky balance at times; however, if the priorities are assessed in the right order, one would seldom run into these difficulties. One needs to be sensitive about the feelings of our colleagues. Again, it is equally important that any team or group of professionals that is going into an area to do consultations or provide workshops keeps in mind the local professionals who need to be pulled into their framework and their expertise used. They need to respect their professional identities and maintain a professional, but friendly and understanding, relationship [4].

We continue to be challenged in this manner and be held responsible to find ways to implement appropriate interventions, seek newer therapies, and advance knowledge by training, supervision, and teaching others. In addition, we need to continue to strive in helping evaluate the various interventions and treatment strategies and disseminate knowledge through written materials and supporting educational materials.

The ethics of professionalism and political neutrality

Several ethical codes have been developed over the years in different parts of the world to guide physicians in their work. These were summarized by Bloch and Chodoff [35]: (1) "whatever houses I may visit I will come for the benefit of the sick, remaining free of all intentional injustice"; (2) "the health of my patient will be my first consideration" and that "'considerations of religion, nationality, race, party politics, or social standing' should not intervene between my duty and my patient"; and 3) the Hippocratic Oath states that a doctor should "keep his patients from harm and injustice." Unlike the Hippocratic Oath, the emphasis in the former Soviet Physicians' Oath did not demand paramount loyalty to the individual but did include a commitment "to be guided by the principles of Communist morality, ever to bear in mind the high calling of the Soviet physician, and of my responsibility to the people and the Soviet statue." Medical students in the Soviet Union were required to take political studies and "to be well acquainted with the principles of Marxism-Leninism" [35]. Communist Party Membership was an absolute requirement if one wished to rise in the medical hierarchy.

In 1983, in response to abuses of psychiatry in the Soviet Union, a more specific injunction in the Declaration of Hawaii was produced by the World Psychiatric Association. Section 7 states that "the psychiatrist must never use his professional possibilities to violate the dignity or human rights of any individual or group and should never let inappropriate personal desire, feelings, prejudices or beliefs interfere with the treatment" [35]. One of the defining characteristics of a profession, as opposed to a trade, is the existence of such codes [36]. All of these codes stress the most important and overriding responsibility of a physician to the well-being of the individual patient responsibility that is to be taken seriously and not to be abdicated under any circumstances. Ultimately, the profession asks for public trust based on these codes.

There is a widely held view among those doing psychosocial work that, in some way, political ignorance confers political neutrality and that this is desirable. It is these assumptions and the vexed relationship between politics and professional practice that presents a huge dilemma and also confusion about the role of the mental health professional engaged in such work. One should consider whether a position of political neutrality is valid or practical when doing psychosocial work with survivors of such events. Although political neutrality theoretically is of the utmost importance, often, the total life situation of a victim requires intervention, including one's legal status, financial situation, and spiritual life. By engaging in these multiple modalities of healing, a clinician may need to practice active nonneutrality [31]. On one hand, political neutrality poses problems that arise when mental health professionals identify themselves with a particular political ideology. The contradiction between the demand for neutrality and a commitment to a person's well-being should be explored, as well as the difficulties and consequences of sustaining a value-free position. A tendency to focus on individual psychology, while ignoring political and social context, may seem to confer neutrality, but may have adverse psychological and political consequences. When faced with problems such as genocide and ethnic cleansing, is neutrality even possible? For those involved in trauma work, political literacy and an acknowledgment of one's subjectivity is essential. Psychosocial programs should examine the long-term political consequences of their work as well as the short-term humanitarian impact.

The Nazi practice of achieving mental hygiene through murder and the ethnic cleansing in the Balkans and other parts of the world are some of the most frightening examples of what can follow when there is close identification of the practice of psychiatry with a particular ideology, as was the practice of psychiatry in the former Soviet Union. Bloch [37] argued that many such abuses were made possible with this politicization of psychiatry. For example, minor behavioral changes were encompassed in the broadening of the diagnosis of schizophrenia. This made it possible to use involuntary hospitalization and treatment as a means of controlling political dissent. In 1983, anticipating expulsion, the Soviet Psychiatric Society withdrew from the World Psychiatric Association. Before readmission in 1989, the Society acknowledged "… that previous political conditions created an environment in which psychiatric abuse occurred for non-medical, including political, reasons" [34].

These are extreme examples; however, they highlight what can happen when doctors, for ideological reasons, put their loyalty to a collective above their loyalty to a patient. Jones [6] argued that such examples seem to suggest that the solution lies in political neutrality. Yet political neutrality tends to suggest ethical neutrality, and the fact is that the practice of medicine cannot be either if it is to act out completely the values underlying the codes of conduct. The American Medical Association stated that "a physician shall respect the law and also recognize a responsibility to participate in activities contributing to an improved community" [34]. In its annotations for the psychiatric profession, the American Psychiatric Association pointed out that civil disobedience in protest against social injustice may be acceptable. All of these statements suggest a need for public action in pursuit of the well-being of the patient, and it is hard to see how any such action can be value-free or apolitical. The existence of ethical codes of conduct actually denotes the existence of a framework of values [36].

Value systems in psychiatry

In the last decade or so there have been remarkable scientific advancements in the field of psychiatry and behavioral sciences. Psychiatric genetics and procedures, such as neuroimaging and functional MRIs, continue to unravel the mysteries of how we think, feel, and behave. Discovery of newer psychotherapeutic agents and evidence-based therapies have contributed to better care of our patients; however, despite these cutting-edge scientific advances, therapeutic decisions in present-day psychiatry are no less value laden, as is reflected in different kinds of care to different populations. Moreover, as London [38] pointed out, therapists have their own personal value systems. In developing a therapeutic alliance with the patient there is always the underlying possibility that the therapists make implicit comparisons between themselves and their values and those of their patients. So how does one suspend one's own beliefs completely and become morally neutral? Is that even possible? This becomes even more pertinent when working in an international setting that is laden with differing religious, geopolitical, ethnic, and cultural values.

To many, aggression, for example, is akin to "fever of unknown origin." Although for decades it was associated primarily with a diagnosis of oppositional defiant disorder or conduct disorder, it is now clear that aggression, especially of the impulsive kind, can be associated with several other *Diagnostic and Statistical Manual of Mental Disorders* (DSM) diagnoses, such as schizophrenia, bipolar disorder, major depression, PTSD, attention-deficit/hyperactivity disorder, and substance use disorder [39]. It also is associated frequently with adverse psychosocial environments, including unsatisfactory family relationships and failure at school. The World Health Organization *International Statistical Classification of Diseases, 10th Revision* guidelines [40] define conduct disorder as "repetitive and persistent pattern of dissocial, aggressive, or defiant conduct [which] should amount to major violations of age appropriate social expectations." This is a description of unacceptable social behavior, as much as it is a psychiatric disorder; however, based on the mental health professional's value system, it is very possible that in many parts of the world, such behaviors are viewed entirely reflecting the person's moral compass. Many youth end up in the juvenile justice system deprived of appropriate therapeutic interventions and treatment. Conversely, others view aggression as a symptom of what many might consider a "bona fide" psychiatric diagnosis. The practical, social, and moral implications of making the diagnosis are clear: the diagnosis may save a child from being excluded from school, because he or she "has a psychiatric problem," and may change sentencing policy in court. Others can argue that doing so provides the youngster with a way to escape responsibility for antisocial acts. This is the same debate that is waged when one country defines aggressive citizens as "freedom fighters," whereas another country views them as "terrorists."

Even if most agree that it is possible, in many areas of psychiatry, to make a diagnosis and decisions about therapy based only on the person's symptoms and signs and our scientific knowledge, one cannot ignore the values that medical and mental health professionals bring to bear. By deliberately ignoring the political and social context in which these symptoms and signs emerge, we may actively contribute to an environment that is harmful to the individual [41].

Dilemmas of psychosocial work

The term "psychosocial" was used first by the sociologist F.W. Moore, who stated that "there are also psychosocial phenomena such as language, customs, rights, religion, etc. arising from the action of social elements with or upon the individual mind" [42]. One might argue that the concept of the term "psychosocial" is deliberately constructed to embrace the social context to make it more acceptable and, hence, circumvent the stigma around mental health. Although some involved in the psychosocial work of trauma may acknowledge social and political causation, they tend to focus on the psychological impact of such trauma and develop and recommend psychological therapies, rather than discuss or engage with the social and political world [6].

This attitude is echoed often in the general public's response to the psychological problems caused by war. For example, in response to the severe sanctions that were levied against Iraq after the first Gulf War, Iraqi children (almost half of the population of Iraq) were becoming even more traumatized because of malnutrition, deprivation, and near-famine conditions [6]. Would such psychosocial efforts restore normality in the population affected without the ability or will to have an impact on political/governmental decisions? These are examples of the many moral and ethical dilemmas that we face in doing psychosocial work.

Mental health professionals working in many war-torn areas of the world often have believed that most of the psychological problems of the victims would be resolved if Western governments would use political and military muscle and lift the siege of the city [43]. The work of local and international aid agencies and nongovernmental organizations also is affected by social and political agendas that have implications of which we should be aware. Even in different parts of the same country, such as the United States, aid efforts after natural disasters, for example, are dictated by local and federal guidelines, which often do not work well together. As a result, there are gaps as well as overlap in services, resulting in the wasting of precious resources. As mental health professionals, we need to be aware of these challenges and make informed choices as to what would be in the best interests of the population at risk.

In developing psychosocial intervention programs, it is extremely important to value the local cultural and religious practices, putting aside one's own biases and prejudice or beliefs. In some cultures, great emphasis is placed on exploring ways to interrupt the cycle of violence, trauma, and war to protect the next generation of children. The nonviolent movement promoted by Mahatma Gandhi in India, which ultimately led to the ousting of British dominance, has been adopted by many. In such situations, emphasis is placed on children learning nonviolent ways of resolving disputes and conflicts. The Government of Sri Lanka, along with United Nations International Children's Emergency Fund (UNICEF), developed one such program, called Education for Conflict Resolution (ECR), taking into account the traditional Hindu and Buddhist values of that country. This method of conflict resolution, views aggression and passivity as two polar extremes. This approach advocates a better and more effective middle ground assertiveness. Buddhism is in synch with this approach and favors this middle path, which was adopted easily by the government, school personnel, trainers, and parents alike. In recent years, the West also has adopted some of these activities that incorporate Eastern ethnic and religious practices, such as the extensive use of meditation and yoga. The ECR program incorporated meditation, although not for religious purposes. The goal was to calm and concentrate the mind to create a sense of inner peace. For example, a typical lesson for school children starts with meditation and then covers issues such as decision making and conflict resolution [6].

After any traumatic event many questions are raised: "Why did this happen?", "Will it happen again?", "Who is responsible?", and "How do we stop it?" Often, as mental health providers, we do not have the answers to such questions. Children often ask "Is God angry at me?" or "Is it my fault that bad things happened?" Avoiding such questions inhibits the possibility of doing good therapeutic work, but there is a dilemma about how best to answer. Therefore, it is important at that time to remain problem focused. In this situation, does honesty and transparency about one's own views help or cause distrust? Personal views should not be imposed nor volunteered at any time. Opaqueness on the part of therapists may increase their own feeling of being in control. A willingness to discuss and acknowledge one's own views and to confront issues of power and authority remain an ethical dilemma. In the case of war or terrorist activities, this becomes even more complicated if you, as the professional, happen to be from a country that is viewed by the traumatized youngsters as their "enemy."

We live in the era of instant messaging, information technology, and cyberspace and are exposed to events as they unfold; we are bound to have some kind of prejudices as to why such events are occurring. It is important to acknowledge one's subjective opinions and feelings, since such prejudices often affect one's perception of and response to the very people whom we try to help. Therefore, it might be better to acknowledge one's subjective opinions. If they are acknowledged, they are easier to put aside. With psychosocial work it is inherent that, one engages with the social issues that impact on a person's mental health. Therefore, one has a duty to be psychologically sensitive, politically literate, and well informed; otherwise, one cannot fully understand the problems or the most effective treatment for one's patients. Moreover, attempts to remain neutral in the face of genocide or terrorist attacks are likely to be construed as tacit collaboration with the aggressor and interfere with effective therapeutic work. This invariably raises the question of how to work with those who one perceives as the perpetrators of such crimes. There is no easy answer to this dilemma, except to say that pretending to moral and political neutrality do everyone a disservice [6].

The challenges of traumatic memories

One of the most frightening and challenging aspects of trauma work is the degree of the victims' ability to sustain their own version of the truth. It becomes even more imperative to stress the need for political literacy. This has been well documented and captured in Simon Wiesenthal's [44] memories of Secret Service men cynically admonishing prisoners:

> "However this war may end, we have won the war against you; none of you will be left to bear witness, but even if someone were to survive, the world will not believe him. ...There will be no certainties because we will destroy the evidence together with you. And even if some proof should remain and some of you survive, people will say that the events you describe are too monstrous to be believed: they will say that they are the exaggerations of Allied propaganda and will believe us who will deny everything and not you. We will be the ones to dictate history."

One can draw some parallels from work with physically and sexually abused children. In many cases, when there are not two witnesses, the perpetrator is not prosecuted because of lack of evidence. This impunity leaves the child with a feeling of not being believed that increases his or her sense of powerlessness and lack of worth. Therapy becomes difficult and often ineffective and the process of forgiveness and reconciliation impossible. One cannot forgive what is not acknowledged [6].

Similarly when working with patients who have suffered political abuses, such as torture, rape, siege, and genocide, therapista often are faced with patients who want to know if their stories are believed, and whether we, as therapists, are able to provide some degree of validation for the events that have destroyed their lives. In making such a judgment about external reality we will be making a political choice. Therefore, neutrality is not a possibility. If we do believe them, they will want to know what actions we and they could take to give such events meaning.

Lykes [45] wrote that "impunity rewrites the past, purging it of the reign of torture, disappearance, and rape." Although it protects the perpetrators, it interferes with the possibility of individual and social reparation. Usually, patients see more value in recounting their stories for the media and publication than telling them in a therapy session, "for it is publication not therapy that creates history" [6].

Ethical responsibility of preventing children from becoming socialized to violence

Destruction forces the uprooting of hundreds of thousands of people, leading to increased unemployment and poverty and overall changes in the complexion of the community. The most pronounced of these community-level changes include shifted priorities of the social welfare, health, and educational systems; loss of community balance and distortion of typical community value systems; and increased prejudice and social rigidity toward other groups.

Three phenomena have been identified in children who are exposed to persistent and extreme violence: fear, aggression, and desensitization. Fear has the potential and capacity to paralyze children and negatively affect their emotional growth. Increases in aggressive behavior or changes in attitudes and values favor the use of aggression to solve conflicts, especially among adolescents. There is some evidence suggesting that exposure to increased levels of violence leads to decreased sensitivity to violence and a greater propensity to tolerate increasing levels of aggression and violence [46]. Reinforcement for aggressive acts, in the form of material and nonmaterial rewards, also increases the probability of aggressive response among youth [47]. In adolescents, advances in abstract thought and self-focus facilitate feelings of disenchantment and a sense of being unappreciated and unwanted, leaving them vulnerable to the influence of militant adults and governments that recruit them as pupils of war, glorifying their acts of terror. Such youth are made to feel important with a purpose in life, albeit a destructive and dangerous one [46].

In such states of violence, children are sometimes armed to fight in insurgent or counterinsurgency forces, exploited in the labor force, and thrust into political and social spheres that are not intended for the young [48]. Sadly, many of these children who are socialized to violence remain violent and unaccepted by society long after wars have ended. For example, in postwar South Africa, now-grown children who in the 1980s entered into sustained military action must suddenly shed their political military past, upon which so much of their identities have formed, and face lost educational and career opportunities, estranged families, and a high risk for substance abuse and criminal activity [48]. Collectively, we bear added burden and responsibility to minimize the moral and ethical dilemmas that young people face under such circumstances, for it is only in doing so that we might hope to end repeated cycles of intergenerational violence.

Summary

A common consensus that children should not suffer because of adult inability to live in peace has become part of a global commitment to human rights. Yet, much compelling evidence exists informing us that children who are exposed to acts of war and terrorism are placed at risk for the development of multiple and sometimes protracted forms of biopsychosocial maladjustment. Children, as the unwitting and innocent recipients of these horrific consequences, are best understood as possessing normal, expected reactions to horribly abnormal events. Full recovery often involves living through a difficult process of relearning on physiologic, psychologic, and social levels how to understand the world without the constant threat of fear, hostility, and danger [46]. This knowledge brings with it an imperative to learn more about how such trauma, from one generation to the next, causes illness and behavioral disorders, lying dormant in the psyche and later spreading as destructively as a latent virus.

Therefore, peace-building may be the central effort in preventing irrational violence that plagues our children all around the world; however, the challenge that we face as mental health professionals is how psychosocial interventions can be implemented while being acutely aware of the many ethical, moral, and professional dilemmas that we encounter. Love and respect for children are key elements to humanitarian and political progress. Many of today's most intractable disputes, for all of the ethnic or religious character that they acquire, are at heart, struggles for resources and for survival. The urgency now is to vastly enhance the means to prevent future conflicts and to better support victims. Today's problems of poverty and violence will never subside unless we invest in the physical, mental, and emotional development of the next generation. Averting future conflicts will require caring for the youngest victims of war, terror and trauma as well as educating them for peace.

References

[1] Joshi PT. Childhood trauma [editorial]. Int Rev Psychiatry 1998;10:173–4.

[2] Joshi PT, O'Donnell DA. Consequences of child exposure to war and terrorism. Clin Child Fam Psychol Rev 2003;6(4):275–92.

[3] Joshi PT, Lewin SM. Disaster, terrorism and children. Psychiatr Ann 2004;34:710–6.

[4] Joshi PT. Guidelines for international trauma work. Int Rev Psychiatry 1998;10:179–85.

[5] United Nations Department of Public Information: DPI/1653/HR/Reprint: 96–23492, October 1996.

[6] Jones L. The question of political neutrality when doing psychosocial work with survivors of political violence. Int Rev Psychiatry 1998;10:230–47.

[7] Mechanic D. The social dimension. In: Bloch S, Chodoff P, editors. Psychiatric ethics. New York: Oxford University Press; 1991. p. 41–52.

[8] Jacobsen K, Landau LB. The dual imperative in refugee research: some methodological and ethical considerations in social science research on forced migration. Disasters 2003;27(3): 185–206.

[9] LaGreca AM, Silverman WK, Vernberg EM, et al. Helping children cope with disasters and terrorism. Washington, DC: American Psychological Association; 2002.

[10] Bjorn GJ, Bjorn A. Ethical aspects when treating traumatized refugee children and their families. Nord J Psychiatry 2004;58:193–8.

[11] American Psychiatric Association. Disaster psychiatry handbook. Washington, DC: American Psychiatric Foundation; 2004.

[12] Kelley SD. A contextualized approach to IRB review for collaborative international research. Ethics Behav 2002;12(4):372–5.

[13] Upvall M, Hashwani S. Negotiating the informed-consent process in developing countries: a comparison of Swaziland and Pakistan. Int Nurs Rev 2001;48:188–92.

[14] Marshall P. Facing ethical dilemmas of international research. Celveland, OH: Department of Bioethics, Case Western Reserve University; 2003.

[15] Schrag B. Commentary on crossing cultural barriers: informed consent in developing countries. Celveland, OH: Ethics Center for Engineering and Science, Case Western Reserve University; 2004.

[16] American Psychiatric Association. Ethics primer. 2001 edition. Arlington (VA): American Psychiatric Association; 2001.

[17] Hurricane Katrina Emergency Health Workforce Act of 2005. Available at: http://www.govtrack.us/congress/bill.xpd?bill=s109-1638. Accessed May 1, 2007.

[18] Mekki-Berrada A, Rousseau C, Bertot J. Research on refugees: means of transmitting suffering and forging social bonds. Int J Ment Health 2001;30(2):41–57.

[19] American Psychological Association Policy and Planning Board. APA's response to international and national disasters and crises: addressing diverse needs. Am Psychol 2006;61(5): 513–21.

[20] Leaning J. Ethics of research in refugee populations. Lancet 2001;357:1432–3.

[21] Kleinman A, Good B. Culture and depression. Berkeley (CA): University of California Press; 1985.

[22] Manson SM. Culture and depression: discovering variations in the experience of illness. In: Lonner WJ, Malpass RS, editors. Psychology and culture. Boston: Allyn & Bacon; 1998. p. 285–90.

[23] Murphy S. A mile away and a world apart: the impact of interdependent and independent views of the self on US-Mexican communications. In: Power JG, Byrd T, editors. U.S.-Mexico border health: issues for regional and migrant populations. Thousand Oaks (CA): Sage Publications; 1998. p. 3–30.

[24] Winch PJ, Alam MA, Afsana A. Local understandings of vulnerability and protection during the neonatal period in Sylhet district Bangladesh: a qualitative study. Lancet 2005;366: 475–85.

[25] Winch PJ, Makemba AM, Kamazima SR, et al. Seasonal variation in the perceived risk of malaria: implications for the promotion of insecticide-impregnated bed nets. Soc Sci Med 1994;39(1):63–75.

[26] Reese L, Gallimore R. Immigrant Latino's cultural models of literacy development: an evolving perspective on home-school discontinuities. American Journal of Education 2001;108:103–36.

[27] Swartz L, Drennan G. The cultural construction of healing in the truth and reconciliation commission: implications for mental health practice. Ethn Health 2000;5(3):205–13.

[28] Chaitin J. I wish he hadn't told me that: methodological and ethical issues in social trauma and conflict research. Qual Health Res 2003;13(8):1145–54.

[29] Pillay BJ. Providing mental health services to survivors: a Kwa Zulu-Natal perspective. Ethn Health 2000;5(3):269–72.

[30] Glantz M, Jamieson D. Societal response to Hurricane Mitch and intra- versus intergenerational equity issues: whose norms should apply? Risk Anal 2000;20(6):869–82.

[31] Peltzer K. A process model of ethnocultural counseling for African survivors of organized violence. Couns Psychol Q 2001;12(4):335–51.

[32] Eagle GT. Promoting peace by integrating western and indigenous healing in treating trauma. Peace and Conflict 1998;4(3):271–82.

[33] Bjorn GJ. Ethics and interpreting in psychotherapy with refugee children and families. Nord J Psychiatry 2005;59:516–21.

[34] Hawryluck L, Gold WL, Robinson S, et al. SARS control and psychological effects of quarantine, Toronto, Canada. Emerg Infect Dis 2004;10(7):1206–12.

[35] Bloch S, Chodoff P, editors. Psychiatric ethics. Oxford (UK): Oxford University Press; 1991.

[36] Dyer A. Psychiatry as a profession. In: Bloch S, Chodoff P, editors. Psychiatric ethics. Oxford (UK): Oxford University Press; 1991. p. 6–76.

[37] Bloch S. Political misuse of psychiatry. In: Bloch S, Chodoff P, editors. Psychiatric ethics. Oxford (UK): Oxford University Press; 1991. p. 492–501.

[38] London, P. The modes and morals of psychotherapy. In: Holt, Rinehart & Winston, editors. New York: 1964. p. 12–13.

[39] Jensen PS, Youngstrom EA, Steiner H, et al. Consensus report on impulsive aggression as a symptom across diagnostic categories in child psychiatry: implications for medication studies. J Am Acad Child Adolesc Psychiatry 2007;16:309–22.

[40] World Health Organization. The ICD-10 classification of mental and behavioral disorders: clinical descriptions and diagnostic guidelines. Geneva (Switzerland): WHO; 1992.

[41] Gilbert GN, Mulkay M. A sociological analysis of scientist's discourse. Cambridge (MA): Cambridge University Press; 1984.

[42] Oxford English dictionary. 2nd edition. vol. xii 1989. Prepared by. JA Simpson, ESC Weiner. Oxford (UK): Clarendon Press.

[43] Jones L. Letter from Sarajevo: on a front line. Br Med J 1995;1052.

[44] Wiesenthal S. The murderers amongst us. New York: McGraw Hill; 1967.

[45] Lykes MB. Human rights and mental health in the United States: lessons from Latin America. J Soc Issues 1990;46:151–65.

[46] Joshi PT, O'Donnell DA, Cullins LM, et al. Children exposed to war and terrorism. In: Feerick MM, Silverman GB, editors. Children exposed to violence. Baltimore, MD: Paul H. Brookes; 2006.

[47] Bandura A. Social learning theory of aggression. J Commun 1978;28:12–29.

[48] Feldman A. X-children and the militarization of everyday life: comparative comments on the politics of youth, victimage and violence in transitional societies. International Journal of Social Welfare 2002;11:286–99.

ELSEVIER
SAUNDERS

Child Adolesc Psychiatric Clin N Am
17 (2008) 187–207

CHILD AND
ADOLESCENT
PSYCHIATRIC CLINICS
OF NORTH AMERICA

Ethics Education

Arden D. Dingle, MD[a],*, Margaret L. Stuber, MD[b]

[a]Child and Adolescent Psychiatry, Emory University School of Medicine,
1256 Briarcliff Road #317 South, Atlanta, GA 30306, USA
[b]UCLA Department of Psychiatry & Biobehavioral Sciences, UCLA Neuropsychiatric
Hospital, 760 Westwood Plaza, Los Angeles, CA 90095-1759, USA

Producing ethical and professional graduates and practitioners has been a fundamental tenet of medical education throughout its history. Ethics is the discipline that describes a code of moral principles or values. The ethics of medicine generally has concerned itself with upholding the beliefs of prioritizing the patient's best interests and societal good while respecting the patient's rights as a person. The ethics of medicine remains an essential area of medical practice, although many now include it in the concept and practice of professionalism, which is a broader term. There are several definitions of professionalism by various medical organizations. All share basic commonalities that describe the qualities and behaviors of a virtuous person who practices medicine. The attributes of professionalism include subordinating one's own interests to those of patients, adhering to high ethical and moral standards, responding to societal needs, being humanistic and accountable, demonstrating a commitment to excellence and scholarship, and being responsible. Recently, medical education has begun to develop and implement more explicit educational standards and benchmarks for these aspects of medical practice. Part of the motivation for these standards has been concern that today's medical students and physicians are not living up to the expectations and trust of the profession and society that physicians will provide the best care possible and put the patient first. Additionally, several educators have documented that trainees tend to develop more cynicism and negative attitudes as they progress through their medical education, with what seems to be a decline in their moral standards. Currently, all accredited American and Canadian medical schools and residencies are required to teach ethics and professionalism and ensure that

* Corresponding author. Child and Adolescent Psychiatry, Emory University School of Medicine, 1256 Briarcliff Road #317 South, Atlanta, GA 30306.
E-mail address: adingle@emory.edu (A.D. Dingle).

1056-4993/08/$ - see front matter © 2008 Elsevier Inc. All rights reserved.
doi:10.1016/j.chc.2007.07.009   childpsych.theclinics.com

their trainees meet defined minimal standards. Practicing physicians also are expected to conform to basic ethical and professional standards, which have been defined by various professional organizations and are required by state licensing agencies and certification agencies. Standard learning objectives, competencies, and maintenance of certification are used to increase accountability in medical education and practice by requiring evidence that students and physicians practice what they have been taught [1–15].

General issues

Several issues complicate the effective teaching of ethics and professionalism within medicine. One issue is that the students are adults, who come to medicine and their specialties with values and beliefs shaped by prior experience and education. Modifying core personal beliefs is challenging. The literature on education indicates that teaching approaches based on the learner's learning style and previous knowledge and experience tend to be most effective; however, most medical education systems are not set up to systematically teach in this manner [16–20].

Another issue is teaching a specific set of standards in an environment in which there is a diversity of values. Certain values may be expressed in the formal curriculum but not reinforced by daily practices (the "informal" or "hidden" curriculum). For example, a medical school and residency may teach the importance of treating patients, regardless of their ability to pay; however, the trainees are taught within a hospital that generally only admits those with insurance or financial resources [21,22].

There also is an inherent ethical and professional conflict in being a student or trainee. The obligation to patients that they receive optimal care may be compromised when residents are learning while providing patient care. Residents may feel compelled to follow a problematic supervisor suggestion for a patient, to follow certain patient care practices that the institution mandates but with which the resident disagrees. Given the stress, fatigue, and vulnerability of residency, trainees may choose not to deal with these issues when they occur [23]. Further, many physicians are confused about the distinctions between ethics and the law, and several tend to be concerned about liability [24]. Students and residents may be dismayed that there often is no "right" ethical answer, although there usually is agreement about behavior that is clearly inappropriate [24].

Finally, it should not be minimized that taking the most ethical or professional path can be inconvenient, financially disadvantageous, time-consuming, frustrating, or complicated. Obtaining adequate informed assent and consent takes more time, providing care to those who cannot pay has financial consequences for private practitioners, being available during off hours can interfere with personal lives, and calling child protective services can complicate the provision of therapy. Generally, individuals have to believe that meeting ethical and professional standards is important enough to mitigate the potential disadvantages.

Levels of training

Undergraduate

The accreditation standards of the Liaison Committee of Medical Education (LCME) of the American Association of Medical Colleges (AAMC) require that medical schools teach medical ethics and human values and that the students must demonstrate "scrupulous ethical principles in caring for patients, and in relating to patients' families and to others involved in patient care." Examples of such principles include honesty; integrity; maintenance of confidentiality; and respect for patients, families, peers, and other professionals. Schools may identify other dimensions of ethical behavior as well. These standards also require that there exist methods to identify potential unethical behavior related to patient care. The LCME also mandates that medical schools have educational objectives and associated outcome measures that assess students' acquisition of the competencies expected of physicians [25]. The AAMC's Medical School Objectives Project identified and defined four necessary attributes of physicians—altruistic, knowledgeable, skillful, and dutiful—and recommended that medical schools use the learning objectives described in its report to shape the undergraduate medical curriculum. The definition of being altruistic strongly emphasizes the acquisition and demonstration of ethical principles as well as exhibiting professionalism. Being dutiful includes a commitment to providing care to those who cannot pay and advocating for traditionally underserved populations [26,27].

Graduate

In the United States, the American Council on Graduate Medical Education (ACGME) and the American Board of Medical Specialties (ABMS) spearheaded the competency movement for graduate medical education by defining core competency areas and then mandating their inclusion into all residency training programs by incorporating these core competencies into the Residency Review Committee program requirements for each specialty [28]. The ACGME Outcomes Project has identified six core competencies that define the essential knowledge, skills, and attitudes for the practice of medicine and represent the minimal standard that physicians are expected to attain for clinical practice. ACGME-accredited residency and fellowship programs are expected to teach their trainees these competencies and ensure that they demonstrate each by graduation. The core competencies are patient care, medical knowledge, practice-based learning and improvement, interpersonal and communication skills, professionalism, and systems-based practice. Although individual programs are expected to define the details of the competencies, there is a growing consensus that patient care and medical knowledge are specialty specific and that the other competencies share many characteristics across fields. The ACGME description is "professionalism, as manifested through a commitment to performing professional responsibilities, adherence to ethical principles, and sensitivity to a diverse patient population" [29]. Therefore, ethical principles must be taught and evaluated, and there must be required interventions for knowledge and actions that do not meet standards, as well as demonstrated improvement before graduation. The Work Group on Training and Education of the American Academy of Child and Adolescent Psychiatry (AACAP) also has developed a suggested template for professionalism and ethical behavior [30] and described possible methods of assessment [31]. Recommended content areas include the AACAP code of ethics, confidentiality, minor's/guardian's rights to receive and refuse treatment, involuntary commitment, research assent and consent principles, and cultural competence principles. Suggested evaluation techniques include supervisor evaluations, patient logs, observation, standardized oral examinations, case conferences, seminars, and the child Psychiatric Residents in Training Examination (PRITE).

Postgraduate

Licensing (state licensing boards) agencies traditionally have required that practicing physicians uphold basic ethical and professional standards. As part of the accountability movement in medical education, the certification boards have gone to a model of time-limited certification [32]. The American Board of Psychiatry (ABPN), a member of ABMS, grants certification in child and adolescent psychiatry for 10 years upon successful completion of an accredited child and adolescent psychiatry residency program and successful completion of written and oral examinations. To be recertified, the ABPN is developing a program of maintenance of certification (MOC). The mission of this program is to ensure that certified child and adolescent psychiatrists adhere to the highest standards in medicine and pursue excellence in all areas of care and practice improvement. The MOC program has four key components that are being phased in gradually: professional standing, self-assessment and lifelong learning, cognitive expertise, and performance in practice. These areas are tied to the ABPN core competencies, which mirror the ACGME core competencies [33,34]. To meet the professional competency, a psychiatrist must demonstrate specific behaviors that indicate:

- Responsible patient care
- Ethical behavior with an emphasis on integrity, honesty, compassion, confidentiality, informed assent/consent, professional conduct, and conflict of interest
- Respect for diversity
- Attention to end-of-life and quality-of-care issues

- Self-assessment and correction of professional conduct
- Review of colleagues' professional conduct
- Awareness and remediation of safety issues
- Awareness and demonstration of standards expressed in AACAP code of ethics and the Health Insurance Portability and Accountability Act (HIPAA)
- Knowledge of special issues related to minors and their guardians in terms of confidentiality, treatment, research, and involuntary commitment as well as cultural competence

In addition to continuing education in professionalism and ethics for practicing physicians, there has been increasing awareness of the importance of successful faculty development and education in these areas [1, 35–40].

Literature

Ethics education in psychiatry has tended to focus on topics relevant to all of medicine (eg, confidentiality, impaired physicians) as well as issues more specific to the specialty (eg, involuntary commitment, boundary violations). All programs include skill development in problem solving about clinical ethical dilemmas, whereas some include a focus on issues specific to the training setting. Eckles and colleagues [41] reviewed the literature on ethics education for medical students from 1978 to 2004. They concluded that the literature failed to provide adequate information on the theoretic foundation of the overall goals of ethics education and lacked studies examining student outcomes, teaching approaches, and teaching effectiveness. Their review suggested a lack of consensus on the relevant core ethical content, processes, and skills necessary for medical practice, although there did seem to be agreement that ethics should be taught throughout all 4 years. Two perspectives seemed to prevail: that medical ethics is a way to produce virtuous physicians and that it is an approach to teach physicians a skill set for analyzing and resolving ethical dilemmas. Significant unresolved issues in ethics education and assessment continue to exist [42]. In surveys of students and residents on ethical and professional issues they reported inadequate education in these areas, identified a need for more training, and expressed interest in more clinically and practice-based teaching. Preferences for teaching by experts, demonstrated by role modeling and supported by the environment, were noted. Surveys of practicing psychiatrists find a mild to moderate interest in further education on ethical and professional issues related to practice. Those physicians in practice longer were less interested [43–48]. Other investigators have found that residents tend to underuse ethical services because of a lack of awareness or discouragement by the faculty [49].

Teaching approaches

Traditionally, professionalism has been taught to medical students within a didactic framework, with an emphasis on learning the appropriate rules, skills, and behaviors and little formal education done in the clinical setting. Residents and practitioners have tended to have less formal curriculum on this topic [10,21,50]. Methods of teaching medical ethics described in the literature have included specific courses (required or elective), lectures, patient consultations, case discussions, clinical round teaching, supervision, small groups, movie-triggered discussions, issue-driven discussions, problem-based learning, simulations, standardized patients, role playing, Web-based approaches, written assignments, written reflections, student papers, and presentations. There has been increasing interest in developing formal medical ethics education for students and residents within the context of professionalism and in clinical settings. Small-group or clinically based instruction seems to be the most effective, especially when it is integrated throughout the curriculum, includes structured feedback, and is tied to professionalism [41,51–60]. Role modeling by faculty and practicing physicians within the institutional environment are critical [17,61–67]. A comprehensive, institutional approach that includes students, residents, and practicing physicians is required to achieve consistency between the formal curriculum and the modeling, which is the "hidden" or informal curriculum [1,42,51,68–74]. Several medical schools have created administrative positions that are responsible for providing leadership and accountability in the areas of professionalism and ethics [1]. A consistent institutional approach also empowers trainees to voice their concerns about ethical problems that they experience or observe clinically [75–78].

Child and adolescent psychiatry

Most of the child and adolescent psychiatry literature on the teaching of ethics has focused on describing the essential content with limited information on teaching approaches or strategies of assessment. Ethical considerations in child and adolescent psychiatry include the need to consider the interests of caretakers as well as those of the patient, which may not coincide; the changing capacity of children and adolescents to reflect and be responsible for their behavior as children's cognitive and moral judgment develop over time; and the need to work with a variety of personnel and institutions (eg, schools, juvenile court, child protective services) to provide reasonable care [79].

Sondheimer and Martucci [79,80] recommended the use of individual case supervision and case-based group discussions with some didactic instruction as teaching approaches for child and adolescent psychiatry residents. Most child and adolescent psychiatry residency training programs have 2 to 6 hours of formal didactics and 2 to 10 clinical conference hours per year devoted to ethics instruction. Topics included advocacy, child protection, confidentiality, consent/assent issues, treatment refusal, conflict of interests, double agentry, boundaries, provider responsibilities, financial aspects of medicine, AACAP code of ethics, autonomy issues, research, history of ethics, and ethical reasoning [81]. The AACAP has a code of ethics adopted in 1980 and updated in 1995, which provides 17 principles by which a child and adolescent psychiatrist should conduct his or her professional activities [34]. Some literature is available on references for ethics in psychiatry with some information on issues related to children and adolescents [82].

Assessment

Initial studies suggest that behavior indicating inadequate levels of responsibility, reliability, self-improvement, initiative, and motivation in medical school are sensitive, if not specific, predictors of problematic professional behavior later [83–85]. There also is some evidence that trainees tend to prioritize the aspects of their education that are evaluated formally [1,86]. Thus, it is essential that ethical and professional behavior be assessed as well as taught in medical schools and residency.

There are not many reliable and valid evaluation methods and instruments to document whether students, residents, and practicing physicians consistently demonstrate ethical and professional behavior. Strategies that assess knowledge, skills, and attitudes are useful, but not adequate, because they may not be indicative of actual behavior with patients and others. Even if behavior is assessed, there is not general consensus about the specific components of ethical, professional behavior. For example, is it professional to turn off one's beeper during nonworking hours if there is an on-call system that is covering? Is it ethical to obtain informed consent from the parents but not assent from the child when prescribing medication to a 9-year-old? What types of behavior constitute reasonable and accurate assessments of empathy or respect? The behavior of a resident or student may be different under the fairly intense monitoring systems of educational systems than it would be when less scrutinized in practice [11,65,87–90].

A variety of assessment strategies have been used to assess ethical and professional reasoning and behavior of students and residents. Written or computer-based examinations have used multiple choice questions, essays, and case vignettes with written justification of answers to assess moral reasoning. Oral or clinically based evaluation methods have used standardized patients in objective structured clinical examinations, simulations, and clinical evaluation exercises, as well as direct faculty observation of patient interactions. Various types of rating forms have been used to collect 360° evaluations on residents from peers, staff, and students. Self-assessment reports, self-reflection, and portfolios are being used at some schools. Standardized patients also have been used to assess the behavior of practicing physicians. Methods that involve direct observation of behavior in clinical settings with feedback to improve learning and performance (formative evaluations) seem to be the most informative approach in training settings [1,42,89,91–108].

Incorporation into child and adolescent psychiatry

Although didactic teaching is important, most teaching of medical ethics and professionalism is done by example. Medical students, general psychiatry residents, child psychiatry fellows, and the faculty learn from one another. Clinical ethical and professionalism challenges presenting in child and adolescent psychiatry can and should be used to teach medical students and residents. In addition, faculty can develop, maintain, and revise opportunities to discuss issues that may not occur until residents are in practice. Examples include being invited to be a speaker for a pharmaceutical company or maintaining one's commitment to the underserved while running a self-pay private practice. Ideally, there would be consensus within the institution, program, faculty, and trainees about what constitutes ethical and professional behavior, at least in terms of the core values. If complete agreement is not possible, there should be an environment that promotes and mandates discussion of various positions and the underlying rationale. For example, if there are different views on acceptable relationships and exchanges between physicians and the pharmaceutical industry, there should be repeated, open dialog about these relationships.

For all levels of training, formal education on ethics and professionalism probably is taught best using case- or issue-based material that is currently relevant to the participants. Basic medical ethical principles that can be used in the analysis of ethical dilemmas include the duties of beneficence (promoting the welfare of the patient), nonmaleficence (not harming the patient), autonomy (respecting the patient's decision making), and justice (treating patient and society fairly). Weighing the relative importance of these values in reaching a decision about what is "right" in an individual situation may be more or less complicated, depending upon the patient and circumstances. The goals of discussion are to help students understand their core values, how to approach the analysis of ethical or professional dilemmas, and how to apply this knowledge practically.

Specific resources are available for some topics, such as ethical issues related to research with children [109], physician's relationships with pharmaceutical industry [110–115], physician–patient sexual misconduct [116], managed care [117], physician impairment [118,119], use of e-mail, providing care over the Internet (cyber-psychiatry), and telemedicine [120].

Ethical and professional concerns that commonly occur in the practice of child and adolescent psychiatry include those related to working with children and adolescents in clinical and research settings. Examples include issues related to decision making, assent/consent, confidentiality, privacy, double agentry/conflict of interests, boundaries, access to care/resources, working with children and adolescents in particular settings, and youth participation in research. Other potential areas include associated physician behavior, such as relationships with pharmaceutical, advocacy, or health care organizations; working with the media; presenting and publishing about cases and research; and monitoring colleagues. Because much of this material is covered elsewhere in this issue, this section briefly reviews some important topics.

Decision making

Informed consent requires that adequate information is provided, the decision is voluntary, and the individual making the choice is competent. Research indicates that 14-year-olds have the same ability to make complicated decisions as do adults [121]. The legal age of consent for medical and psychiatric care varies by state in the United States. Under certain circumstances, such as family planning or drug treatment, some states allow adolescents to consent for treatment at a younger age. Adolescents also may become legally emancipated, making them legally able to make decisions like competent adults. The criteria to become an emancipated minor differ between states, although they generally require marriage or the ability to care for oneself financially. For most children and adolescents, competence to give consent is related to the assessment of the patient's decision-making abilities in context (capability). Factors to consider include the patient's developmental status, the medical or psychiatric diagnosis, benefits and risks of treatment/no treatment/alternative treatment options, consequences of possible decisions, and the minor's ability to make and express a decision. Contextual variables include cultural and community background, health care literacy, family involvement, resources, and possible clinician biases. Complicating the ethical considerations is that the minor often is not the one initiating the evaluation or treatment. Also, many of the psychopharmacological treatments lack rigorous data supporting their efficacy and effectiveness for children and adolescents or information on their potential neurodevelopmental impact. When parental consent is required for an intervention, children and adolescents are expected to be able to give assent. It also is variable when youth are legally or ethically allowed to refuse treatment, despite parental consent to the treatment, and when they can consent to treatment against their parents' wishes [119,122–126]. Finally, some children and adolescents may have restrictions on their ability to assent or consent, depending on their circumstances. For example, children and adolescents in state custody often cannot decide with whom to live, and those who are incarcerated may not be able to make decisions about treatment [119,120,122–131].

Confidentiality/privacy

Confidentiality and privacy are essential aspects of medical care, especially in psychiatry. When providing care for children and adolescents, providers must balance the patient's desires to keep information between him- or herself and the physician and the caretakers' requests to be informed. Many children and adolescents are unaware of what information their legal guardians can access. In addition to respecting the patient's decision making, these components of care are integral to trust and the therapeutic alliance. Child and adolescent psychiatrists also can face the dilemma of deciding whether the patient's revelations really constitute a serious problem, such as abuse, or are more representative of psychologic issues. State laws vary on what providers are permitted to keep confidential and private, although all mandate the disclosure of imminent serious harm to self or others. Federal regulations, as set forth in HIPAA, also govern what information may be disclosed. Often, children and adolescents fail to realize the amount and type of information that may be shared to facilitate heath care, billing, and insurance coverage [119,124].

Conflict of interests/double agentry

Child and adolescent psychiatrists may have conflicts of interest related to their responsibilities to other agencies, such as schools, juvenile court, department of juvenile justice, child protective services, managed care organizations, or their employers (eg, hospitals, clinics) [120]. Other situations that may produce conflict of interests are child custody disputes, research situations, or priorities other than the child's best interests [120,125,129–132]. In such cases, the general rules of confidentiality and primacy of the patient's interests are altered by the role and responsibilities of the child and adolescent psychiatrist.

Boundaries/relationships

Ethical issues can arise when there is not an agreement between the therapist, patient, and guardians about the goals of treatment. This can happen when the psychiatrist's goals are in conflict with the patient's or family's cultural or religious beliefs (eg, when a child is brought in to "fix" his/her homosexuality) or when the clinician's countertransference or personal issues get in the way of treatment (eg, desire to protect or save the child). Boundaries between the therapist and family can be difficult to manage. Whether to give or accept gifts, attend various activities (eg, graduations, baseball games, bar mitzvahs), or to see relatives or friends of the patient may be more or less complicated, depending on the location and type of practice (eg, a small town). Sexual relationships between physicians and patients obviously are unethical and unprofessional and usually would be illegal; however, the boundaries on relationships—sexual and nonsexual—with the patient's caretakers and other involved adults should be discussed. Other boundaries to be discussed are sexual or intimate relationships between residents and faculty, other residents, or staff, all of which have the potential to impact the learning environment and patient care [116,119,133].

Special populations

Juvenile justice

Although there is agreement that youth lack the ability to be fully criminally responsible for developmental reasons (diminished capacity), states vary on the ages at which children and adolescents are considered responsible, with different minimal and maximal ages for juvenile court involvement. Several states have additional age requirements for certain types of crimes. All states have mechanisms to transfer juveniles between juvenile and adult criminal courts. There has been increasing interest in examining competency to stand trial, even for those in juvenile court. Providing clinical assessments and treatment for children and adolescents involved in the juvenile or adult justice system is complicated by several factors. In addition to the youth, decisions have to consider the guardians, lawyers, and the court or the department of juvenile justice. Children or adolescents may feel coerced into participating in treatment. Nonmaleficence and beneficence may be compromised by conflicts with the system or societal interests. Additional issues may include confidentiality, stigma, reasons/rationale for treatment, interactions with monitoring or advocacy groups, involving these youth in research, and dealing with institutional practices that are potentially abusive. Maintaining one's professional commitment to advocate for youth also may be complicated, depending on one's role and responsibilities within this system. Forensic work, such as competency evaluations or serving as an expert witness for the court, has clear boundaries; however, it becomes much more complex if the child and adolescent psychiatrist is asked to have clinical and forensic roles with the same patient. Although not recommended, this situation may not be avoidable [120,127,128].

Research

Children and adolescents are considered to be a vulnerable group of research subjects. They may not be competent to voluntarily participate, their guardians may have reasons other than the child's best interests for consenting, youth may have institutional or state guardians who have a less than ideal investment in the child's best interests, and historically, youth have not been treated well as research subjects. Federal regulations on having children and adolescents participate in research require a delineation of the risk and benefit involved, with most research projects falling into the category of minimal risk or potential benefit to the individual participant. Parents must give informed consent, and children and adolescents (depending on state law) must assent. Most of the discussion on research related to children and adolescents has concentrated on safety or welfare issues, rather than on children's rights [125,129–131].

Access to care/resources

Access to care continues to be a major issue for children and adolescents, particularly for adequate mental health treatment. Problems include a lack of parity of insurance coverage for psychiatric illness; managed care; uninsured youth; poverty; a lack of awareness and recognition of mental illness in children and adolescents; inadequate private and public funding for a continuum of services; shortage of child and adolescent psychiatrists, with several regions of the country not having any; and the number of child and adolescent psychiatrists in private practice who do not accept any forms of insurance [134].

Rapid biotechnological medical advances have raised new ethical dilemmas as well as strains on limited resources. These include the impact of assisted reproductive technology, improved life-sustaining technology, and highly sensitive, expensive tests that may lead to unnecessary interventions [135]. For example, MRIs on healthy pediatric volunteers have detected incidental abnormal findings, raising significant ethical and management issues [136]. Current evidence indicates that the expression of most psychiatric disorders is due to an interaction between genetic vulnerability (usually multiple genes) and environment. This knowledge has ethical implications for the practice of child and adolescent psychiatry in several areas. If tests verifying the genes responsible for various psychiatric disorders become available, this would allow screening prenatally as well as before adoption, marriage, or insurance coverage. Clinicians will have to learn how to consider how helpful this information might be in predicting the following [137]:

What is a child's chances of having a particular disorder?
How impairing is the disorder?
What level of risk makes certain decisions reasonable (eg, abortion, not adopting)?
Are there beneficial aspects to this gene constellation (eg, creativity)?
Do interventions exist that could decrease the likelihood of the disorder being expressed or minimize the symptoms?
Would this information impact treatment (eg, serotonin transport gene)?
What are the personal and societal implications of being positive (eg, self-image, insurance access)?
What are the potentials for misunderstandings and discrimination?
What are the duties of physicians?

Educational methods

Generally, ethical and professional topics are best taught and assessed in context. For most medical students and physicians, this approach means using case or clinical research material to discuss and explore the relevant issues. Given the limited access to child and adolescent psychiatry that most medical students have, the emphasis for undergraduate education probably should be on understanding the unique aspects of consent, assent, confidentiality and privacy; access to care/resources; and research participation, with other subjects being reviewed as relevant to clinical cases. Psychiatry residents would benefit from a review of these areas and education on the issues related to double agentry, conflicts of interest, boundaries, and working in different clinical settings. Child and adolescent psychiatry residents and practitioners should have exposure and an understanding of all of the issues listed in this section. Additionally, there should be an emphasis on learning and being able to use problem-solving or analytic strategies to identify and manage ethical and professional concerns at all levels of education. Including the consideration of relevant ethical and professional material as an expected part of clinical care and professional activities, particularly during undergraduate and graduate education, makes it more likely that these aspects of practice will be evaluated routinely at all levels of practice.

Evaluating the ethical and professional knowledge and behavior of students, residents, and physicians probably is best done as one aspect of an assessment of their performance. In addition to reinforcing the importance of these areas to physician practice, it also tends to be easier to implement because it does not become an additional form to complete, assignment to grade, or activity to observe. Using this type of framework for the evaluation means that many of the assessment techniques commonly used for students, residents, and physicians (eg, general written examinations; supervisor feedback; case presentation and write-ups; observation of interactions with patients, families, and staff; feedback from peers and colleagues) can be used to assess these behaviors. It is essential to have general agreement about what constitutes acceptable ethical and professional behavior and how it should be assessed.

Resources for teaching ethics and professionalism

There are several child and adolescent psychiatry textbooks that include information on relevant ethical and professional issues, and many recently published articles related to ethical and professional concerns in psychiatry and child and adolescent psychiatry. There is an increasing literature on defining, teaching, and assessing ethics and professionalism within medical educational programs and residency training programs as well as for practitioners. Given that many of the attributes of ethical, responsible physicians are not specialty specific, literature from other specialties can be useful, particularly in developing assessment and remediation approaches.

A variety of psychiatric- and child-related organizations have presentations on relevant ethical and professional issues during their annual meetings and provide information through print and electronic forums. The

Web pages of various educational and psychiatric organizations offer additional information on ethics and professionalism. The emphasis on many of the Web sites tends to be on definitions, specific content of ethical issues, and descriptions of ethical and professional behavior, but increasingly, there are resources describing teaching and assessment approaches. The AAMC Web page (www.aamc.org) has several sources of information to help educators with these topics. Another resource is MedEdPortal, a Web-based service that provides peer-reviewed curriculum for undergraduate, graduate, and postgraduate medical education [138]. The Group on Educational Affairs has provided an annotated bibliography of references dealing with the assessment of professionalism [91]. The AAMC and National Board of Medical Examiners cosponsored a conference on "Embedding Professionalism in Medical Education: Assessment as a Tool for Implementation." The report from this conference discusses behaviors that exemplify professional behavior by students as well as reasons for and approaches to the assessment of these behaviors [8]. The ACGME Web site (www.acgme.org) provides information on the core competencies, strategies, and methods of assessment, methods of implementation, and possible resources. The Web site (www.aadprt.org) of the American Association of Directors of Psychiatric Training has recommended resources and sample curriculum and assessment tools from several programs. The American Psychiatric Association has its code of ethics (www.apa.org) as well as information on educational content and strategies. The AACAP posts its code of ethics (www.aacap.org) on its Web page and has the practice parameters on various clinical issues that include the relevant ethical and professional issues. The American Medical Association has several resources on its Web page (www.ama-assn.org), including a code of ethics, variety of publications, discussion forums, and a collaborative project with several medical schools to develop teaching and assessment approaches (Strategies for Teaching and Evaluating Professionalism, STEP). The Association for Academic Psychiatry has an on-line electronic journal, *Medical Education Online* (www.med-ed-online.org), with articles related to ethics education. The ABPN disseminates information about certification, its core competencies, and the MOC program on its Web site (www.abpn.com), with links to other relevant sites, and in its newsletter, the *ABPN Diplomate*.

Future directions

With the impetus of the LCME, ACGME, and the ABMS, medical schools, residencies, and the credentialing boards will be developing and implementing formal methods of teaching and assessing medical ethics and professionalism. Clearer standards and a dedication to practical teaching will be required for accreditation of programs. Better, validated tools for assessment will result, as well as remediation programs that work. Child and adolescent psychiatry can work with and learn from the work in other specialty areas.

The most challenging and important component of ethical training will continue to be having excellent role models and an institutional commitment to professionalism. One approach to this has been the Relationship-Centered Care initiative at a growing number of medical schools across the United States [73,139,140]. The National Institutes of Health also have invested in 5 years of funding to a consortium of nine medical schools to respond to a recent Institute of Medicine report. The report called for medical schools to strengthen their teaching of social and behavioral sciences [141]. This group will contribute to the teaching of professionalism, including assessment of the impact of the context of care on the clinical training of medical students and residents.

Summary

Learning and maintaining an ability to see, analyze, and make decisions in ethical dilemmas is a key set of skills for all medical students, residents, and physicians. These are critical components of what is considered to be professionalism in medicine. A growing number of resources are available for child and adolescent psychiatrists and for the medical students and residents whom they teach and supervise. Effective teaching requires a combination of case discussion, reflection, and modeling, in the context of ongoing positive reinforcement and constructive feedback. Only in this way do students experience a consistency between the formal curriculum and the informal or "hidden" curriculum, which is the culture of medicine. Being an ethical child and adolescent psychiatrist requires knowledge of certain ethical principles as well as the skills to use them to analyze a situation, an attitude that this is an important thing to do, and ongoing ethical behavior.

Providing educational experiences that promote an understanding of ethical and professional standards and produce behavior consistent with these values remains a challenge. Although the concerns of society and the field of medicine about the ethical and professional attitudes and actions of students and physicians is distressing, these concerns have promoted a renewed interest in developing effective educational and assessment strategies. The competency movement also has contributed by identifying professionalism and ethical behavior as core attributes of students and physicians, requiring explicit documentation of knowledge and its effective use, and tying the teaching and learning to assessment. Developing and implementing systematic quality educational and evaluation methods that can be used across the various levels of training and practice are in the early stages, but they have the potential to improve our educational systems significantly.

References

[1] Cohen J. Professionalism in medical education, an American perspective: from evidence to accountability. Med Educ 2006;40:607–17.

[2] Medical Professional Project. Medical professionalism in the new millennium: a physician charter. Lancet 2002;359:520–2.

[3] Inui TS. A flag in the wind: educating for professionalism in medicine. Washington DC: Association of American Medical Colleges; 2003.

[4] Cohen JJ. Our compact with tomorrow's doctors. President's address. Presented at the Annual Meeting of the Association of American Medical Colleges. Washington DC; November 4, 2001.

[5] AAMC. Compact between resident physicians and their teachers. Available at: http://www.aamc.org/meded/residentcompact/residentcompact.pdf. Accessed April 4, 2007.

[6] Cruess SR, Johnston S, Cruess RL. "Profession": a working definition for medical educators. Teach Learn Med 2004;16(1):74–6.

[7] Frohna A. Medical students' professionalism. Med Teach 2006;28(1):1–2.

[8] AAMC, NBME. Embedding professionalism in medical education: assessment as a tool for implementation. Invitational conference. Baltimore, May 15–17, 2002.

[9] Hilton SR, Slotnick HB. Proto-professionalism: how professionalism occurs across the continuum of medical education. Med Educ 2005;39:58–65.

[10] Huddle TS. Teaching professionalism: is medical morality a competency? Acad Med 2005; 80(10):885–91.

[11] Misch DA. Evaluating physicians' professionalism and humanism: the case for humanism "connoisseurs". Acad Med 2002;77(6):489–95.

[12] Talbott JA, Mallott DB. Professionalism, medical humanism, and clinical bioethics: the new wave–does psychiatry have a role? J Psychiatr Pract 2006;12(6):384–90.

[13] Wear D, Kuczewski MG. The professionalism movement: can we pause? Am J Bioeth 2004; 4(2):1–10.

[14] Hafferty FW. Professionalism–the next wave. N Engl J Med 2006;355(20):2151–2.

[15] Stern DT, Papadakis M. The developing physician–becoming a professional. N Engl J Med 2006;355(20):1794–9.

[16] Armstrong E, Parsa-Parsi R. How can physicians' learning styles drive educational planning? Acad Med 2005;80(7):680–4.

[17] Duff P. Teaching and assessing professionalism. Obstet Gynecol 2004;104:1362–6.

[18] Puliyel MM, Puliyel JM, Puliyel U. Drawing on adult learning theory to teach personal and professional values. Med Teach 1999;21(5):513–5.

[19] Arseneau R, Rodenberg D. A developmental perspective on teaching. In: Pratt D, editor. Five perspectives on teaching in adult and higher education. Melbourne (FL): Krieger Publishing; 1998.

[20] Mann KV. Thinking about learning: implications for principle-based professional education. J Contin Educ Health Prof 2002;22:69–76.

[21] Coulehan J. Today's professionalism: engaging the mind but not the heart. Acad Med 2005; 80:892–8.

[22] Hafferty F. Beyond curriculum reform: confronting medicine's hidden curriculum. Acad Med 1995;73:403–7.

[23] Hoop JG. Hidden ethical dilemmas in psychiatric residency training: the psychiatry resident as dual agent. Acad Psychiatry 2004;28(3):183–9.

[24] Appelbaum PS. Legalism, postmodernism, and the vicissitudes of teaching ethics. Acad Psychiatry 2004;28:164–7.

[25] LCME. Functions and structure of a medical school: standards for accreditation on medical education programs leading to the M.D. Degree. Washington DC: Association of American Medical Colleges; 2004.

[26] MSOP. Report I learning objectives for medical student education guidelines for medical schools. Washington DC: American Association of Medical Colleges; 1998.

[27] The Medical School Objectives Writing Group. Learning objectives for medical student education—guidelines for medical schools: report I of the Medical School Objectives Project. Acad Med 1999;74:13–8.

[28] Schieber SC, Kramer TAM, Adamowski SE, editors. Core competencies for psychiatric practice: what clinicians need to know. Washington DC: American Psychiatric Publishing, Inc.; 2003.

[29] ACGME. Outcome project: ACGME general competencies version 1.3 (9.28.99); 2000. Available at: http://www.acgme.org/Outcome/. Accessed April 4, 2007.

[30] Sexson SB, Sargent J, Zima B, et al. Sample core competencies in child and adolescent psychiatry training: a starting point. Acad Psychiatry 2001;25(4):201–13.

[31] Sargent J, Sexson S, Cuffe S, et al. Assessment of competency in child and adolescent psychiatry training. Acad Psychiatry 2004;28(1):18–26.

[32] ABMS. Annual report of the American Board of Medical Specialties 2005. Evanston (IL): American Board of Medical Specialties; 2005.

[33] American Board of Psychiatry and Neurology. Maintenance and certification in child and adolescent psychiatry. Available at: http://www.abpn.com/moc_cap.htm. Accessed April 4, 2007.

[34] AACAP. AACAP code of ethics. Washington DC: American Academy of Child and Adolescent Psychiatry; 1995.

[35] Cruess R, Cruess S. Teaching professionalism: general principles. Med Teach 2006;28: 1–4.

[36] Srinivasan M, Lizelman D, Seshadri R, et al. Developing an OSTE to address lapses in learners' professional behavior and an instrument to code educators' responses. Acad Med 2004;79(9):888–96.

[37] Mohamed M, Punwani M, Clay M, et al. Protecting the residency training environment: a resident's perspective on the ethical boundaries in the faculty-resident relationship. Acad Psychiatry 2005;29(4):368–73.

[38] Riess H, Fishel AK. The necessity of continuing education for psychotherapy supervisors. Acad Psychiatry 2000;24(3):147–55.

[39] Green SA. The ethical commitments of academic faculty in psychiatric education. Academic Psychiatry 2006;30:48–54.

[40] Roberts LW, Coverdale J, Louie A. Professionalism and the ethics-related roles of academic psychiatrists. Acad Psychiatry 2005;29(5):413–5.

[41] Eckles RE, Meslin EM, Gaffney M, et al. Medical ethics education: where are we? Where should we be going? A review. Acad Med 2005;80(12):1143–52.

[42] Goldie J. Review of ethics curricula in undergraduate medical education. Med Educ 2000; 34:108–19.

[43] Roberts LW, Hammond KAG, Geppert CMA, et al. The positive role of professionalism and ethics training in medical education: a comparison of medical student and resident perspectives. Acad Psychiatry 2004;28:170–82.

[44] Roberts LW, Johnson ME, Brems C, et al. Preferences of Alaska and New Mexico psychiatrists regarding professionalism and ethics training. Acad Psychiatry 2006;30(3):200–4.

[45] Roberts LW, Warner TD, Hammond KAG, et al. Becoming a good doctor: perceived need for ethics training focused on practical and professional development topics. Acad Psychiatry 2005;29(3):301–9.

[46] Roberts LW, McCarty T, Lyketsos C, et al. What and how psychiatry residents at ten training programs wish to learn about ethics. Acad Psychiatry 1996;20(3):131–43.

[47] Ratanawongsa N, Bolen S, Howell EE, et al. Residents' perceptions of professionalism in training and practice: barriers, promotors, and duty hour requirements. J Gen Intern Med 2005;21:758–63.

[48] Al-Umran KU, Al-Shaikh BA, Al-Awary BH, et al. Medical ethics and tomorrow's physicians: an aspect of coverage in the formal curriculum. Med Teach 2006;28(2):182–4.

[49] Gacki-Smith J, Gordon EJ. Residents access to ethics consultations: knowledge, use and perceptions. Acad Med 2005;80:168–75.

[50] Whitcomb ME. Medical professionalism: can it be taught? Acad Med 2005;80:883–4.

[51] Goldstein E, Maestas RR, Fryer-Edwards K, et al. Professionalism in medical education: an institutional challenge. Acad Med 2006;81(10):871–6.

[52] Goldie J, Schwartz L, McConnachie A, et al. Impact of new course on students' potential behaviour on encountering ethical dilemmas. Med Educ 2001;35:295–302.

[53] Goldie J, Schwartz L, Morrison J. A process evaluation of medical ethics education in the first year of a new medical curriculum. Med Educ 2000;34:468–73.

[54] Goldie J, Schwartz L, McConnachie A, et al. The impact of a modern medical curriculum on students' proposed behaviour on meeting ethical dilemmas. Med Educ 2004;38:942–9.

[55] Smith S, Fryer-Edwards K, Diekema DS, et al. Finding effective strategies for teaching ethics: a comparison trial of two interventions. Acad Med 2004;79(3):265–71.

[56] Schnapp WB, Stone S, Norman JV, et al. Teaching ethics in psychiatry. A problem-based learning approach. Acad Psychiatry 1996;20(3):144–9.

[57] Rubin E, Edelson R, Servis M. Literature as an introduction to psychiatric ethics. Acad Psychiatry 1998;22(1):41–6.

[58] Neitzke G, Fehr F. Teacher's responsibility: a Socratic dialogue about teaching medical ethics. Med Teach 2003;25(1):92–3.

[59] Roberts LW, McCarty T, Roberts BB, et al. Clinical ethics teaching in psychiatric supervision. Acad Psychiatry 1996;20(3):176–88.

[60] Hassenfeld IN, Grumet B. Fifteen years of teaching psychiatric law and ethics to residents. Acad Psychiatry 1996;20(3):165–75.

[61] Ber R, Alroy G. Teaching professionalism with aid of trigger films. Med Teach 2002;24(5): 528–31.

[62] Stephenson A, Higgs R, Sugarman J. Teaching professional development in medical schools. Lancet 2001;357:867–70.

[63] Sklar DP, Doezema D, McLaughlin S, et al. Teaching communications and professionalism through writing and humanities: reflections of ten years of experience. Acad Emerg Med 2002;9(11):1360–4.

[64] Harris GD. Professionalism: part II–teaching and assessing the learner's professionalism. Fam Med 2004;36(6):390–2.

[65] Johnston S. See one, do one, teach one: developing professionalism across the generations. Clin Orthop Relat Res 2006;449:186–92.

[66] Krych EH, Voort JLV. Medical students speak: a two-voice comment on learning professionalism in medicine. Clin Anat 2006;19:415–8.

[67] Welling RE, Boberg JT. Professionalism. Arch Surg 2003;138:262–4.

[68] Ludmerer KM. Instilling professionalism in medical education. JAMA 1999;282:881–2.

[69] Swick HM, Philip S, Danoff D, et al. Teaching professionalism in the undergraduate curriculum. JAMA 1999;282(9):830–2.

[70] Markakis KM, Beckman HB, Suchman AL, et al. The path to professionalism: cultivating humanistic values and attitudes in residency training. Acad Med 2000;75:141–50.

[71] Hafferty F, Franks R. The hidden curriculum, ethics teaching and the structure of medical curriculum. Acad Med 1994;69:861–71.

[72] Stephenson AE, Adshead LE, Higgs RH. The teaching of professional attitudes within UK medical schools: reported difficulties and good practice. Med Educ 2006;40:1072–80.

[73] Suchman AL, Williamson PR, Litzelman DK, et al. Toward an informal curriculum that teaches professionalism. Transforming the social environment of a medical school. J Gen Intern Med 2004;19(5 Pt 2):501–4.

[74] Lazarus CJ, Chauvin SW, Rodenhauser P, et al. The program for professional values and ethics in medical education. Teach Learn Med 2000;12(4):208–11.

[75] Caldicott CV, Faber-Langendoen K. Deception, discrimination, and fear of reprisal: lessons in ethics from third-year medical students. Acad Med 2005;80(9):866–73.

[76] Satterwhite R, Satterwhite W, Enarson C. An ethical paradox: the effect of unethical conduct on medical students' values. J Med Ethics 2000;26:462–5.

[77] Gordon J. Progressing professionalism. Med Educ 2006;40:936–8.

[78] Schildmann J, Cushing A, Doyal L, et al. Informed consent in clinical practice: pre-registration house officers' knowledge, difficulties and the need for postgraduate training. Med Teach 2005;27(7):649–51.

[79] Sondheimer A, Martucci LC. An approach to teaching ethics in child and adolescent psychiatry. J Am Acad Child Adolesc Psychiatry 1992;31(3):415–22.

[80] Sondheimer A. Ethics and child and adolescent psychiatry. Acad Psychiatry 1996;20(3): 150–7.

[81] Sondheimer A. Teaching ethics and forensic psychiatry: a national survey of child and adolescent psychiatry training programs. Acad Psychiatry 1998;22(4):240–52.

[82] Anzia DJ, Puma JL. An annotated bibliography of psychiatric medical ethics. Acad Psychiatry 1991;15(1):1–17.

[83] Papadakis M, Hodgson C, Teherani A, et al. Unprofessional behavior in medical school is associated with subsequent disciplinary action by state medical board. Acad Med 2004;79: 244–9.

[84] Papadakis M, Teherani A, Banch M, et al. Disciplinary action by medical schools and prior behaviour in medical school. N Engl J Med 2005;353:2673–82.

[85] Kirk L, Blank L. Professional behavior: a learner's permit for licensure. N Engl J Med 2005; 353:2709–11.

[86] Goldie J, Schwartz L, McConnachie A, et al. The impact of three years' ethics teaching, in an integrated medical curriculum, on students' proposed behaviour on meeting ethical dilemmas. Med Educ 2002;36:489–97.

[87] Veloski J, Fields S, Boex J, et al. Measuring professionalism: a review of studies with instruments reported in the literature between 1982 and 2002. Acad Med 2005;80:366–70.

[88] Stern D, editor. Measuring medical professionalism. New York: Oxford University Press; 2006.

[89] Wong JG, Cheung EP. Ethics assessment in medical students. Med Teach 2003;25(1):5–8.

[90] Jha V, Bekker H, Duffy S, et al. Perceptions of professionalism in medicine: a qualitative study. Med Educ 2006;40:1027–36.

[91] Charles P, Cleary L, Dudding B, et al. Assessment of professionalism: annotated bibliography. Association of American Medical Colleges; Washington DC: 2004.

[92] Singer P, Robb A, Cohen R, et al. Performance-based assessment of clinical ethics using an objective structured examination. Acad Med 1996;71:495–8.

[93] Norcini JJ, Blank LL, Duffy FD, et al. The Mini-CEX: a method for assessing clinical skills. Ann Intern Med 2003;138(6):476–81.

[94] Cohen R. Assessing professionalism and medical error. Med Teach 2001;23(2):145–51.

[95] Gisondi MA, Smith-Coggins R, Harter PM, et al. Assessment of resident professionalism using high-fidelity simulation of ethical dilemmas. Acad Emerg Med 2004;11(9): 931–7.

[96] Goldie J, Schwartz L, McConnachie A, et al. Can students' reasons for choosing set answers to ethical vignettes be reliably rated? Development and testing of a method. Med Teach 2004;26(8):713–8.

[97] Srinivasan M, Franks P, Meredith LS, et al. Connoisseurs of care? Unannounced standardized patients' rating of physicians. Med Care 2006;44(12):1092–8.

[98] Gordon J. Assessing students' personal and professional development using portfolios and interviews. Med Educ 2003;37:335–40.

[99] Hemmler PA, Hawkins R, Jackson JL, et al. Assessing how well three evaluation methods detect deficiencies in medical students' professionalism in two settings of an internal medicine clerkship. Acad Med 2000;75(2):167–73.

[100] Hren D, Vujaklija A, Ivanisevic R, et al. Students' moral reasoning, Machiavellianism and socially desirable responding: implications for teaching ethics and research integrity. Med Educ 2006;40:269–77.

[101] Risdon C, Baptiste S. Evaluating pre-clerkship professionalism in longitudinal small groups. Med Educ 2006;40:1123–47.

[102] Ozuah PO, Reznik M, Braganza SF. Reliability of adolescent standardised patients in assessing professionalism. Med Educ 2006;40:481.

[103] Murray E, Gruppen L, Canton P, et al. The accountability of clinical education: its definition and assessment. Med Educ 2000;34:871–9.

[104] Mazor KM, Zanetti ML, Alper EJ, et al. Assessing professionalism in the context of an objective structured clinical examination: an in-depth study of the rating process. Med Educ 2007;41(4):331–40.

[105] Lynch DC, Surdyk PM, Eiser AR. Assessing professionalism: a review of the literature. 2004;26(4):366–73.

[106] Swick SD, Hall S, Beresin E. Assessing the ACGME competencies in psychiatry training programs. Acad Psychiatry 2006;30(4):330–51.

[107] Bennett AJ, Roman B, Arnold LM, et al. Professionalism deficits among medical students: models of identification and intervention. Acad Psychiatry 2005;29(5):426–32.

[108] Jarvis RM, O'Sullivan PS, McClain T, et al. Can one portfolio measure the six ACGME general competencies? Acad Psychiatry 2004;28(3):190–6.

[109] Roberts LW, Solomon Z, Roberts BB, et al. Ethics in psychiatric research. Acad Psychiatry 1998;22(1):1–20.

[110] Jibson MD. Medical education and the pharmaceutical industry. Acad Psychiatry 2006; 30(1):36–9.

[111] Geppert CMA. Medical education and the pharmaceutical industry: a review of ethical guidelines and their implications for psychiatric training. Acad Psychiatry 2007;31(1):32–9.

[112] Lazarus A. The role of pharmaceutical industry in medical education in psychiatry. Acad Psychiatry 2006;30(1):40–4.

[113] Chan CH. The pharmaceutical role. Acad Psychiatry 2006;30(1):45–7.

[114] Randall ML, Rosenbaum JR, Rohrbaugh RM, et al. Attitudes and behaviors of psychiatry residents toward pharmaceutical representatives before and after an educational intervention. Acad Psychiatry 2006;29(1):33–9.

[115] Varley CK, Jibson MD, McCarthy M, et al. A survey of the interactions between psychiatry residency programs and the pharmaceutical industry. Acad Psychiatry 2005;29(1):40–6.

[116] Roman B, Kay J. Residency education on the prevention of physician-patient sexual misconduct. Acad Psychiatry 1997;21(1):26–34.

[117] Wright SM, Carrese JA. Ethical issues in the managed care setting: a new curriculum for primary care physicians. Med Teach 2001;23(1):71–5.

[118] Broquet KE, Rockey PH. Teaching residents and program directors about physician impairment. Acad Psychiatry 2004;28(3):221–5.

[119] Koocher GP. Ethics in child psychotherapy. Child Adolesc Psychiatr Clin N Am 1995;4(4): 779–91.

[120] Ratner RA. Ethics in child and adolescent forensic psychiatry. Child Adolesc Psychiatr Clin N Am 2002;11:887–904.

[121] Weithorn L, Campbell S. The competency of children and adolescents to make informed treatment decisions. Child Dev 1982;53:1589–98.

[122] English A, Kenney KE. State minor consent laws: a summary. 2nd edition. Chapel Hill (NC): Center for Adolescent Health & the Law; 2003.

[123] Campbell AT. Consent, competence, and confidentiality related to psychiatric conditions in adolescent medicine practice. Adolesc Med Clin 2006;11:25–47.

[124] Diaz A, Neal WP, Nucci AT, et al. Legal and ethical issues facing adolescent health care professionals. Mt Sinai J Med 2004;71(3):181–5.

[125] Coffey BJ. Ethical issues in child and adolescent psychopharmacology. Child Adolesc Psychiatr Clin N Am 1995;4(4):793–807.

[126] Ash P, Jurkovic G, Harrison S. Observation, interview, and mental status assessment of competence for independent decision-making. In: Noshpitz J, editor. Handbook of child psychiatry and the law, vol. 5. 2nd edition. New York: John Wiley and Sons, Inc.; 1997. p. 518–25.

[127] Zerby SA, Thomas CR. Legal issues, rights and ethics for mental health in juvenile justice. Child Adolesc Psychiatr Clin N Am 2006;15:373–90.

[128] Penn J, Thomas CR. Practice parameter for the assessment and treatment of youth in juvenile detention and correctional facilities. Washington DC: American Academy of Child and Adolescent Psychiatry; 2005.

[129] Glantz LH. Conducting research with children: legal and ethical issues. J Am Acad Child Adolesc Psychiatry 1996;34(10):1283–91.

[130] Levine R. Children as research subjects: ethical and legal considerations. Child Adolesc Psychiatr Clin N Am 1995;4(4):853–68.

[131] Vitiello B, Jensen P, Hoagwood K. Integrating science and ethics in child and adolescent psychiatry. Biol Psychiatry 1999;46:1044–9.

[132] AACAP. Practice parameters for child custody evaluation. J Am Acad Child Adolesc Psychiatry 1997;36(10 Suppl):57S–68S.

[133] Schetky D. Boundaries in child and adolescent psychiatry. Child Adolesc Psychiatr Clin N Am 1995;4(4):769–78.

[134] Geraty R, Hendren R, Flaa C. Ethical perspectives on managed care as it relates to child and adolescent psychiatry. J Am Acad Child Adolesc Psychiatry 1992;31(3):398–402.

[135] Gonnella JS, Hojat M. Biotechnology and ethics in medical education of the new millennium: physician roles and responsibilities. Med Teach 2001;23(4):371–7.

[136] Kumra S, Ashtari M, Anderson B, et al. Ethical and practical considerations in the management of incidental findings in pediatric MRI studies. J Am Acad Child Adolesc Psychiatry 2006;45(8):1000–6.

[137] Applebaum PS. Ethical issues in psychiatric genetics. J Psychiatr Pract 2004;10(6):343–51.

[138] AAMC. MedEdPortal: American Association of Medical Colleges; 2007. Available at: www.aamc.org/mededportal.

[139] Haidet P, Kelly PA, Bentley S, et al. Not the same everywhere. Patient-centered learning environments at nine medical schools. J Gen Intern Med 2006;21(5):405–9.

[140] Litzelman DK, Cottingham AH. The new formal competency-based curriculum and informal curriculum at Indiana University School of Medicine: overview and five-year analysis. Acad Med 2007;82(4):410–21.

[141] Cuff PA, Vanselow NA, editors. Improving medical education: enhancing the behavioral and social science content of medical school curricula. Washington DC: National Academies Press; 2004.

ELSEVIER
SAUNDERS

Child Adolesc Psychiatric Clin N Am
17 (2008) 209–224

CHILD AND
ADOLESCENT
PSYCHIATRIC CLINICS
OF NORTH AMERICA

The Role of the Child and Adolescent Psychiatrist on Health Care Institutional Ethics Committees

Sandra B. Sexson, MD[a],*, William R. Sexson, MD[b]

[a]Division of Child, Adolescent and Family Psychiatry, Department of Psychiatry and Health Behavior, Medical College of Georgia, 997 St. Sebastian Way, Augusta, GA 30912-3800, USA
[b]Emory Center for Ethics, Emory University School of Medicine, Suite 201, 49 Jesse Hill Jr. Drive, Atlanta, GA 30303, USA

Over the past 3 decades, institutional ethics committees (IECs) have developed across the United States in health care institutions: general hospitals, pediatric hospitals, and inpatient psychiatric institutions. Following the Joint Commission on Accreditation of Healthcare Organizations' 1992 requirement that hospitals develop a method for addressing ethical issues in the health care setting, the IEC became the preferred medium through which most health care institutions endeavored to meet this requirement. Early in the history of the development of these IECs in the general hospital, psychiatrists, particularly those practicing in consultation/liaison roles, were integrally involved in service on and in leadership roles of IECs [1–5]. In child psychiatry, the pediatric consultation/liaison psychiatrist has long been familiar with consultation questions and clinical situations that overlap with ethical challenges [6,7]. Although there is considerable literature regarding the general psychiatrist's contributions to IECs, little has been written regarding the role of the child and adolescent psychiatrist (CAP) on the IEC of the general hospital that has a large pediatric population, the pediatric hospital, or the child and adolescent psychiatric facility. This article explores the potential contributions that CAPs may make—by virtue of their training, expertise, and frequent practice on the cusp between clinical psychiatric and bioethical dilemmas—within the context of an IEC in several health care settings.

* Corresponding author.
E-mail address: ssexson@mcg.edu (S.B. Sexson).

1056-4993/08/$ - see front matter © 2008 Elsevier Inc. All rights reserved.
doi:10.1016/j.chc.2007.07.006   *childpsych.theclinics.com*

The institutional ethics committee

IECs were developed initially to consider decisions regarding end-of-life issues related to limiting or withdrawing care for severely neurologically compromised adults. Issues regarding the treatment or withdrawal thereof for severely disabled infants and children soon became paramount [8]. The role of the IEC has expanded over the past several decades. Today, the IEC generally accomplishes its various roles through at least three major areas of activities, including (1) education of hospital professional and administrative staff, other employees, and even patients and families, whenever appropriate, in the concepts of bioethics; (2) hospital policy oversight regarding issues with ethical implications, which may include drafting policy as well as reviewing existing policy; and, perhaps, most significantly, (3) clinical ethics case consultation aimed at resolving conflicts regarding treatment decisions and comprehensive care of the patient and family [8]. More recently, IECs have assumed roles in organizational ethics as well [8]. Evolving requirements from various professional and regulatory agencies (eg, The Center for Medicare and Medicaid Services; The Joint Commission; and local, state, and national professional societies) influence the role of IECs to address several goals within the institution, including legal, compliance, fiduciary, and professional aspects of health care provision. Generally, IEC recommendations are advisory in nature, and the IEC has no direct patient care responsibility [8].

As part of their mission statement, some IECs have the mandate to be a "moral community" with diverse cultural and educational background that can express the ethical views of the professions, the community, and the individuals that it represents and serves. The committee does this by being readily available, well versed in ethical concepts, and allowing open access and equality of voice to those asking questions as well as those helping to resolve ethical tension. Points of ethical tension or conflict do not generally represent a "right" or "wrong" view of a particular issue, but rather represent inherently conflicting views of what is the good and right thing to do in a particular situation. The mandate usually is summarized in a mission statement of the IEC similar to the one below:

> "The ethics committee is an interdisciplinary group, a moral community, which acts to represent the highest calling of the institution by assuring access, consideration and equality of voice to all who seek our help and to all who speak. Its mission is to enhance both the ethical environment of the hospital and the care we provide to its patients and to the community. The committee fulfills these roles through education, policy development and case consultation" (WR Sexson, MD, Grady Health System Institutional Ethics Committee Mission Statement, 2007).

Several essential traits are common to most IECs that help them to facilitate achievement of their mission:

Clear mandate
Clear reporting structure

Diverse representation
Transparency
Availability
Ethical competency
Equality of voice
Avoidance of conflict of interest

Committee members must be aware of these traits and should participate actively in assuring committee success by reinforcing these traits as they perform their functions within the committee.

Within the health care institution setting, the clear mandate can be expressed in the mission statement. The inevitable tension generated by differing ethical opinions makes it imperative that the IEC have a clear reporting structure, usually through the medical staff structure—but at times through the institution's administrative structure—and be unambiguously established in such a way as to avoid coercion based on conflicts of interest within the system. In its role in fulfilling the public trust, the IEC must assure adequate transparency, such that the process of decision-making is open to input and discourse and provides an acceptable mechanism for addressing points of ethical tension through diverse moral voices that minimize the potential for bias and discrimination.

Membership on the IEC must be diversely representative (Box 1). An essential aspect of committee discourse relates to the diversity and equality of the voices on the committee. Although many institutional committees fall within the medical staff reporting structure, it is essential that consideration be given to other disciplines from within the hospital that should be represented. Similarly, consideration should be given to making committee membership more broadly representative of the community. Personal characteristics necessary for optimal committee functioning include integrity, tolerance of diversity, the ability to consider opposing viewpoints through open discussion and debate, acknowledging the value of the contributions of each member, the ability to accept negotiated decisions, and the absolute necessity for maintaining confidentiality. Optimally, IECs also should have representatives with expertise in the fields of clinical ethics and law and health policy as well as experience in such issues as group and family process, interpersonal communication skills, and mediation.

Membership on an active, mature IEC is demanding and requires a major commitment of time and effort. The IEC must be rapidly and openly available to anyone requesting a consult on a 24/7 basis. Membership requires basic ethics training to achieve ethical competence and extra training in IEC functions beyond the specific primary expertise of the member (Box 2).

The optimal functioning of an IEC requires an equality of voice. Widely diverse membership may engender different individual comfort levels at speaking or voicing opinions in the context of a full committee meeting.

Box 1. Potential considerations for representative membership on a pediatrics institutional ethics committee

General pediatricians
Representative pediatric subspecialists
   Could include CAP here
Nurses
   Floor
   ICU
   Outpatient
Chaplain
Attorneys (not hospital lawyers, except in *ex officio* capacity, because of conflict of interest)
Administrators
   Nursing
   Other
Community-at-large members
Patient family members
A patient representative (eg, a college-aged individual who has cystic fibrosis and has had multiple health care–related experiences)

An essential aspect of a functioning committee as a moral community is for all of the committee to assure and reinforce the importance—and equality—of each person's voice within the discussion. There may be committee members who have greater knowledge of the moral or medical subject matter with which an individual case deals. Hence, the voices of these individuals may carry greater influence as the entire committee decides on recommendations; however, the "equality" of voice does demand that all voices are heard and respected. Regular acknowledgment of this important mandate verbally during IEC meetings is imperative.

Finally, avoidance of conflict of interest on the part of each committee member as well as on the part of the IEC as a whole is imperative. Every committee member comes to the table with a set of knowledge, biases, priorities, and functions that may lead to potential conflicts of interest. Disclosing these potential conflicts on a regular basis and empowering the diverse IEC members to confront conflicts openly and aggressively when they arise are necessary to limit bias in the discussions and the recommendations of the IEC. Persons with single-issue social or personal agendas related to health care ethics are unlikely to be able to contribute to an IEC where tolerance of opposing viewpoints is crucial. A balance of health care and community representatives allows a process that achieves the breadth of perspective that truly facilitates open moral discourse.

Box 2. Suggested committee member training

Premembership interview to emphasize role and commitment
Basic ethics training for the new member
Ethical principles
Common committee functions
Review of applicable institution policy
Review of frequent reasons for consultation
Review of approach to consultation
Practice case consultation

Competence in specific topics for new and continuing membership
Legal
Health policy
Religion and spirituality
Cultural issues
Emotional contributions to decision-making under stress
Decision-making capacity
End-of-life issues
Mentorship

How can a CAP contribute specifically to these mandates for an IEC? First, by virtue of their training, CAPs are comfortable within a multidisciplinary setting, acknowledging the value of voices from various backgrounds. Their training also focuses on recognition of conflicts or "blind spots" within themselves as well as in those with whom they work, a valuable asset in working with potential bias and conflicts of interest within the group process of committee deliberations. In their everyday practices, CAPs work intensively with families, integrating spiritual and cultural principles into their formulation of the biopsychosocial understanding of the clinical problem. Additionally, their core expertise allows them to evaluate for decision-making capacity and identify emotional aspects of decision making under stress as well as identifying the actual origin of the stress rather than the assumption of the source of stress, a far too common mistake in the health care process. A case example is a mother of premature triplets. When one of the triplets did not respond to standard treatment, the health care team presented the mother with the problem and recommended limitation of care. The mother was distraught and very much opposed to this move. The team recognized her stress and assumed that it was related primarily to the potential loss of her baby and being guilt-ridden because she had been unable to carry her babies to a term delivery. Child psychiatric consultation revealed that the mother's greatest stress was that she was most fearful that the staff was making this recommendation because they were mad at her for not always being as cooperative as she thought they expected her to be. She was afraid that her behavior was leading to the recommendation for limitation of care. Once this fear could be discussed openly and addressed sensitively as well as cognitively, the mother was able to see the futility of continuation of the intensive medical interventions for this baby and approach the baby's death in a humane, supportive environment. Her relationship with the staff in the care of her remaining two infants also improved. This case demonstrates the CAP's ability to identify the true source of stress, which could be addressed to help this mother make a better informed decision regarding her child's care during this emotionally charged situation.

The education function of the institutional ethics committee

One of the three major activities of an IEC revolves around education. The educational mandate is first for the members of the IEC and more broadly for health care professionals, hospital administrators, hospital employees and, when appropriate, patients and families. The range of topics typically addressed by an IEC is diverse. Table 1 identifies some of the educational topics addressed by one IEC (Grady Health System), categorizing topics certainly within the training expertise of the CAP. Many CAPs have special interest and expertise in many of the other educational topics as well. It is in the context of multidisciplinary rounds and case conferences, an area in which CAPs have considerable expertise, that most of the general educational needs are identified. Health care teams then typically ask for lectures on identified topics. This IEC averages around 400 hours annually of case conference, multidisciplinary rounds, and lectures throughout the hospital and community. With the increase in educational venues, case consultation for challenging ethical issues occurs more frequently and much earlier in the course of the conflict.

Ethics policy

Another function of the IEC involves the development and review of institutional policies that involve ethics issues. IECs may be asked by administration to draft policies on certain issues with ethical import for the institution. Additionally, an IEC may, in the course of its educational and case consultation functions, identify issues of such ethical import to warrant institutional policy and initiate draft policies for consideration by the institution. Box 3 lists some of the areas in which IECs typically weigh in on health care policy. It is in the context of ethical policy along with education that the institution develops the infrastructure through which ethical problems and tensions can be addressed at the bedside by health care providers

Table 1
Ethics education topics 2004–2006 Grady Health System Institutional Ethics Committee

Topic taught	Training for ethics committee members	Training for health care system and community persons	Within training expertise of CAP
Decision-making capacity	X	X	X
Communication issues	X		X
Research ethics	X	X	
Allow a natural death versus do not resuscitate	X	X	
Conflict of interest		X	
Organizational ethics	X		
Scarce resources and resource Allocation		X	
Informed consent	X	X	X
Legal cases that form the basis of current United States ethics	X		
Social work "diligent" search for family	X		
End-of-life issues		(Case conferences and multidisciplinary rounds weekly in various units)	X
HIV and the law consent disclosure	X	X	X
Culture and decision making		X	X
Advanced directives		X	
Emergency consent	X	X	
End-of-life care "orchestrating a good death," deceleration, do not resuscitate		X	X
Stem cell research		X	
Medical errors		X	
Professionalism	X	X	X
Palliative care	X	X	
Communicating dad news		X	X
Surrogate decision makers	X	X	
Substituted judgment	X		
Spirituality, religion, and miracles		X	X

or through IEC consultation. The participating CAP can reinforce the importance of the consideration of emotional and interpersonal issues related to many of these difficult decisions faced by health care providers and their patients and their patients' families.

Box 3. Institutional policies commonly reviewed/drafted by institutional ethics committees

Do not resuscitate (DNR)
    Advanced directives
    DNR when there is no decision maker present
    DNR when the patient cannot make his/her own decisions
Limitation or withdrawal of various treatments
    Fluid
    Nutrition
Brain death
Organ donation
    Including "donation after cardiac death"
Consent
    Informed consent
    Emergency consent
Refusal of care
Ability of physicians and hospital employees to object to taking
    care of certain patients
    Categorical patients (eg, patients seeking abortion)
    "Firing a patient" because of conflict
Statements regarding institutional business ethics
Medical errors

Case consultation

Commonly occurring ethical issues

Generally, there is an amazing consistency and repetition of ethical issues that generate most ethics consults between institutions and across age groups (Table 2). The need for ethical consultation generally occurs because of an individual's or family's beliefs and understanding that are incongruous with that of the health care providers or the institution. IEC case consultation is the ultimate avenue by which individual ethical questions are answered, using the institutional infrastructure provided by ethics education and institutional policy. Many of the situations that generate ethical issues and ethics consultations are issues with which CAPs are familiar in their everyday clinical work.

Ethical issues versus ethical questions: defining the point of ethical tension in case consultation

There is a difference between an ethical issue and an ethical question. Issues are broad topics about which we may have strong moral and ethical

Table 2
Commonly occurring ethical issues and the potential contribution of the child and adolescent psychiatrist

Ethical issue	Commonly seen in children's hospital	Commonly seen in the general hospital	Within the clinical expertise of the CAP
Communication issues/ failures	X	X	X
Death	X	X	X, particularly developmental and psychologic aspects of death and dying
Components of "decision-making capacity" versus "competence"		X	X
Consent			X
For clinical care	X	X	
For research	X	X	
Medical decision making in the patient without decision-making capacity		X	X
Guardianship	X	X	X
Brain death	X	X	
Organ donation and "donation after cardiac death"	X	X	X, eg, developmental and psychologic aspects
Relationship between organizational ethics and patient-centered ethics	X	X	
Requests for medically futile care	X	X	
Moral agency and the role of patients and doctors in medical decision making	X	X	X
Cultural and ethics implications for ethical decisions	X	X	X
Decision making under stress	X	X	X
Disclosure of errors	X	X	
Inappropriate hope versus malevolent treatment	X	X	X
Paternalism versus autonomy	X	X	X
Assent versus consent	X		X
Portability of advanced directives and "What did the patient really mean?"		X	

feelings. The ethical question that a committee must answer is a specific question about an individual in a particular situation. One of the key functions of the ethics committee as it hears case consultation is to delineate the ethical question and decide the "point of ethical tension." The point of ethical tension represents the ethical question voiced in terms of competing potentially ethically appropriate views. It was pointed out by a mentor of one of the authors (WRS) that, "Most of us are smart enough to answer any question we are smart enough to ask" (A. Brann, MD, personal communication, 1975). A committee cannot answer a question unless it can frame the question that it is being asked.

In the health care setting, ethical tension is seen most frequently when there is a disagreement between the patient (or patient's family) and the health care team. This is demonstrated easily in a 2 × 2 table (Fig. 1).

Abortion, for example, is an ethical issue. Whether a 17-year-old emancipated minor who is dying of pregnancy-induced heart failure should get an abortion raises a specific ethical question. If the health care providers and the adolescent woman agree, there may be no ethical tension, but disagreement leads to a situation that may result in IEC consultation. The point of ethical tension may be articulated by this ethical question: "Is it ethically acceptable to force an abortion on this 17-year-old emancipated minor to save her life?" Another ethical issue involves the typically accepted practice of parental autonomy in decision making for their children in the best interest of the child. An ethical question may arise when a parent, for religious, cultural, or idiosyncratic reasons, will not consent to a well-accepted life saving procedure for his/her child, such as a blood transfusion. Clearly, there is disagreement between the health care team and the parents. The ethical question may become whether the hospital and health care team should ask for legal permission to provide this treatment to the child against parental consent. The CAP may be particularly effective in helping the health care team and the family to understand the issues involved and facilitate communication that can help to avoid conflict or illuminate the issues that can inform the ultimate recommendation by the IEC. Sometimes, defining the question helps the health care team to understand the longer-term implications of making a decision to override parental autonomy. An example is a case in which a child who has leukemia usually would need to receive blood transfusions in the course of the treatment. The parents, because of religious beliefs, were opposed to blood products of any kind. After consultation with the IEC, in which a CAP was involved, the health care team understood better the intense struggle that the parents were having between

YES/*YES*	YES/*NO*
NO/*YES*	NO/*NO*

The difficulty arises typically only in the shaded boxes where there is disagreement.

Medical Team Recommendation (YES or NO)
Patient/Family Response (YES or NO)

Fig. 1. Situations most likely to produce ethical tension in health care settings.

wanting to help their child while truly believing that such permission would doom their child to eternal damnation. The team agreed to work hard to avoid transfusions if at all possible. The family was appreciative and much more cooperative, having been reassured that the team was trying to provide care within the boundaries of their religious beliefs. The child was managed without blood transfusion, but should it have become necessary, the team believed that the family would have understood better their need to get a court order for treatment. Ongoing follow-up in this kind of case is essential to maintain open communication and to assure that this point of ethical tension continues to be addressed.

Communications and ethics consultation: case examples

One of the most common problems generating ethics consultation relates to failure of communication. This failure usually occurs unintentionally as a consequence of the way that we communicate under stress as well as each person's own comfort level with his/her abilities and goals (Box 4). Failure in communication is a common origin for psychiatric consultations as well, and effective communication is one of the primary skill sets incorporated into a CAP's training. The CAP has specialized expertise in communication, in general, and is well trained in recognizing emotional and psychologic issues that stand in the way of effective communication. The CAP also is specifically trained to appreciate spiritual and cultural issues that may confound effective communication between the patient/family and the health care team.

One case example of a communication issue related to informed consent is that of a 15-year-old girl who would not give assent for cardiac transplant after the surgeon had described the procedure and the recovery process to her. The parents favored the life-saving measure, but the health care team was not comfortable proceeding without the patient's assent, expressing concern that compliance with follow-up treatment was unlikely. An IEC consult was requested. The CAP on the committee questioned whether the adolescent was informed adequately. In the process of the consultation, the IEC team discussed with the girl her concerns about the transplant. Her overriding fear was that of the pain and suffering that she would have to undergo during and following the surgery; however, when confronted openly with the question of whether she would choose to die rather than have the surgery, she immediately said that she did not want to die. Her resistance to assent involved her—and perhaps the health care team's—focus more on the short-term aspects of her care rather than the long-term aspects. Once she had incorporated her choices in a fully informed and understood way, she was willing to give assent for the surgery.

Another example is a case that failed to recognize cultural issues related to failure to comply with a required treatment regimen. A 10-year-old Guatemalan immigrant who had resistant tuberculosis failed to respond to

---

Box 4. Communication issues frequently causing ethics consultation

Patient/family-related communication issues
Difficulty in hearing bad news
Stress-induced decrease in effective levels of communication
Failure or discomfort in communicating effectively issues that
    may impact the decision-making process
      Emotional issues
      Spiritual issues
      Cultural issues
Failure to participate in defining the long- and short-term goals of
    care
Failure to recognize the dynamic nature of disease

Physician/health care worker communication issues
Use of medical jargon
Difficulty in communicating bad news
Failure to communicate on the appropriate level for the patient/
    family's best understanding
Failure to recognize emotional, spiritual, and cultural issues that
    may impact communication
Failure to recognize that the patient/family's emotional, spiritual,
    and cultural issues may take precedence over scientific and
    statistical information in decision making
Failure to listen to the patient/family
Failure to define the long- and short-term goals of care
Failure to communicate the dynamic nature of the disease

---

treatment. Ultimately, it was discovered that his parents were not adherent to his medication regimen. Because of the seriousness of the disease as well as the public health concern, the health care team sought outpatient IEC consultation regarding the advisability of involving child protective services in this case of what the team considered medical neglect. The family and child appeared to be well attached, and in all other areas the family seemed to take care of the child appropriately. The CAP on the committee questioned whether there might be some cultural or religious issue that prevented the family from adhering to the medical regimen. Further interviewing by the IEC consultation team revealed that the parents were fearful of giving the medication to their child because it was "red," a color that they associated with the devil. Once the medication was formulated into a clear capsule, the family was compliant with the treatment regimen and involvement with child protective services was avoided.

Another case involved failure to communicate the long-term goals of care. A 13-year-old African American boy who lived with his guardian, his maternal grandmother, to whom he was well attached, had severe Crohn's disease that required colectomy. The adolescent refused to comply with postoperative treatment and behaved in such an oppositional and confrontive way that the staff no longer wanted to treat him. A psychiatric consultation was requested. The psychiatrist recommended inpatient psychiatric care to help the boy deal with his profound oppositionality and his adjustment to the colostomy; however, care could be attained only if the grandmother gave up custody of the adolescent to child protective services so that they could access funding for this intensive treatment. The IEC was consulted regarding whether such a plan should be undertaken when neither the grandmother nor the adolescent wanted this intervention. During the committee deliberations, the CAP on the committee raised the issue of whether the adolescent was fully aware of his choices. IEC consultation to the boy and his grandmother concretely described the choices that were available, which led to the adolescent's agreement to—and ultimately, demonstration of his willingness to comply with—treatment recommendations to avoid being removed from his grandmother's custody. The boy was discharged home with the grandmother with close follow-up to monitor adherence to his medical treatment. Psychiatric outpatient treatment was recommended.

Finally, in another case, which involved emotional and communication issues, assistance was requested by the family. The parents of a 30-month-old boy who had severe congenital heart disease and heart failure requiring heart transplant sought consultation with the IEC. The child had been hospitalized in the ICU since he was 18 months old, requiring intensive and intrusive medical management to keep him alive while he waited for a cardiac donor. Initially, the parents were in favor of this course of treatment; however, over time it was found that the child had major antibodies that made him incompatible with each heart that became available. The treatment became more and more invasive. The staff was attached to the child. When the parents began to bring up the futility of the ongoing interventions, the health care team became upset and threatened to involve child protective services. The parents requested consultation to the IEC because of their perception of the futility of the ongoing care, a difficult thing for a family to do because the outcome is likely to result in their child's death.

During IEC deliberations, the CAP on the IEC raised the question regarding the health care team's difficulty in seeing the futility of this case because of their months of work and intense attachment to this amiable little boy. The IEC consultation team was able to work with the health care team and the family to facilitate communication between them. Over time, the health care team members were able to recognize their emotional conflicts in this case and achieve consensus with the family about palliative care that would allow the child and the family some more positive time together, while still in the ICU. The most aggressive components of the child's care were limited or discontinued while the family stayed at his bedside, and he died 3 days later. In this case, the CAP's knowledge of defense mechanisms and countertransference issues (blind spots) helped the IEC and, ultimately, the health care team acknowledge their blind spot in recognizing the futility of ongoing intensive care for this child and his family and create a setting where they and the family could support a more humane death for the child.

Summary

Over the past 30 years, IECs have become the vehicle for addressing ethical issues in health care institutions. General psychiatrists, particularly those who practice in the general hospital as consultants to their medical and surgical colleagues, have been involved in the evolution of the functioning IEC [1–5,9,10]. Not much has been written regarding the involvement of CAPs at the interface between ethics and psychiatry [6]; however, CAPs have characteristics similar to those of general psychiatrists that prepare them well for service on IECs. Like the general psychiatrist, the CAP who consults with pediatricians has defined expertise in many of the consultation questions that come to the IEC (see Table 2). Communication issues, issues of informed consent and decision-making capacity, and emotional, psychiatric, and developmental aspects that are common to many complex medical care and end-of-life care issues are within the purview of expertise of most practicing CAPs. Additionally, child psychiatrists, like general psychiatrists, are able to recognize the emotional and psychiatric issues that confound many ethics consultations because of IECs' tendency to underestimate the importance of these issues in resolving ethical problems [3]. The voice of the CAP on an IEC may better inform the IEC regarding decision-making issues that involve family members and surrogate decision makers. Steinberg [3] also emphasizes that psychiatrists, including CAPs, have many skills that are common to optimal ethicist function. The CAP is well trained in interviewing, empathic listening, nonjudgmental approaches to complex human questions, and the ability to elicit information and move to conflict resolution, all attributes that help the ethicist to deal with complex and competing concerns. Additionally, the CAP has in-depth understanding of the child's and adolescent's ability to understand illness from a developmental perspective along with special expertise in family dynamics, skills that inform interactions of the IEC with children, adolescents, and their families. CAPs, by the very nature of their practice, are comfortable working in a multidisciplinary setting, recognizing the value of all of the voices in evaluating a problem and recommending a resolution. CAPs are trained in facilitating group process while managing difficult issues within the group and identifying blind spots within themselves, group members, and the group itself that might lead to misunderstandings regarding the case and inappropriate or unfair recommendations. This particular expertise is especially helpful in recognizing subtle potential bias and conflicts of interest within the group process of committee deliberations. Finally, CAPs are required to have training in cultural, spiritual, and religious issues that may contribute to the biopsychosocial understanding of the clinical and bioethical problem. Beyond expertise regarding ethics consultation, the CAP is uniquely trained to educate committee members and health care institution staff regarding many ethical issues of importance (see Table 1). Still, being a CAP does not make one an ethicist. The practicing CAP must be committed to ethics training that will augment his/her clinical skills. As a contributing member of the IEC, the CAP must be educated in the field of ethical thought and principles, achieve a knowledge of common legal and ethical issues, and develop an ability to identify points of ethical tension and determine the ethical questions. Working within this specific "moral community" of the institution may require additional understanding of the ethical consultation process; however, like the CAP's adult psychiatric colleagues, CAPs are uniquely trained and competent to become valued contributors to their institutions' IECs because of the similar nature of many aspects of the work of the CAP who consults to pediatrics and much of the work of IECs. Each IEC member brings common and unique strengths to the deliberations and work of the IEC. The unique strengths of the typical CAP include such things as developmental understanding, enhanced understanding of communication styles and failures, an understanding of specific psychiatric factors, and cultural expertise. By acquiring expertise in the other aspects of ethical theory and legal issues related to ethics work, CAPs can function easily within the IEC to the betterment of the patient and the processes within the institution.

References

[1] Engel CC. Psychiatrists and the General Hospital Ethics Committee. Gen Hosp Psychiatry 1992;14:29–35.
[2] Powell T. Consultation-liaison psychiatry and clinical ethics. Representative cases. Psychosomatics 1997;38(4):321–6.
[3] Steinberg M. Psychiatry and bioethics: an exploration of the relationship. Psychosomatics 1997;38(4):313–20.
[4] Tweeddale MG. Teaching old dogs new tricks–a personal perspective on a decade of efforts by a clinical ethics committee to promote awareness of medical ethics. J Med Ethics 2001; 27(Suppl 1):i41–3.
[5] Youngner SJ. Consultation-liaison psychiatry and clinical ethics: historical parallels and diversions. Psychosomatics 1997;38(4):309–12.
[6] Krener P. Ethical issues in pediatric consultation-liaison. Child Adolesc Psychiatr Clin N Am 1995;4(4):723–45.
[7] Sexson SB, Rubenow J. Organ transplantation in the child and adolescent—psychological aspects. In: Craven JR, Rodin G, editors. Psychiatric aspects of organ transplant. Oxford (UK): Oxford University Press; 1992. p. 33–49.

[8] Committee on Bioethics. American Academy of Pediatrics: institutional ethics committees. Pediatrics 2001;107(1):205–9.

[9] Leeman CP, Blum J, Lederberg MS. A combined ethics and psychiatric consultation. Gen Hosp Psychiatry 2001;23:73–6.

[10] Geppert C, Cohen MA. Consultation-liaison psychiatrists on bioethics committees: opportunities for academic leadership. Acad Psychiatry 2006;30(5):416–21.

ELSEVIER
SAUNDERS

Child Adolesc Psychiatric Clin N Am
17 (2008) 225–236

CHILD AND
ADOLESCENT
PSYCHIATRIC CLINICS
OF NORTH AMERICA

The Ethics Committees of the American Academy of Child and Adolescent Psychiatry and the American Psychiatric Association: History, Process, Education, and Advocacy

Adrian N. Sondheimer, MD[a],*,
William M. Klykylo, MD[b]

[a]Division of Child and Adolescent Psychiatry, UMDNJ–New Jersey Medical School,
BHSB Room 1416, 183 South Orange Avenue, Newark, NJ 07103, USA
[b]Division of Child and Adolescent Psychiatry, Wright State University Boonshoft School
of Medicine, POB 927, Dayton, OH 45401, USA

History

The history of mental disturbance and its commonly associated questions—what is it, what causes it, how might it be defined, by whom, who treats it, and how is it to be treated—goes back millennia, whereas the modern history of organized psychiatry in the United States dates back to the early 1800s. Mentally disturbed individuals of that time were housed in large community institutions of the ill that could number in the many thousands, and physician administrators oversaw their care. In 1844, 13 administrative superintendents of these institutions combined forces to form the Association of Medical Superintendents of American Institutions for the Insane [1]. Over the course of the next 70 years, their numbers and those of assistant physicians grew; in 1921, the extant group established the American Psychiatric Association (APA) [2].

Medical training, via the impact of the Flexner [3] report of 1910, had become formalized only a short while before. Training in psychiatry had largely functioned as an apprenticeship system, and did not itself become considerably more formalized until the mid-1930s [4]. Psychiatric training

* Corresponding author. 315 East Northfield Road, Livingston, NJ 07039.
E-mail address: adriansondheimer@aol.com (A.N. Sondheimer).

1056-4993/08/$ - see front matter © 2008 Elsevier Inc. All rights reserved.
doi:10.1016/j.chc.2007.08.001 *childpsych.theclinics.com*

and practice of the time was subject to the prevailing explanations for manifestations of disturbed behaviors and the corresponding rationales for their treatments. In the mid-nineteenth through the mid-twentieth century, with little in the way of scientific documentation for purported etiologic causations of mental illness, practitioners generally wavered between attempts to provide humane care and those designed to maintain order in institutions [5]. Postulated somatic causations for illness presentations resulted in the use of "biological" treatments (eg, hydrotherapy, hypothermia, insulin- and electro-shock therapy). Subsequently, during several decades surrounding the mid-twentieth century, individuals' intrapsychic processes, as formulated by Freud and his successors, rapidly gained ascendance as both explanations for disturbance and as foci for treatment. These developments contributed to a large increase in the number of psychiatrists practicing in office-based, nonhospital settings [6]. Beginning in the 1960s awareness of family dynamics and the surrounding cultural context loomed larger, and these developments were followed in turn by the profession's emphasis on greater diagnostic specificity, exemplified by the advent of the DSM-III in 1980. Both the concurrent and subsequent explosion in numbers of novel pharmacologic entities and the understandings of their application to treatment, coupled with the coming to the fore of problem-focused verbal therapeutics, most prominently that of cognitive-behavioral therapy, have dominated the last two decades of psychiatric practice. Looming in the future is the potential impact of advances in molecular biology, which will likely encourage clinical basing of diagnostics and therapeutic interactions on the knowledge of an individual's genetic endowment.

Ethics

Why this brief review of 150 years of psychiatric history? Because, as psychiatric knowledge increased and became more systematized, practitioners progressively became more aware of their encounters with moral dilemmas. The need to address these dilemmas as a profession became more obvious and pressing, fostered in particular by the impact of psychoanalytic theory, with its emphasis on unconscious as well as conscious motivations for the behaviors of both individual patients and practitioners. Grossly immoral state-sponsored psychiatric and medical practices, most visible during the totalitarian eras of Nazi Germany and the post–World War II Soviet Union, similarly alerted the psychiatric profession to the dangers of morally distorted, politically supported, unethical practices at the governmental level.

Ethics is a discipline of thought and study; medical ethics is a study of ethics as applied to the field of medicine [7]. As a focus of philosophical investigation, the study of ethics lends itself to explorations of both the extraordinarily broad variety of human behaviors as well as its minutiae. Bringing this area of study down to earth (relatively speaking) from philosophical ivory tower heights, however, often necessitates the creation of administrative structures that harness the theory via the creation of bodies that exercise the knowledge in a systematic fashion. Thus, the need to address the issues surrounding the moral basis of the professional behaviors of psychiatric practitioners led to the creation of the APA's ethics committee in 1944, and to the production of the APA's Code of Ethics in 1973 [8].

American Psychiatric Association

American Psychiatric Association ethics committee structure and functions

The Ethics Committee of the APA is composed of six voting members, one of whom is an APA past president, and another a member in training. The committee customarily recommends for membership those who have served either as chairperson or as members of a district branch ethics committee. The Ethics Committee is assigned two primary specific functions by the organization. The first is to process and resolve ethical complaints; the second is to develop educational materials for the membership.

American Psychiatric Association ethics committee procedures for handling complaints of unethical conduct

The Ethics Committee must ensure that ethical complaints are handled in accordance with the relevant APA bylaws and with *The Principles of Medical Ethics With Annotations Especially Applicable to Psychiatry* [9]. The most recent edition of the *Principles* was published in 2006, the prior revision was published in 2001, and some 12 editions and revisions have appeared since the original publication in 1973. The APA was the first national organization to develop a code of ethics specifically for psychiatrists [10], and it in turn was based upon *The Principles of Medical Ethics* of the American Medical Association [11].

Although the APA Ethics Committee may itself initially respond to complaints, complaints are usually first addressed by the ethics committees of the district branches, with oversight by the national committee. Complaints of unethical behavior must be presented in writing and signed by the complainant. The APA *Principles* [9] contain a detailed sequence of procedures, including fact-finding, enforcement, and educational options, in response to a complaint against an APA member. The committee can act only on complaints against members of the organization. Complainants against nonmembers are referred by the APA ethics committee to state medical boards.

Following a complaint, a district branch may order a hearing, at which both the complainant and respondent have due process rights, including representation by counsel. Extrinsic evidence, such as reports, records or depositions, may be presented. Upon completion of the hearing and review of its findings, the district branch ethics committee may decide that: (1) the respondent did not act unethically; (2) the case should be concluded without a finding; or (3) the respondent acted unethically. If the district branch conducts such an investigation and finds a complaint unwarranted, it must so notify the complainant, who may ask for a review by the national committee. If the district branch determines that further action is warranted, it must notify the Secretary of the APA.

In this last case, the committee recommends an appropriate sanction. Sanctions recommended by the committee may include reprimand, suspension from the APA for up to 5 years, or expulsion. If a case is concluded without a finding, the committee may still require supervised educational remediation for the respondent as a condition of continued membership. In any case, the findings and recommendations of the district branch must be reviewed by the APA Ethics Committee before implementation. The respondent may appeal the outcome to the APA Ethics Committee or another body, the Ethics Appeal Board, which is composed of senior APA leaders. A decision to expel a member must be ratified by a two-thirds vote of the Board of Trustees.

All expulsions and resignations from the APA during the course of an ethics investigation must be reported in *Psychiatric News*, the monthly newspaper of the APA. Expulsions are rare events; only two were reported between 2000 and 2006, out of a membership averaging upwards of 35,000 psychiatrists. In that same time period, four resignations were received during the process of an ethics investigation (per WMK's review of *American Psychiatric News*, 2000–2006).

Educational activities of the American Psychiatric Association ethics committee

Beyond the education of members regarding their individual ethical conduct, the Ethics Committee has a series of charges related to generic education of the profession. These include the obligations to "respond to members' inquiries about ethical issues and [separately] publish *The Opinions of the Ethics Committee on The Principles of Medical Ethics With Annotations Especially Applicable to Psychiatry*" [12]. Eight editions of the *Opinions* have appeared since 1979. A most recent edition (2001) contains discussions of approximately 150 items in a question-and-answer format, reflecting the range of member enquiries directed to the committee. The range is broad, almost from "A to Z"; more specifically, it begins with "abandonment" and ends with "warning others." Furthermore, the committee was charged with publishing *An Ethics Primer* [13]. This succinct work, developed by and with contributions from the committee members, is intended primarily for residents and those teaching ethics. The *Primer* is self-described as a practical compilation of ethical thinking regarding the most frequently encountered problems facing all psychiatrists. Residents and less-experienced practitioners are likely to find some of the material novel.

To stimulate collaboration in educational approaches, the Committee is charged to "maintain contact with the 'ethics network', ie, the chairpersons of district branch ethics committees, by means of mailings, meetings, and workshops," and to work with other components of the APA to develop educational materials. The Committee also administers the Carol Davis Ethics Award. Carol Davis served for 30 years as the Director of the APA Office of Ethics, and the award is given annually in her honor for the best district branch newsletter article on ethics.

Children

Children have always differed from adults. For millenia, high infant mortality rates aside, they developed into adults, only later. As a rule the youngsters looked different (generally smaller), were not as strong physically, seemed to their elders to have much to learn, and though the developmental phases were not identified as such they progressed more rapidly through their stages (ie, infancy, toddlerhood, pre-apprentice and apprenticeship phases) than did the adults through theirs. These phenomena, and their rapid changes, have continued to hold true to date, though the nomenclature of the later stages has more recently changed to pre-school, school age, and adolescence. Two historians of childhood posited that awareness of children as developmentally distinct from adults did not truly begin to be formally acknowledged and addressed in the West until the seventeenth century [14], and that the attitudes of European adults toward children before that time were often fundamentally hostile [15]. While these perspectives are open to significant question and criticism [16], it seems quite true that societies in general traditionally concentrated first on the needs of adults, and only later on those of their children. Despite this general rule, however, there are those adults who have been and are primarily drawn to a focus on the needs of youngsters. Within medicine, those interests led to the establishment of pediatrics as a unique specialty in the mid to late 1800s [17].

Child and adolescent psychiatry

One-half century later, a melange of 50 professionals possessing varied backgrounds—some with primary experience in pediatrics, others who functioned as psychoanalysts, and still others who were psychiatrists and members of the APA—whose primary interest was invested in children with mental disturbance organized a core group that ultimately resulted in the formation of the American Academy of Child Psychiatry (AACP), incorporated in 1959 [18]. During the time the AACP organization evolved and grew, the American public simultaneously and progressively paid more attention to the needs and issues of its children. For example, within the justice system, the US Supreme Court's decision in the case of In re Gault [19] led to legal protections and representation for minors that had heretofore been reserved for adults. The National Child Abuse Prevention and Treatment Act of 1974 legislatively acknowledged the needs for protection of suffering children that until then had largely been ignored. The tenor of these external changes in laws, values, and policies in turn impacted the Academy members. As their experience with exposure to potentially dangerous situations, cases of abuse and neglect, mundane clinical affairs, and information exchange between parties were mutually shared and discussed, the need to create an ethical code for the AACP became apparent. Owing to these ethical challenges, the AACP, (which subsequently specifically added the word "adolescent" to its title, thus the current AACAP), established a five-member committee in 1975 headed by Norbert Enzer, MD, charged with producing a code of ethics for the organization.

AACAP code of ethics

The code of ethics was intended to provide principles and guidelines to practitioners dealing with child and adolescent psychiatric patients, by explicitly describing professional standards. Implicitly, it thus could supply assurance to the public of the profession's integrity. The AACAP Code endorsed the codes of ethics of the American Medical Association and the APA, but it identified as well separate significant issues germane to children that exist in addition to those concerns or behaviors relevant primarily to adults [20]. More specifically, the Code discusses and is informed by the following unique concerns: care is sought for children by adults, eg, parents, guardians and/or agencies; the rights, needs and desires of children may conflict or coincide with those of parents, guardians and society; children's maturation occurs over time, affecting the youngsters' abilities to choose and judge rationally; decisions concerning children often require implementation by adults; children's dependency and vulnerability obligate adult responsibility for their welfare; children's dependency on adults leave the youngsters vulnerable to abuse and/or coercion; research involving children as subjects must take into account their immature decision-making capacities; and, despite their immaturity, children are deserving of respect as autonomous individuals. The Code of Ethics, implicitly or explicitly, addresses all of these factors, and it places obligations on child and adolescent psychiatrists (CAPs) to foster the welfare of their child patients while simultaneously fully acknowledging the importance of family relationships. It emphasizes that physician decisions about children should not be influenced by sources of compensation; advocacy for children both as individuals and as a group is obligatory; considerations of confidentiality and avenues of access to care may differ between adolescents and younger children; and similarly, maturational and chronological age may affect the ability of children to assent/consent to treatment. The Code addresses the paramount issue of ensuring children's safety, and the possible divulging of confidences by a CAP to ensure their welfare. Similarly, it respects the refusal of a child, who possesses sufficient cognitive understanding, to participate in research and professional educational opportunities. (At the time of this publication, the AACAP Code of Ethics was in the process of revision. Readers are referred to the AACAP Web site [www.aacap.org] for the most updated version of Code of Ethics.)

Functioning and activities of the AACAP ethics committee

Essentially simultaneous with the adoption of the Code of Ethics by the AACP in 1980, the organization established an ethics committee with Norbert Enzer as its first chair. The committee subsequently advocated for the profession to educate itself and its trainees in the consideration and discussion of ethical issues. Consequently, in the years that followed, it specifically addressed dilemmas related to children and research; expressed views on public policy matters; and, in 1995, created an addendum entitled "Annotations to the Code" under the guidance of Diane Schetky, MD. The addendum focused on the effect of the changing economic environment on medical practice, as exemplified by the appearance of "managed care" and its impact specifically on CAP provision of health care [21].

The past quarter century has witnessed considerable growth in the child psychiatric knowledge base and expanded therapeutic approaches, in turn engendering continuous emergence of new ethical dilemmas. The AACAP Ethics Committee, chaired by eight individuals since Dr. Enzer's tenure, responded to these challenges by progressively enlarging the committee's scope of activities. In a manner similar to that of the APA's ethics committee, the AACAP committee has largely concentrated on an educational role for the membership. It should be noted that, in part, it has pursued this direction because, in contrast to the APA committee, the AACAP committee is not charged with a regulatory role. Thus, the committee does not formally process complaints against members concerning alleged unethical conduct, because the AACAP does not have adequate staffing or financial resources to do so. Therefore, complainants are referred to the APA and/or state licensing boards to address such complaints. Relevant AACAP by-laws stipulate that membership in the AACAP is automatically withdrawn from a member upon loss of state medical licensure in the event that the loss rests on a finding of an ethics violation.

The committee's educational and advocacy efforts include Diane Schetky's ethics column, which has appeared bimonthly in the AACAP's *Academy News* for the past two decades. The range of topics is wide, and includes dealing with the death of a patient [22], responses to the impact of managed care [23], boundary concerns [24,25], administration of the death penalty to youths [26], and children of same-sex marriages [27]. In addition, under Dr. Schetky's direction, an AACAP Task Force set guidelines to stringently govern relationships between the AACAP and corporate sponsors [28]. During the mid-1990s, an ethics clinical consultation breakfast was initiated at the AACAP annual meeting, which has since continued on a yearly basis. In this venue, Academy members pose ethical problems they have encountered and, in turn, receive feedback from the "faculty" and the other participants. Several journal articles focused on the teaching of ethics to child and adolescent psychiatry trainees [29–31], and various symposia were presented at the annual meeting concerning ethical considerations as they interface with child psychiatric institutional administration, electronic information transmission, religious behaviors and cultural mores, insurance and business practices, and health care provision.

Individual AACAP members, professionals in related fields, medical students, and interested citizens have forwarded queries and received confidential responses from the committee focusing on such ethical concerns as:

inadequate research supervision;
noninclusive and/or biased custodial evaluations;
child psychiatry practice without formal training;
poor or potentially harmful patient care;
unorthodox treatment approaches for highly disturbed children;
advertising via the Internet for adoption of children placed in foster care;
abandonment of children by professionals in the context of threatening parents
impact of TV on the very young;
potential adoption of former patients;
requests for funding of research from families of patients; and
treatment by a CAP of the psychiatrist's own child.

In a manner analogous to the APA's ethics committee's published "Opinions," the AACAP ethics committee recently has begun to provide written responses to case-based ethical issues in the semimonthly AACAP Academy News. Comprehensive responses describing the reasoning process are published, which include quotes from or phrases provided by some of the members. To illustrate, the first three cases in this series review the ethics of the proposed provision by a CAP of condoms to a patient [32], use of video monitoring on adolescent inpatient units [33], and state mandated reporting of abuse and neglect [34].

Ethical issues of the near and intermediate-term future

Finally, it is useful to speculate about ethical issues on the horizon that are likely to raise serious discussion. The AACAP ethics committee is likely in turn to eventually address them, in its role as one of the organization's internal advocates. Three matters immediately come to mind: (1) the impact of the pharmaceutical industry on CAP research and practice; (2) the effects of genomics on CAP practice; and (3) concerns about proposed treatments of psychiatric prodromes.

With regard to the pharmaceutical industry, "Big Pharma" funds the majority of CAP psychopharmacologic research and many of the researchers investigating newly formulated medications; by contrast, studies funded by the federal or state governments represent a relatively small minority of the total. Further, pharma underwrites many of the costs of professional meetings, lectures and dinners, and provides practitioners with medications and other "freebies." All of these practices can lead to various conflicts of interest for researchers, practitioners, and editors of professional journals, which in turn could negatively impact optimal patient care and the public trust [35–37]. (See Schetky's article elsewhere in this issue for a discussion of ethical issues associated with pharmaceutical companies.)

Major increases in knowledge gleaned from advances in technology at the biomolecular level facilitate honing in on the genetic underpinnings for psychiatric disease [38]. Whether the findings are single gene mutations, as in the case of Huntington's disease, or multifactorial and polygenic, as is currently postulated for the autism spectrum and most other major child and adult onset psychiatric illnesses, future findings are likely to raise ethical questions that heretofore have not been addressed. Such dilemmas include concerns about the degree of confidentiality and ownership accruing to an individual's genetic information, the impact of this knowledge on an individual's access to health insurance and employment, and the utility, versus the possible deleterious impact, of the determination of potential vulnerability to a disease process for which no known cure exists. Furthermore, assent/consent to or requests for genetic testing on the part of children, when such consents or requests are ordinarily made by adult guardians, pose unique ethical dilemmas in addition to concerns about children's rights to ownership of the information upon attainment of the age of majority [39,40].

The promising advances in genetic understandings relate directly to the third case, that of the treatments of prodromes. For example, several academic centers have undertaken investigations, frequently centering on adolescents, of treatment parameters of schizophreniform prodromes, with the hope of warding off or minimizing the often debilitating impacts of the full-blown disease. Yet, uncertainty concerning the likelihood of eventual full or actual expression of the disease is a serious concern, prodromal treatment necessarily requires the uses of medications (eg, neuroleptics) that themselves can initiate severe deleterious effects, and the science that might give these treatments legitimacy (ie, genetic studies) has yet to reach the point at which one could predict the eventual development of the illness with confidence [41–44].

Summary

Psychiatry has a history. What was once an inchoate awareness of mental disturbance over time has become more systematized. Pertinent administrative organizations developed and, in the United States, they took the forms of, among others, the present day APA and AACAP. Simultaneously, questions regarding the ethics of professional practices, treatments, and approaches to research gained prominence in the twentieth century, stimulated significantly by the impact of psychoanalytic thought and, separately, egregious state-sponsored medical practices. Investigations of ethical questions residing in the psychiatric sphere were similarly incorporated into the prevailing administrative structures, resulting in the creation of the ethics committees of the APA and later of the AACAP. Both committees are charged with educating their memberships concerning ethical matters and, to provide guidelines for professional behaviors, with updating their respective organizations' Codes of Ethics. In addition, the APA ethics committee is charged, in the event a complaint about a member's ethics is formally lodged with the committee, with the responsibility of judging that member and the degree of substance to the allegation. Finally, the ethics committees, in addition to commenting on matters of current concern, fulfill their educational and advocacy functions by anticipating future ethical concerns as well.

Acknowledgment

This article is written with expressions of deep gratitude to Norbert Enzer, MD, whose efforts have formed the bedrock for the AACAP's focus on ethical matters. Impaired health precluded Dr. Enzer's participation in the actual writing of the article, but his verbal contributions and his review and editing of the manuscript were essential, and his spirit lives in the words. With best wishes for improved health!

References

[1] Colp R Jr. History of psychiatry. In: Sadock B, Sadock V, editors. Comprehensive textbook of psychiatry. 8th edition. Philadelphia: Lippincott Williams & Wilkins; 2005. p. 4013–47.

[2] Baxter W. American psychiatry celebrates 150 years of caring. Psychiatr Clin North Am 1994;17:683–93.

[3] Flexner A. Medical Education in the United States and Canada. Bulletin Number 4. New York: Carnegie Foundation for the Advancement of Teaching; 1910.

[4] Scheiber S. Graduate psychiatric education. In: Sadock B, Sadock V, editors. Comprehensive textbook of psychiatry. 8th edition. Philadelphia: Lippincott Williams & Wilkins; 2005. p. 3931–43.

[5] Musto D. A historical perspective. In: Bloch S, Chodoff P, Green S, editors. Psychiatric ethics. 3rd edition. New York: Oxford University Press; 1999. p. 7–23.

[6] Huey L, Cole S, Trestman R, et al. Public and community psychiatry. In: Sadock B, Sadock V, editors. Comprehensive textbook of psychiatry. 8th edition. Philadelphia: Lippincott Williams & Wilkins; 2005. p. 3845–63.

[7] Beauchamp T, Childress J. Principles of biomedical ethics. New York: Oxford University Press; 2001.

[8] Lazarus JA. Ethics in the American Psychiatric Association after World War II. In: Menninger R, Nemiah J, editors. American Psychiatry after World War II. Washington, DC: American Psychiatric Association Press; 2000. p. 546.

[9] American Psychiatric Association. The principles of medical ethics with annotations especially applicable to psychiatry. Available at: http://www.psych.org/psych_pract/ethics/ppaethics.pdf. Accessed March 19, 2007.

[10] Bloch S, Pargiter R. Codes of ethics in psychiatry. In: Bloch S, Chodoff P, Green S, editors. Psychiatric ethics. 3rd edition. Oxford: Oxford University Press; 1999. p. 81–103.

[11] American Medical Association. The principles of medical ethics of the American Medical Association. Available at: http://www.ama-assn.org/ama/pub/category/2512.html. Accessed March 19, 2007.

[12] American Psychiatric Association. The opinions of the ethics committee on the principles of medical ethics with annotations especially applicable to psychiatry. Available at: http://www.psych.org/psych_pract/ethics/ethics_opinions52201.pdf. Accessed March 19, 2007.

[13] Wahl D, Milone R. Ethics primer of the American Psychiatric Association. Washington, DC: American Psychiatric Association; 2001.

[14] Aries P. Centuries of childhood. New York: Random House; 1962.

[15] DeMause L. The evolution of childhood. In: Demause L, editor. History of childhood. New York: Harper and Row; 1974.

[16] Kroll J, Bachrach B. Child care and child abuse in early medieval Europe. J Am Acad Child Adolesc Psychiatry 1986;25:562–8.

[17] Luecke P Jr. The history of pediatrics at Baylor University Medical Center. Proc (Bayl Univ Med Cent) 2004;17:56–60.

[18] Certificate of Incorporation of American Academy of Child Psychiatry, Inc. AACAP Archives, Washington DC. Registered with Prentice-Hall Corporation System Inc., Dover, DE, April 30, 1959.

[19] Malmquist C. Overview of juvenile law. In: Schetky D, Benedek E, editors. Principles and practice of child and adolescent forensic psychiatry. Washington, DC: American Psychiatric Publishing Inc.,; 2002. p. 259–66.

[20] Enzer N. Ethics in child psychiatry—an overview. In: Schetky D, Benedek E, editors. Emerging issues in child psychiatry and the law. New York: Brunner/Mazel; 1985. p. 3–21.

[21] American Academy of Child and Adolescent Psychiatry. Code of Ethics. Available at: http://www.AACAP.org/galleries/AboutUs/CodeOfEthics.PDF. Accessed March 26, 2007.

[22] Schetky D. Bringing closure when a patient dies. AACAP News 1996;27(6):8.

[23] Schetky D. Silent grief. AACAP News 1998;29(2):47.

[24] Schetky D. Too close for comfort. AACAP News 1998;29(5):185.

[25] Schetky D. Boundaries in child and adolescent psychiatry. Child Adolesc Psychiatr Clin North Am 1995;4(4):769–78.

[26] Schetky D. Juveniles and the death penalty. AACAP News 2000;31(4):158, 168.

[27] Schetky D. Same sex marriage: who speaks for the children? AACAP News 2005;36(4):162, 171.

[28] American Academy of Child and Adolescent Psychiatry. Guidelines for commercial contribution to the AACAP. Available at: http://www.aacap.org/galleries/AboutUs/GuidelinesforCommercialContributiontotheAACAP. Accessed March 26, 2007.

[29] Sondheimer A, Martucci L. An approach to teaching ethics in child and adolescent psychiatry. J Am Acad Child Adolesc Psychiatry 1992;31:415–22.

[30] Sondheimer A. Ethics and child and adolescent psychiatry: curricular design and clinical teaching. Acad Psychiatry 1996;20:150–7.

[31] Sondheimer A. Teaching ethics and forensic psychiatry: a National Survey of Child and Adolescent Psychiatry Training Programs. Acad Psychiatry 1998;22:240–52.

[32] Sondheimer A. Condoms for kids? AACAP News 2006;37(6):334–5.

[33] Sondheimer A. Big brother and the child inpatient unit. AACAP News 2007;38(1):20–1.

[34] Sondheimer A. To report or not to—that and other questions. AACAP News 2007;38(5): 252–3.

[35] Lewis D, Michels R, Pine D, et al. Conflict of interest. Am J Psychiatry 2006;163:571–3.

[36] Perlis R, Perlis C, Wu Y, et al. Industry sponsorship and financial conflict of interest in the reporting of clinical trials in psychiatry. Am J Psychiatry 2005;162:1957–60.

[37] Wazana A, Primeau F. Ethical considerations in the relationship between physicians and the pharmaceutical industry. Psychiatr Clin North Am 2002;25:647–63.

[38] Farmer A, Owen M. Genomics: the next psychiatric revolution? Br J Psychiatry 1996;169: 135–8.

[39] Burke W, Diekema D. Ethical issues arising from the participation of children in genetic research. J Pediatr 2006;149(Suppl):S34–8.

[40] Thomas S. Genomics: the implications for ethics and education. Br Med Bull 1999;55: 429–45.

[41] Haroun N, Dunn L, Haroun A, et al. Risk and protection in prodromal schizophrenia: ethical implications for clinical practice and future research. Schizophr Bull 2006;32:166–78.

[42] Corcoran C, Malaspina D, Hercher L. Prodromal interventions for schizophrenia vulnerability: the risks of being "at risk". Schizophr Res 2005;73:173–84.

[43] Cornblatt B, Lencz T, Kane J. Treatment of the schizophrenia prodrome: is it presently ethical? Schizophr Res 2001;51:31–8.

[44] Gosden R. Prepsychotic treatment for schizophrenia: preventive medicine, social control, or drug marketing strategy? Ethical Hum Sci Serv 1999;1:165–77.

ELSEVIER
SAUNDERS

Child Adolesc Psychiatric Clin N Am
17 (2008) 237–244

CHILD AND
ADOLESCENT
PSYCHIATRIC CLINICS
OF NORTH AMERICA

Index

Note: Page numbers of article titles are in **boldface** type.

1056-4993/08/$ - see front matter © 2008 Elsevier Inc. All rights reserved.
doi:10.1016/S1056-4993(07)00111-3   *childpsych.theclinics.com*

Refugee(s), international and political, disasters and, ethical issues related to, 172–173

Relationship(s), in incorporation into child and adolescent psychiatry, 198

Religion, as factor in prescribing psychotropic medications, 102–103

Research
conducting of, ethical issues related to, 175–176
fradulent, publication of, in child and adolescent psychiatry publishing, 153
in incorporation into child and adolescent psychiatry, 197
inhumane, in child and adolescent psychiatry publishing, 153

Resource(s), in incorporation into child and adolescent psychiatry, 198

S

Scientific merit, effect on psychiatric research on children and adolescents, 131–134

Secrecy
defined, 32
privacy vs., in child and adolescent psychotherapy, 32
"Small community," practice in, challenges of, in child and adolescent psychotherapy, 30–31

Social impact, of new media, 73–74

Software, in new media, 72

Special interest groups, physicians and, conflicts of interest between, **113–125.** See also *Conflict of interest, between physicians and pharmaceutical industry and special interest groups.*

State wards, prescribing medications for children in, 103–104

T

The Bemont Report, 129

The Doubtful Guest, 53

"Therapeutic misconception," 143

Thoroughness, of medical records and professional communication, 38–39

Trauma, illness and, conceptualization of, ethical issues related to, 173–174

Traumatic memories, challenges of, ethical issues related to, 181–182

U

Unethical publishing, understanding of, 156–157

US Department of Health and Human Services, 129

US Food and Drug Administration, 129

US National Commission for the Protection of Human Subjects of Biomedical and Behavioral Research, 129

User interface, in new media, 73

V

Value systems, in psychiatry, ethical issues related to, 178–179

Violence, ethical responsibility of preventing children from becoming socialized to, 182–183

Virtual worlds, Internet sites of interest, 91

Virtue ethics, 8–9

W

Willowbrook State Hospital, 128

World Medical Association, Declaration of Helsinki of, 128

Moving?

Make sure your subscription moves with you!

To notify us of your new address, find your **Clinics Account Number** (located on your mailing label above your name), and contact customer service at:

E-mail: elspcs@elsevier.com

800-654-2452 (subscribers in the U.S. & Canada)
407-345-4000 (subscribers outside of the U.S. & Canada)

Fax number: 407-363-9661

Elsevier Periodicals Customer Service
6277 Sea Harbor Drive
Orlando, FL 32887-4800

*To ensure uninterrupted delivery of your subscription, please notify us at least 4 weeks in advance of move.